WORKBOOK TO ACCO

Medical Assisting

Administrative and Clinical Competencies

WORKBOOK TO ACCOMPANY

Medical Assisting

Administrative and Clinical Competencies

Eighth Edition

Michelle Blesi, MA, BA, AA, CMA (AAMA)
Program Director, Medical Assisting
Century College – East Campus
White Bear Lake, MN

Virginia Busey Ferrari, MHA, BA, CEHRS

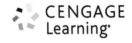
CENGAGE
Learning·

Australia • Brazil • Mexico • Singapore • United Kingdom • United States

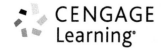

Workbook to Accompany Medical Assisting: Administrative and Clinical Competencies, Eighth Edition

Michelle Blesi

SVP, GM Skills & Global Product Management: Dawn Gerrain

Product Director: Matthew Seeley

Product Team Manager: Stephen Smith

Senior Director, Development: Marah Bellegarde

Product Development Manager: Juliet Steiner

Content Developer: Lauren Whalen

Product Assistant: Mark Turner

Vice President, Marketing Services: Jennifer Ann Baker

Marketing Coordinator: Courtney Cozzy

Senior Production Director: Wendy Troeger

Production Director: Andrew Crouth

Content Project Manager: Thomas Heffernan

Senior Art Director: Jack Pendleton

Manager, Digital Production: Jamilynne Myers

Media Producer: Jim Gilbert

Cover image(s): iStock.com/ monkeybusinessimages/Greyfebruary, © Shutterstock.com/Real Deal Photo/ Goncharuk Maksim

Library of Congress Control Number: 2015946688

ISBN: 978-1-305-11085-4

Cengage Learning
20 Channel Center Street
Boston, MA 02210
USA

Cengage Learning is a leading provider of customized learning solutions with employees residing in nearly 40 different countries and sales in more than 125 countries around the world. Find your local representative at **www.cengage.com.**

Cengage Learning products are represented in Canada by Nelson Education, Ltd.

To learn more about Cengage Learning, visit **www.cengage.com**

Purchase any of our products at your local college store or at our preferred online store **www.cengagebrain.com**

Printed in the United States of America
Print Number: 02   Print Year: 2017

PART 1: CHAPTER WORKSHEETS

PART 2: COMPETENCY CHECKLISTS

Part 1

CHAPTER WORKSHEETS

SECTION 1

Medical Assisting Foundations

Health Care Roles and Responsibilities

The Medical Assistant

Words to Know Challenge

Spelling: Each line contains three spellings of a word. Underline the correctly spelled word.

1. <u>accreditation</u>   acreditation   accretitation
2. alltruism   alltrueism   <u>altruism</u>
3. inate   <u>innate</u>   innat
4. empathatic   <u>empathetic</u>   empithetic
5. addvocate   <u>advocate</u>   advocat
6. <u>confidential</u>   confidental   confidinal
7. <u>generalist</u>   gineralist   generelist
8. providar   providir   <u>provider</u>
9. partnarship   partnirship   <u>partnership</u>
10. <u>certified</u>   certifeid   cerdified

Matching: Match the term in column I to its definition in column II.

COLUMN I		COLUMN II
___	1. Patient-centered medical home	A. Skills necessary regardless of whether working in a clinical or administrative capacity
___	2. Clinical skills	B. When an individual provider makes all the decisions for the practice
___	3. General skills	C. A team-based model of care led by a personal provider who provides continuous and coordinated care throughout a patient's lifetime to maximize health outcomes
___	4. Time management	D. Two or more providers who have a legal agreement to share in the total business operation of the practice
___	5. Solo practice	E. One who assists the patient, or acts on his or her behalf.
___	6. Urgent care center	F. An assortment of skills, tools, and practices by which to manage time during daily activities and when accomplishing specific projects
___	7. Partnership	G. Skills that vary by state laws and are an extension of the provider's responsibilities of assessment, examination, diagnosis, and treatment
___	8. Advocate	H. Ambulatory care centers that take care of patients with acute illness or injury and those with minor emergencies; used quite often when patients cannot see their own provider

Chapter Review

Short Answer

1. To become a successful medical assistant, you must acquire a specific _____ (theory) and _____ (procedures) while also demonstrating specific _____ .

2. What are the three broad areas of medical assisting?

   a. _____

   b. _____

   c. _____

3. What role should the medical assistant take on concerning communications when working with patients?

   _____

   _____

   _____

4. The chapter listed 10 administrative skills performed by medical assistants; name 6.

   _____

   _____

   _____

5. The chapter listed 11 clinical skills performed by medical assistants; name any 6.

   _____

   _____

   _____

   _____

6. List four environments in which medical assistants work.

   _____

   _____

   _____

7. According to the United States Department of Labor, employment for medical assistants is expected to grow by _____ through 2022.

8. List six traits of professionalism.

   _____

   _____

   _____

9. List five traits of a professional medical assistant.

   _____

   _____

   _____

10. Match the following organizational abbreviations with the responses listed in the chart.

    American Association of Medical Assistants (AAMA)

    American Medical Technologists (AMT)

    National Center for Competency Testing (NCCT)

    National Healthcareer Association (NHA)

    American Academy of Professional Coders (AAPC)

Fill in the Blank: Fill in the organization that corresponds to the response.

Organization Abbreviation	Response
_____	CPC
_____	The only avenue for credentialing with this organization is by graduating from either a CAAHEP- or ABHES-accredited institution
_____	Provides the CMA credential with the organization's initials in parenthesis beside it
_____	Offers training and certification in the areas of medical billing and coding
_____	Provides the National Certified Medical Assistant (NCMA) credential
_____	Provides the Certified Medical Administrative Specialist (CMAS) credential
_____	This organization started in 1955
_____	Provides the Registered Medical Assistant (RMA) credential
_____	Must take credentialing exam at an approved Prometric center
_____	After receiving the Authorization to Test letter, applicants can take the test at any PearsonVUE testing center
_____	Must receive the candidate's application within two weeks of the requested test date
_____	Provides eight certification exams for allied health care specialties

Chapter Application

Case Studies with Critical Thinking Questions

Scenario 1

The following tasks are all occurring at the same time. Prioritize the following tasks by putting numbers 1–4 next to each statement. (1 is the task you will do first, and 4 is the task you will do last.)

1. ____ The doctor asks you to perform an ECG on the patient in room 2 as he goes into room 3.

2. ____ Room 1 is open and ready for a patient.

3. ____ The receptionist calls back to tell you that you have a patient who would like you to call her back regarding lab results.

4. ____ The doctor is going into room 3 to perform a short procedure and needs you to assist him.

Scenario 2

You are competing with two other candidates for a medical assisting position at a large family practice center. All three of you are new graduates of the same medical assisting program. You all did well in your program and had a good rapport with the other students. Out of the three, you are the only one who is credentialed. During the interview, the supervisor asks you why she should hire you over the other two candidates.

1. What would you say?

_____

_____

_____

Role-Play Activity

Bella is a coworker you have grown very fond of. As a matter of fact, she is well respected by everyone in the office. You happen to see her come out of the drug room and slip some drug samples in her purse. You approach her about it, and she says that she received permission from Dr. Castle to take some samples home to her husband. The next week, you see Bella take some more samples; this time she takes several packets of the medicine from the drug cabinet. Once again, you confront her. She states that the doctor told her that it was okay to take as many samples as she wanted because the drug rep always leaves a lot more samples than necessary. The next day, the office manager calls a meeting and states that several samples of the drug that Bella took are missing from the drug cabinet, and she encourages anyone who has knowledge of the disappearance to come forward. Following the meeting, Bella stops you and begs you not to say anything to anyone. Role-play what you would say to Bella.

_____

_____

_____

Competency Practice

1. **Demonstrate Professional Behavior.** With a partner, practice role-playing the various procedure steps that are identified in Procedure 1–1.

2. **Demonstrate Professional Behavior.** Professionalism is a skill you will use daily as a medical assistant. Write a one- to two-page essay, using the various procedure steps in Procedure 1–1 or any of the following scenarios.

   a. Describe how the patient might associate a medical assistant with poor appearance as having a lack of knowledge.

   b. Describe and discuss how being tardy and returning late from breaks will affect your success as a medical assistant.

   c. Discuss the ramifications of not using active listening skills in the field.

   d. Identify tasks that are considered in bounds for a medical assistant and tasks that are considered out of your self-boundaries. What are consequences of performing tasks outside of your scope of duty?

   e. How does a poor attitude reflect on you in the workplace?

   _____

CHAPTER 2

The Health Care Team and the Medical Environment, Past and Present

Words to Know Challenge

Spelling: Each line contains three spellings of a word. Underline the correctly spelled word.

1. cadoceus	<u>caduceus</u>	caducious
2. docterate	<u>doctorate</u>	doctarate
3. <u>apprenticeship</u>	appretaship	apprentiship
4. epademic	epedemic	<u>epidemic</u>
5. <u>homeopathy</u>	homeopaty	homepathy
6. hospitilist	<u>hospitalist</u>	hospitelist
7. <u>biofeedback</u>	bioofeedback	biofeedbak
8. <u>naturopathy</u>	natropathy	nateropathy
9. plage	plauge	<u>plague</u>
10. receprocity	reciprcety	<u>reciprocity</u>

Fill in the Blank: Complete the following sentences with correctly spelled words from the Spelling section.

1. A _____ works with patients admitted to the hospital.

2. An _____ is a period of time during which one is bound by agreement to learn some trade or craft.

3. _____ indicates that one state recognizes the licensing requirements of another state as being similar to its own.

4. Someone who holds a _____ has attained advanced knowledge through higher education in a discipline such as nursing, mathematics, or education.

5. A medical symbol depicted by a staff with a serpent coiled around its shaft is referred to as a _____.

6. A _____ is a potentially infectious, life-threatening disease, usually transmitted by bites of rodent fleas.

7. _____ is a method that enables a person, usually with the help of electronic equipment, to learn to control otherwise involuntary bodily functions.

8. _____ is a 200-year-old system based on the Law of Similars.

9. _____ is a multidisciplinary approach to health care based on the belief that the body has power to heal itself.

10. An _____ is a disease affecting large numbers of individuals in a population.

Chapter Review

Short Answer

1. Physicians now must take all three steps of what exam before being eligible for full licensure as a physician?

_____

2. List the members of the three guilds of medicine during the seventeenth century.

_____

_____

_____

3. **List and describe five types of nurses.**

_____

_____

_____

_____

_____

_____

_____

4. Why is it important for medical assistants to know the role of other health care providers?

_____

_____

_____

5. In ancient civilizations, people thought disease was due to _____ brought on as punishment for disobedience to the gods.

6. Egyptians used leeches to remove _____ and produce _____, which helps _____.

7. The Hindus in India were known for the world's _____.

8. What did the Romans discover regarding sanitation, and what did they do about it?

_____

_____

_____

9. How did the Christian church feel about illness during medieval history, and what did it suggest for treatment?

_____

_____

_____

10. What is a possible theory for the origin of the caduceus symbol?

_____

_____

_____

11. How did the red and white barber poles originate?

_____

_____

_____

12. In the following table, match the following medical historians with their contributions.

Florence Nightingale	Clara Barton	Elizabeth Blackwell
Louis Pasteur	Wilhelm Roentgen	Marie Curie
George Papanicolaou	Fredrick Banting	Robert Jarvik
Joseph Lister	Antony Van Leuwenhoek	Hippocrates
Patrick Steptoe	Edward Jenner	Rene Laennec
Andreas Vesalius	Sir Alexander Fleming	A. B. Sabin

Historian	Contribution
_____	Designed the first permanently implantable artificial heart
_____	Built microscopes, allowing him to see red blood cells for the first time
_____	Known for the first vaccination
_____	Invented the stethoscope
_____	Known as the father of medicine
_____	Founder of modern nursing
_____	Founder of aseptic technique
_____	Discovered X-rays
_____	Discovered that mold could stop the growth of bacteria, which later contributed to the discovery of penicillin
_____	Originator of the Pap test
_____	Discovered and isolated insulin
_____	Credited with the pasteurization process
_____	First female physician in the United States
_____	Founded the Red Cross
_____	Developed the first attenuated vaccine for polio
_____	Credited with the world's first successful in vitro fertilization
_____	First woman scientist; discovered radium
_____	Anatomist that wrote one of the most influential anatomy books of its kind

13. Match the patient's symptoms or disease to the type of specialist he or she might see.
    Podiatrist, Pediatrician, Chiropractor, Dentist, Ophthalmologist, Pulmonary specialist, Sports medicine specialist, Dermatologist, Allergist, Gynecologist, Optometrist, Nuclear medicine specialist, Plastic surgeon, Otorhinolaryngologist, Anesthesiologist, Urologist, Gerontologist, and Endocrinologist

Specialist	Symptoms or Disease
_____	Whiplash injury
_____	Tooth pain
_____	Impotence or urinary problems
_____	Emphysema patient
_____	Sports injury
_____	Someone who needs radiation treatment for cancer
_____	Patient with glaucoma
_____	Patient with diabetes
_____	Patient who suffers from hay fever
_____	Patient needing an epidural prior to delivery of her baby
_____	An 87-year-old patient
_____	Female with a possible STD
_____	Patient with foot pain
_____	Patient with a suspicious mole
_____	Well-baby check
_____	Patient wanting to make facial improvements
_____	Patient with persistent hoarseness
_____	Patient with vision problems

14. Match the description with the appropriate organization or legislation.
    FDA, NIH, WHO, Medicaid, Medicare, CLIA, Uniform Anatomical Gift Act,
    OSHA, Controlled Substances Act, HIPAA, Patient Protection and Affordable Care Act,
    Hill-Burton Act, Medicare Part D

Organization or Legislation	Description
_____	National insurance for persons over the age of 65, the disabled, or those suffering from end-stage renal disease
_____	Establishes guidelines for operating laboratories
_____	Regulates the foods we purchase and drugs we consume and is part of the Department of Health and Human Services
_____	An organization that protects employees in the workplace
_____	An act that allows living individuals to indicate their desire for their organs to be gifted at the time of death
_____	An act that expands access to health insurance

Organization or Legislation	Description
_____	A prescription drug plan for seniors to make drugs more affordable
_____	One of the world's foremost medical research centers
_____	Legislation responsible for improving construction of hospitals
_____	A specialized agency of the United Nations that cooperates to control and eradicate disease worldwide
_____	A federal organization that provides for the medical care of the indigent
_____	Legislation that helps control the abuse of drugs
_____	Intended to limit health administration costs and provide for patient privacy

Chapter Application

Case Study with Critical Thinking Questions

Mrs. Dobson has been struggling with pain over the past six weeks. She was in an automobile accident and suffered some injuries to her back. The patient is tired of the pain and is searching for some alternatives to traditional medicine. She asks whether you are an advocate of acupuncture and goes on to state that a friend had acupuncture for some pain she was having and feels much better now. You know that your physician is not a huge fan of acupuncture but is not totally opposed to it either.

1. How would you respond to the patient's question?

   _____
   _____
   _____

2. What are some of the other complementary therapies the provider may suggest, and what do they entail?

   _____

Connecting to the Right Team Member

Connecting patients to the right health care professional is part of the medical assistant's job. Today, you are asked to connect several patients to the correct professional. Fill in the blanks with the appropriate professional.

1. The patient's results from her hearing test were very poor today. The doctor asks you to set up an appointment with Susan Klein, an _____ for the Orange Valley Speech and Hearing Center.

2. A patient calls on the phone regarding her bill. You connect her to Mike Brown, the clinic's _____.

3. Your doctor instructs you to call the EMS for a patient exhibiting chest pain. You will probably need to give the _____ a list of the patient's current medications upon arrival.

4. You send two tubes of blood to the lab. The _____ calls to alert you that the patient's lab results are at a critical level and that the doctor needs to be notified right away.

5. The doctor would like you to set the patient up for an appointment with a _____ to assist the patient with walking, following her stroke.

6. The _____ answered the phone when you called the pharmacy to renew a prescription for Mrs. Wong. She immediately transferred you to the pharmacist.

7. Dr. Prime asked you to contact Missy, _____, regarding the last set of radiographs she took on Mr. Hodges.

8. Dr. Smith asks you to call Jason Brown, a _____ with Visiting Health Professionals, to schedule some breathing tests and treatments on Mrs. Kesterson in her home.

9. Dr. Somadi just completed an exam on Mr. Waterson, who is a diabetic. She would like you to set up an appointment for the patient to see a _____ to educate him about proper food selection.

Role-Play Activities

Delivering messages to other health care professionals is a common responsibility of medical assistants. It is important to have all the details correct. Practice your communication skills by sharing the following message with one of your classmates.

1. The doctor asks you to set up a pelvic ultrasound for Mrs. Jennings, who is pregnant for the first time. The doctor suspects something wrong with the baby because it is measuring at only 12 weeks and should be measuring at 20 weeks. The patient is not scheduled to have an ultrasound today, but the doctor wants the sonographer to skip the patients that are in front of her and perform the ultrasound immediately.

Medical Law
and Ethics

CHAPTER 3

Legal Issues

Words to Know Challenge

Spelling: Each line contains three spellings of a word. Underline the correctly spelled word.

1. misdeamenor · misdemenor · misdemeanor
2. negligence · negligense · negilgense
3. plantif · plaintiff · plaintif
4. respondeat superior · respondent superior · respondat superior
5. libal · lible · libel
6. gardian · guardian · guardan
7. fellany · fellony · felony
8. jurisdiction · juridiction · juresdiction

Matching: Match the term in column I to its definition in column II.

COLUMN I	COLUMN II
___ 1. Manslaughter	A. Spoken defamation of character
___ 2. Damages	B. Taking money or property belonging to another without the presence of the victim
___ 3. Punitive damages	C. The unlawful killing without malice of a human being
___ 4. Slander	D. Unlawfully taking money or goods of another from his or her person or in immediate presence by force or intimidation
___ 5. Burglary	E. Written defamation of character
___ 6. Robbery	F. Having the mental competency to make health care decisions
___ 7. Prosecution	G. Damages recovered in payment for actual injury or economic loss
___ 8. Felony	H. Damages awarded in a lawsuit as a punishment and example to others for malicious or fraudulent acts

(continues)

____ 9. Statute

____ 10. Defendant

____ 11. Federal law

____ 12. Libel

____ 13. Capacity

I. Legislation enacted by Congress

J. A written federal or state law enacted by Congress or a state legislature

K. The party sued in a civil lawsuit or the party charged with a crime in a criminal prosecution

L. Crimes committed by people who intend to do significant harm to others, either through depriving them of their property or injuring them personally

M. In criminal law, the government attorney charging and trying the case against a person accused of a crime

Chapter Review

Short Answer

1. Why is it important for medical assistants to be familiar with the law?

_____

_____

_____

_____

2. What are the four elements that must be present in a given situation to prove that a provider or professional practice is guilty of negligence?

_____

_____

_____

3. A contract may be either implied or express. Define what *implied* and *express* mean.

_____

_____

_____

4. Explain the difference between medical malpractice and negligence.

_____

_____

_____

_____

_____

5. Crimes are divided into two categories. Identify and explain the difference between the two.

_____

_____

_____

6. Explain the concept of "standard of proof," and list the standard of proof in criminal law and civil law.

_____

_____

_____

7. List and explain the essential elements of a contract.

_____

_____

_____

_____

8. Read the following examples listed. Which are examples of express contracts and which are examples of implied contracts?

   a A physician treats a patient in the emergency room for a fractured collarbone   _____

   b. You hire your neighbor to clean your house, and you confirm the deal with a handshake   _____

   c. A patient in your provider's office rolls up his sleeve to have his blood drawn   _____

   d. Written agreement   _____

   e. A provider telling a patient that treatment results are guaranteed   _____

9. What is the Patient Self-Determination Act?

_____

_____

_____

Chapter Application

Case Studies with Critical Thinking Questions

Scenario 1

You have just finished seeing Daniel Cho in the office. You are documenting information in his chart. You have accidentally recorded some incorrect lab results.

1. Is it appropriate to change the chart entry? _____

_____

_____

2. What steps must you take to write in the correct information? _____

_____

_____

Scenario 2

You receive samples in your office from pharmaceutical representatives. Rosalee Dunning cannot afford the cost of her blood pressure medication. She comes to you for samples.

1. May you give her samples? Why or why not?

_____

_____

_____

Scenario 3

Mr. Wing has not paid the past-due fees owed your provider. Repeated letters have been sent. The amount owed is now in excess of $1200. You sent a final collection letter stating that he needs to make arrangements with your office to pay on the past-due amount. You receive no monies and no response. Your provider wants to terminate services to Mr. Wing.

1. What steps must you perform so your provider is not responsible for abandonment? _____

_____

_____

Competency Practice

1. **Perform Compliance Reporting Bases on Public Health Statutes**

   Using the detailed instructions and rationales outlined in Procedure 3–1 as a guideline, perform compliance reporting based on public health statutes and report a patient with tuberculosis.

2. **Report an Illegal Activity in the Health Care Setting Following Proper Protocol**

   Using the following scenario and the detailed instructions and rationales outlined in Procedure 3–2 as a guideline, report illegal activity.

   Scenario: In 2014, the Veterans Administration health care system made headlines when the use of secret wait lists to hide delays was discovered (Newsmax.com). Several "whistleblowers" came forward to disclose this illegal activity. Log on to the Internet and review various news articles regarding the scandal. Using this (or a similar) scenario, report illegal activity per proper protocol (e.g., hidden wait lists, colleague taking drug samples from the office for personal use, colleague taking cash from the patient co-pay receipts, provider or colleague injecting wrong medication into a patient, medical assistant or provider routinely billing for services not performed, and HIPAA violations, etc.).

3. **Apply HIPAA Rules in Regard to Privacy and Release of Information**

   Using the detailed instructions and rationales outlined in Procedure 3–3 as a guideline, release patient information to an insurance company requesting documentation for a life insurance policy.

4. **Locate a State's Legal Scope of Practice for Medical Assistants**

   Using the detailed instructions and rationales outlined in Procedure 3–4 as a guideline, go online to research the scope of practice for a different state than chosen in the textbook procedure. Contrast and compare the similarities and differences between the states. In a one- to two-page essay, describe your findings and discuss the scope of practice as if you were employed in each state.

CHAPTER 4

Ethical Issues

Words to Know Challenge

Spelling: Each line contains three spellings of a word. Underline the correctly spelled word.

1. <u>autonomy</u>   automony   autonnomy
2. vallues   valuse   <u>values</u>
3. extrinics   <u>extrinsic</u>   extinsic
4. benificense   benificence   <u>beneficence</u>
5. <u>ethics</u>   ethiks   ethix
6. <u>distributive justice</u>   distribitive justice   distributative justice
7. morral   morale   <u>moral</u>
8. intrinics   <u>intrinsic</u>   intrinsac

Fill in the Blank: Complete the following sentences with correctly spelled words from the Spelling section.

1. In the context of health care, when we recognize the _____ of the patient, we are recognizing that the patient has the right to make decisions about his or her life, death, and health.

2. _____ issues stem from a belief system in which one makes judgments about right and wrong.

3. There are a variety of approaches to the concept of _____; one of the approaches is an egalitarian approach (everyone gets an equal share).

4. Pride in knowing one is upholding the high standards of the organization is an example of an _____ reward.

5. Receiving an end-of-year bonus for achieving the highest patient satisfaction scores is an example of an _____ reward.

6. Organizational ethics represent the _____ by which the organization conducts its business.

7. The concept of _____ requires people to do what is in the best interests of others.

8. The rules of conduct with respect to a particular class of actions are known as _____.

Chapter Review

Short Answer

1. List at least six ethical issues in health care.

_____
_____
_____
_____

2. List at least five examples of cultural communication considerations.

_____
_____
_____

3. List at least five examples of good intercultural communication skills.

_____
_____
_____

4. Describe an ethical dilemma.

_____
_____
_____

5. List three professional organizations that have a code of ethics relating to the medical field.

_____
_____
_____

6. List four characteristics of an organization that encourages ethical behavior.

_____
_____
_____

7. Identify where to report the following illegal and unsafe activities and behaviors that affect the health, safety, and welfare of others: criminal conduct, improper disclosure of patient information, provider misconduct, office staff misconduct.

- _____
_____
- _____
_____
_____
_____
_____
- _____
_____
_____
_____
_____
_____
_____
- _____
_____
_____

Matching: Match the ethical issues in column I with their descriptions in column II.

	COLUMN I		COLUMN II
____	1. Cryonics	A.	Surgical procedure in which tissue or whole organ is transferred from one species to another
____	2. Human cloning	B.	Attempts either to slow down or reverse the processes of aging to maximize life span
____	3. Xenotransplantation	C.	Killing an individual so that he or she will not suffer pain
____	4. Suicide	D.	Brain surgery carried out to ease the complications associated with mental or behavioral problems
____	5. Life extension	E.	Resorting to medical equipment to keep an individual alive
____	6. Eugenics	F.	Creating a genetically identical copy of a human
____	7. Euthanasia	G.	A process whereby the body of a seriously ill or deceased individual is frozen to stop the decomposition of tissues
____	8. Psychosurgery	H.	The act of killing oneself
____	9. Surrogacy	I.	Improving genetic qualities by means of selective breeding
____	10. Life support	J.	A process whereby a woman agrees to carry and deliver a child for a contracted party

Chapter Application

Case Studies with Critical Thinking Questions

Scenario 1

Jennifer observes one of the other medical assistants taking samples of a narcotic pain reliever and placing them in her pocket. When Jennifer confronts her coworker, the coworker states that everyone else takes samples, so she is taking some, too.

1. Is this a legal, ethical, or moral issue? _____

_____

_____

2. Should Jennifer report this to her supervisor? _____

_____

_____

3. What could be the outcome for the medical assistant who took the samples? _____

_____

_____

Scenario 2

Gabrielle, a medical assistant, sees Roberto in the medical office where she works. Roberto works for Gabrielle's husband. Roberto and his wife Sally are also personal friends of Gabrielle and her husband Mark. Roberto has been out of work for the past few weeks because of severe back problems. That night at dinner, Mark asks her if Roberto will be able to return to work and when.

1. Is this a legal, ethical, or moral issue? _____

_____

_____

2. What should Gabrielle do in this situation? _____

_____

_____

Scenario 3

You are standing at the time clock and notice another employee clocking out not only herself but also a fellow employee. You know for a fact that this other employee was not at work today. You check the time card and notice the other employee has "punched in" at the beginning of the day as well as recorded time for lunch. Because you work for a large company and the time cards are not completed at the facility, there is no way anyone at payroll will know whether this person worked.

1. Is this a legal, ethical, or moral issue? _____
_____
_____

2. Who would you report this to? _____
_____
_____

Critical Thinking

1. **Ethics and diversity:** Medical assistants are reminded to strive to provide the same quality of care to all their patients regardless of race or ethnicity and eliminate biased behavior toward any group of patients different from themselves. In the following space, explain why caring for a culturally diverse clientele is an ethical issue.
_____
_____
_____
_____

2. **Personal versus professional ethics:** Whatever your personal perspective might be with regard to ethical matters, you must adapt your personal views to comply with the ethical standards of your profession and the organization in which you are employed.
   a. Assess your personal belief system and upbringing. List two sources that have influenced your own personal ethics the most. _____
   _____
   _____

   b. Review the "Ethics Check Questions" presented in this chapter, and list the three questions to ask yourself when considering ethical issues: _____
   _____
   _____

   c. Now, compare the AAMA Code of Ethics and Creed with the AMT Standards of Practice. What similarities and differences do you see? _____
   _____
   _____

3. **Your view #1:** Select one of the topics in Table 4–1 not previously selected (or another ethical issue related to health care of your choosing), and discuss your personal opinion of the topic. Relate the opinion to the concepts discussed in the chapter (autonomy, beneficence, and distributive justice) if possible.
_____
_____
_____

4. **Your view #2:** Reflecting on the ethics of the four approaches to Distributive Justice, consider how you would allocate health care resources. In a one- to two-page essay, justify your conclusion with fact and opinion.
_____
_____
_____

Competency Practice

1. **Develop a Plan for Separation of Personal and Professional Ethics.**

   Use the detailed instructions and rationales outlined in Procedure 4–1 as a guideline and go online to research a health care organization near you that has some form of a mission, vision, and values statement. In a one- to two-page essay, describe your findings and discuss ethical conduct and action that you would express if you were an employee of that organization and then create a plan to separate your personal and professional ethics. (Some examples might include Northwest Health [www.nwhc.org], Ohio Health, [www.ohiohealth.com], or Sutter Health [www.sutterhealth.org].)

2. **Demonstrate Appropriate Responses to Ethical Issues.**

   Using the detailed instructions and rationales outlined in Procedure 4–2 as a guideline, respond appropriately to the following scenario(s):

   a. Fraternization between employees in the same chain of command is prohibited. Are there ethical issues with fraternization between coworkers?

   b. Is it ever appropriate to accept gifts from patients or clients?

   c. A family member of a terminally ill patient has requested information on end-of-life options. What is your ethical responsibility?

3

Professional Communications

Verbal and Nonverbal Communications

Words to Know Challenge

Spelling: Each line contains three spellings of a word. Underline the correctly spelled word.

1. <u>active listening</u>   activ listening   active listining
2. persepsion   perseption   <u>perception</u>
3. deniul   <u>denial</u>   danial
4. <u>empirically</u>   emperically   imperically
5. contrudict   contredict   <u>contradict</u>
6. intalectualization   <u>intellectualization</u>   intallectualization
7. mallinger   <u>malinger</u>   milinger
8. regresion   regerssion   <u>regression</u>
9. sublimination   <u>sublimation</u>   subliamation
10. compinsation   <u>compensation</u>   compensasion
11. <u>incongruent</u>   encongruent   incongrunent
12. <u>suppression</u>   supression   suppresion
13. rashonization   rationisation   <u>rationalization</u>

31

Matching: Match the term in column I to its definition in column II.

	COLUMN I	COLUMN II
____	1. Articulate	To impart, as an idea; to transfer
____	2. Conceptualize	To explain, translate; to determine the meaning
____	3. Convey	To join together, as in a joint
____	4. Distort	A defense mechanism of trying to blame another for one's own inadequacies
____	5. Interpret	To force painful ideas or impulses into the subconscious
____	6. Intuition	To misinterpret; to twist into unusual shape
____	7. Projection	To form a concept, thought, notion, or understanding
____	8. Repression	The immediate knowing or learning of something without the conscious use of reasoning

Chapter Review

Short Answer

1. Identify and describe the components of the standard communication model.

   _____
   _____
   _____

2. There are several styles and types of verbal communication. In general, people process and communicate information in three basic ways. Identify and describe the three ways.

   _____
   _____
   _____

3. List six examples of nonverbal communication.

   _____
   _____
   _____

4. Explain perception and state its importance in communication.

   _____
   _____
   _____
   _____

5. Why do people use defense mechanisms?

   _____
   _____
   _____

6. The following chart lists the commonly used behavioral defense mechanisms. Next to each defense mechanism, give an example of it. The first two rows have been filled in for you as examples.

Defense Mechanism	Example
Repression	Not crying at a funeral because you've buried the emotions so deeply in the back of your mind.
Displacement	Yelling at your spouse for no reason after having a hard day at the office.
Suppression	
Projection	
Rationalization	
Intellectualization	
Sublimation	
Compensation	
Temporary withdrawal	
Daydreaming	
Malingering	
Denial	
Regression	
Procrastination	

7. Explain what could happen to a person who habitually uses one or more of the defense mechanisms listed in this chapter.

_____
_____
_____

8. List the five stages of understanding needs according to Maslow's hierarchical model. Then identify which of the stages is the one in which the person tends to be a problem solver and places a great deal of emphasis on family and long-term relationships.

_____
_____
_____

9. Dr. Elisabeth Kübler-Ross described five stages of grieving. List the five stages.

_____
_____
_____

10. Describe the difference between positive and negative coping skills.

_____

_____

_____

11. List seven adaptive coping skills and seven nonadaptive coping skills.

    a. Adaptive: _____

_____

_____

    b. Nonadaptive: _____

_____

_____

Labeling

Identify the sections of the following communication process model:

a. _____

b. _____

c. _____

d. _____

e. _____

Chapter Application

Case Studies with Critical Thinking Questions

Scenario 1

A middle-aged woman is being seen in the office for insomnia and hot flashes. She says she cannot understand why these things are happening to her. She has always been a good sleeper, and she is always cold. She says that her friends tell her she is going through menopause, but she doesn't think she is old enough for that and refuses to believe them.

a. What type of coping skill is she using? _____

_____

_____

b. Which of these coping skills is this patient using? _____

_____

_____

c. What can you do to help her accept her condition? _____

_____

_____

Scenario 2

You have had an extremely frustrating day at work but have managed to keep your emotions in check and get through the day. You have been very professional with both patients and coworkers even though you wanted to explode. When you get home, your kids ask you what you are making for dinner, and you direct all your pent-up anger toward them.

a. Which defense mechanism are you using? _____

_____

_____

b. What can you do about reducing the stress at work? _____

_____

_____

c. Which part of you did you use to respond to your children? _____

_____

_____

Competency Practice

1. **Respond to Nonverbal Communication.** With a partner, role-play responding to nonverbal communication. Practice calling the patient back from the waiting room and escorting them to an exam room. Once in the privacy of the room, obtain the reason why the patient is there to see the provider (chief complaint). Use Procedure 5–1 as a guide.

Role-Play Activities

1. Research the boundaries and customs of several ethnic groups, and prepare a brief report of your findings. Choose one of the ethnic groups you researched and, with a partner, demonstrate the correct communication techniques (especially nonverbal ones) you would employ when working with a patient from that ethnic group.

Applying Communication Skills

Words to Know Challenge

Spelling: Each line contains three spellings of a word. Underline the correctly spelled word.

1. adovocasy   avdocacey   advocacy
2. analitical   analytical   annalytical
3. ascertive   assertive   asertive
4. job description   job descripsion   job discription
5. evalation   evolution   evaluation

Matching: Now, using the preceding correctly spelled terms, write each word next to the correct definition.

1. _____ confident; BOLD

2. _____ assessment; judgment concerning worth, quality, significance, or value of situation, person, or product

3. _____ promoting and protecting the rights of patients, frequently through a legal process

4. _____ characterized by a method of analysis, a statement of point-by-point contact

5. _____ set of clear expectations or duties to be performed

Chapter Review

Short Answer

1. What are the steps in applying critical thinking skills to a particular problem?

_____

_____

_____

_____

2. Fill in the following grid, identifying resources and adaptations when working with special-needs patients.

Patients with special needs	
Culturally diverse patients	
Pediatric patients	
Geriatric patients	
Difficult or uncooperative patients	

3. Often, your provider will ask you to provide patient education. List three patient education formats.

_____

_____

_____

4. Describe the steps to follow when providing patient education.

_____

_____

_____

5. What is a patient advocate? Identify situations in which patients might benefit from intervention by a medical assistant.

_____

_____

_____

6. What does it mean to be assertive when communicating in the medical office?

_____

_____

_____

7. Describe relationships among the medical assistant, the employer, and coworkers and how to resolve conflict.

_____

_____

_____

8. Explain methods of communicating information in the medical office.

_____

_____

_____

9. State the purpose of:

A. Staff meeting: _____

_____

_____

B. An employee evaluation: _____

_____

_____

Fill in the Blank: Complete the following sentences with terms from this chapter.

1. Taking a step-by-step approach helps one look realistically and logically at a problem. This method encourages _____ thinking and confident decision making.

2. We use many coping skills and defense mechanisms to deal with difficult or stressful situations. Another approach to handling interpersonal problems and concerns is to use _____ skills.

3. The tone of your voice goes a long way. Using a genuinely warm and caring tone is referred to as _____ to enhance the meaning of phrases.

4. _____ in the ambulatory setting keeps patients healthier and medical conditions from worsening and can reduce the need for hospitalization. This can include verbal instructions, printed materials, or electronic format.

5. _____ means to afford the opportunity to examine behaviors and interactions, act as a verbal mirror, and restate what the patient has said for clarification by all parties.

Chapter Application

Case Study with Critical Thinking Questions

During the past two weeks, Jennifer has noticed that her coworker, Maryn, has been making some charting errors. Jennifer is very concerned about patient care and does not want any of the patients to suffer because of these errors.

1. Who should Jennifer talk with about her concerns? _____

_____

_____

2. What could happen if Jennifer takes the issue on herself and talks to Maryn without consulting the manager?

_____

_____

_____

Competency Practice

1. **Coach Patients Regarding Health Maintenance, Disease Prevention, and Treatment Plans while Considering Cultural Diversity, Developmental Life Stages, and Communication Barriers.** The provider has asked you to coach a patient regarding education on managing diabetes. Read the following patient education handout on managing diabetes and role-play a coaching session with a partner. Be sure to use language the patient can understand as well as appropriate techniques of effective verbal and nonverbal communication. Finally, using the following progress note template, document the patient education session in the patient's medical record. Use Procedure 6–1 as a guide.

DOUGLASVILLE MEDICINE ASSOCIATES
5076 BRAND BLVD
DOUGLASVILLE, NY 01234
(123)456-7890

DIABETES

<u>*Overview:*</u> Diabetes is a chronic disease of metabolism in which blood glucose levels are elevated. According to a 2005 government study, 20.8 million children and adults, or 7% of the U.S. total population, has diabetes. It is estimated that at least 6.2 million of those individuals have yet to be diagnosed.

There are three types of diabetes:

- *Type 1*: 5-10% of Americans diagnosed have this type of diabetes in which the body does not produce enough insulin. Insulin is a hormone that allows glucose to enter the cells of the body to be used as fuel. This type of diabetes is often seen in children.

- *Type 2*: This type of diabetes comes from a resistance to insulin. In other words, the body produces enough insulin, but does not use it effectively. Most Americans diagnosed with diabetes have Type 2. This type of diabetes is often seen in adults.

- *Gestational:* 4% of all pregnant women develop this type.

There is also a condition called pre-diabetes in which the blood glucose levels are elevated, but not high enough for a diagnosis of Type 2 diabetes. Approximately 41 million Americans have pre-diabetes.

Possible Complications from Diabetes:

- Heart attack
- Stroke
- Kidney disease, which can lead to kidney failure and the need for dialysis
- High blood pressure
- Male Impotence

Treatment

Type 2 diabetes can often be managed by diet, exercise, oral hypoglycemics, and/or insulin. It is important to maintain good blood pressure control and to lower cholesterol levels.

What kind of foods should you eat?

Healthy food choices are important in controlling your glucose levels. The Diabetic Food Pyramid is a helpful tool in determining what to eat. Here are some helpful tips based on the pyramid:

- Eat lots of fruits and vegetables: However, be aware of the sugar content in some fruits.
- Eat whole grains rather than processed grains, like brown rice and whole wheat pasta.

- Eat dried beans.
- Include fish in your diet at least 2–3 times per week.
- Eat lean meats.
- Choose non-fat dairy products.
- Drink lots of water and choose sugar-free "diet" drinks.
- Use liquid oils for cooking.
- Cut down on desserts and high-calorie foods like chips.
- Watch your portion sizes.

Other Practices to Control Diabetes

See your physician on a regular basis and consistently monitor your blood glucose. Record results onto a log and share your results with your physician. It is important to keep weight regulated and to alert the physician when symptoms worsen or new symptoms appear. Have regular eye exams and podiatric (foot) exams. Even though diabetes can be a debilitating disease, you can play an active role in delaying the onset of debilitating factors or even the prevention of certain factors.

Resources:
www.diabetes.org (American Diabetes Association)
http://diabetes.niddk.nih.gov/index.htm (National Diabetes Information Clearinghouse)

PROGRESS NOTE

Patient Name: _____ DOB _____

DATE/TIME	PROGRESS NOTES	ALLERGIES

Medical Terminology

CHAPTER 7

Introduction to Medical Terminology

Words to Know Challenge

Spelling: Each line contains three spellings of a word. Underline the correctly spelled word.

1. pleural
   pleral
   plural

2. word rout
   word root
   werd root

3. prifix
   prefix
   preficks

4. combining form
   combinning form
   combineing form

5. suffixes
   suffices
   suffixs

6. singler
   cingular
   singular

Fill in the Blank: Complete the following sentences with Words to Know from this chapter.

1. A word part found at the beginning of a medical term is a _____.

2. _____ means referring to one.

3. *Neur/o*, *cardi/o*, and *cyan/o* are all examples of _____.

4. *Diagnoses* is the _____ form of the word *diagnosis*.

5. A _____ is a word part added to the end of a word to complete the term.

6. A _____ is the foundation of a medical term and usually describes part of the body.

Chapter Review

Short Answer

1. From which two languages are most medical terms derived?

   _____

   _____

   _____

2. In relation to a medical term:
   a. Does the prefix go on the left or on the right? _____
   b. Does the suffix go on the left or on the right? _____

3. Describe the procedure to follow when taking a medical term apart to define it.

   _____

   _____

   _____

4. What is the difference between a word root and a combining form?

   _____

   _____

   _____

5. Explain why spelling is so important in medical terminology.

   _____

   _____

   _____

6. Explain the difference between a singular and a plural term and provide an example of each.

   _____

   _____

   _____

Matching: Determine whether each word in column I is singular (A) or plural (B).

COLUMN I	COLUMN II
_____ 1. bacilli	A. Singular
_____ 2. vertebra	B. Plural
_____ 3. diagnoses	
_____ 4. phalanges	
_____ 5. atrium	
_____ 6. vertebrae	
_____ 7. apex	
_____ 8. bacillus	
_____ 9. appendices	
_____ 10. diagnosis	
_____ 11. phalanx	
_____ 12. atria	
_____ 13. appendix	
_____ 14. apices	

Labeling

For each of the following words, identify the word parts. The first one has been filled in for you as an example.

Word	Prefix	Word Root or Combining Form	Suffix
prenatal	pre-	nat	-al
bradycardia	_____	_____	_____
dyspepsia	_____	_____	_____
leukemia	_____	_____	_____
polyneuropathy	_____	_____	_____

Dissecting and Building Medical Terms

Using Tables 7–1, 7–2, and 7–3 in the text chapter, fill in the missing spaces on this chart. The first one has been filled in for you as an example.

leukocyte	white blood cell
urology	_____
_____	instrument used for cutting bone
_____	person who studies the kidney
cardiomyopathy	_____
_____	without breathing
bradykinesia	_____

Chapter Application

Case Study with Critical Thinking Questions

One of your office responsibilities is to schedule patients for procedures. Today, you are working on charts that have been completed by the transcriptionist and need outside referrals. You contact the hospital to schedule a colposcopy for a patient and speak to Sarah the customer service representative (CSR). Sarah (CSR) asks you for the age of the patient, last monthly period, and tentative diagnosis. You tell Sarah the patient is 55 years old, has no record of a last monthly period, and the diagnosis is positive occult blood in the stool. Sarah asks you whether your data is correct and says the information you have provided is not a reason for a colposcopy. Then Sarah asks you what the patient's name is, to which you reply, "Jack Kelley." Sarah tells you there must be a mistake because a colposcopy is a procedure performed only on females.

1. Using Tables 7–2 and 7–3 in your text, determine the definition of colposcopy and write it here:

   _____

   _____

   _____

2. Using Tables 7–2 and 7–3 in your text, determine the definition of colonoscopy and write it here:

   _____

   _____

   _____

3. Based on your answers to the previous question, what is the correct procedure Mr. Jack Kelley should be scheduled for and why? (You may consult the Internet or a medical dictionary if necessary.)

   _____

   _____

Research Activity

1. Using the Internet or a medical dictionary, find five terms that have Latin or Greek meanings. Explain what the original terms from the original language were and how the ancient physicians assigned such meanings. (Think back to the example in the chapter about the uterus and the word *hysterical*.)

	Term	Origin
a.		
b.		
c.		
d.		
e.		

Understanding and Building Medical Terms of Body Systems

Words to Know Challenge

Spelling: Each line contains three spellings of a word. Underline the correctly spelled word.

1. cholecystolithiases   cholecistolithiasis   cholecystolithiasis
2. femural   femeral   femoral
3. alopesia   alopecia   allopesia
4. ascites   acsites   ascitis
5. myacardium   myocardium   miocardium
6. dialysis   dialisis   dyalysis
7. visera   vicsera   viscera
8. lukocyte   leukocite   leukocyte
9. hyperglycemia   hyperglicemia   hyperglicymia
10. polineuralgia   polyneuralgia   polynuralgia
11. diafragm   diaphram   diaphragm
12. hystologist   hystoligist   histologist
13. atrium   attrium   atriam
14. septim   septume   septum
15. ventrical   ventricle   ventricall
16. gastroentestinal   gastrointestinal   gastrointestinal
17. jaundise   jandice   jaundice
18. micturition   micturation   micsurition
19. neumonitis   pneumonitis   pnumonitis

Matching: Match the terms in column I to their meanings in column II.

COLUMN I	COLUMN II
____ 1. Feces	A. A red blood cell
____ 2. Dermatology	B. Vein that carries deoxygenated blood from the upper half of the body
____ 3. Alimentary canal	C. A nerve cell
____ 4. External	D. Cells and fibers forming a body structure
____ 5. Bicuspid	E. Internal organs
____ 6. Erythrocyte	F. Stool, bowel movement
____ 7. Chyme	G. Specializes in eye diseases and disorders
____ 8. Neuron	H. Pertaining to digestion
____ 9. Bolus	I. Mitral valve
____ 10. Superior vena cava	J. Inflammation of sebaceous glands, producing pimples
____ 11. Inferior vena cava	K. Loss of hair, baldness
____ 12. Nephron	L. Study of the skin
____ 13. Tissue	M. The intestinal tract
____ 14. Pyelonephritis	N. A mass of masticated food ready to be swallowed
____ 15. Digestive	O. Inflammation of the kidney, pelvis, and nephrons
____ 16. Alopecia	P. Mixture of partially digested food and digestive secretions
____ 17. Acne vulgaris	Q. Structural and functional unit of kidney
____ 18. Ophthalmologist	R. Vein that carries deoxygenated blood from the lower half of the body
____ 19. Viscera	S. The outermost part of the body

Chapter Review

Fill in the Blank: Complete the following sentences with the correct terms.

1. Mrs. Holton fell and fractured the thighbone of her leg. This body part is known as the _____.

2. A _____ is a person engaged in the study of the microscopic structure of tissue.

3. The _____ is the muscle of breathing that separates the thorax from the abdomen.

4. Mrs. Silva developed a yellowish discoloration of the sclera and skin known as _____.

5. High blood sugar is known as _____.

6. A physician who specializes in diagnosing and treating disorders and diseases of the skin works in the field of _____.

7. Cindy's physician noted her skin condition characterized by inflammation of sebaceous glands that produced pimples and therefore diagnosed her with _____.

8. The upper chamber of the heart is known as the _____.

9. An inflammation of the cervix of the uterus is known as _____.

10. A(n) _____ is a white blood cell, and a(n) _____ is a red blood cell.

11. Mr. Romero was found to have inflammation of the lungs and therefore was diagnosed with _____, also known as pneumonia.

12. The muscle layer of the heart is known as the _____.

13. Mr. Noto will undergo a valve replacement of his bicuspid, also known as the _____ valve.

14. The membranous wall dividing two cavities, as within the heart, is known as a _____.

15. The functional cells of the nervous system are known as _____.

16. Mr. Smothers will undergo _____, which is the process of removing the products of urine from the blood by passage of the solutes through a membrane.

17. One of the two lower chambers of the heart is known as a _____.

18. The skin, hair, nails, and sweat glands comprise the _____ system.

19. The valve in the right side of the heart, made up of three cusps or leaflets, is known as the _____ valve.

Matching: Match the abbreviations in column I to their meanings in column II and write which body system each abbreviation refers to. The first one has been completed for you as a guide.

COLUMN I		COLUMN II
____ 1. ECG	cardiovascular	A. Chronic obstructive pulmonary disease
____ 2. UA	_____	B. Osteoarthritis
____ 3. GU	_____	C. Electrocardiogram
____ 4. TMJ	_____	D. Gynecology
____ 5. OA	_____	E. Electroencephalogram
____ 6. OU	_____	F. Urinalysis
____ 7. COPD	_____	G. Each eye
____ 8. IV	_____	H. Genitourinary
____ 9. GYN	_____	I. Urinary tract infection
____ 10. EEG	_____	J. Intravenous
____ 11. UTI	_____	K. Temporomandibular joint

Chapter Application

Case Study with Critical Thinking Questions

You are preparing to complete the school training for the medical assistant program and will be starting your clinical practicum soon at a family practice facility. You have been struggling with the pronunciation of medical terms in your classes and are concerned that you are going to make mistakes when you get out in the field and will be looked down upon by your preceptors.

1. What can you do to practice your medical terminology? _____
   _____
   _____
   _____

2. How should you handle the situation if you come across words you are unsure how to pronounce when you are in the clinical setting? _____
   _____
   _____
   _____

Building Medical Terms: Using the definitions provided, build the following medical terms.
(*Hint*: Use the tables from both Chapters 7 and 8 to help you recall all the word parts.)

1. Surgical removal of the appendix: _____

   _____

2. Inflammation of the voice box: _____

   _____

3. An abnormal condition with bluish discoloration: _____

   _____

4. An instrument used to measure breathing: _____

   _____

5. A condition of gallstones in the gallbladder: _____

   _____

6. The process of making an incision into the skull: _____

   _____

7. A condition of scanty urine (production): _____

   _____

8. Inflammation of the lungs: _____

   _____

9. Newborn: _____

   _____

10. Surgical puncture into the chest cavity: _____

    _____

11. A condition of blood clots: _____

    _____

12. Pertaining to the first segment of the small intestine: _____

    _____

13. A fatty tumor: _____

    _____

14. The process of viewing the bladder with a lighted instrument: _____

    _____

15. Difficulty speaking: _____

    _____

16. A deficiency of white blood cells: _____

_____

_____

17. A condition of hardening: _____

_____

_____

18. Pertaining to the kneecap: _____

_____

_____

19. Inflammation of the eyelid: _____

_____

_____

20. Removal of a testis: _____

_____

_____

Defining Medical Terms: Use the definitions of the word parts to define each of the following medical terms. Remember the rules from the text.

(*Hint*: Use the tables from both Chapters 7 and 8 to help you recall all the word parts.)

1. Myectomy: _____

_____

_____

2. Melanoma: _____

_____

_____

3. Meningitis: _____

_____

_____

4. Phlebotomy: _____

_____

_____

5. Atherosclerosis: _____

_____

_____

6. Pyelonephritis: _____

_____

_____

7. Bronchiectasis: _____

_____

_____

8. Lymphedema: _____

_____

_____

9. Splenomegaly: _____

_____

_____

10. Tracheostomy: _____

_____

_____

11. Anencephaly: _____

_____

_____

12. Aerobic: _____

_____

_____

13. Esophagitis: _____

_____

_____

14. Neuralgia: _____

_____

_____

15. Audiometry: _____

_____

_____

16. Carcinogenesis: _____

_____

_____

17. Cardiorrhaphy: _____

_____

_____

18. Polyneuropathy: _____

_____

_____

19. Hematuria: _____

_____

_____

20. Hyperthyroidism: _____

_____

_____

21. Colonoscopy: _____

_____

_____

22. Hypoglycemia: _____

_____

_____

SECTION 2

Structure and Function of the Body

Anatomy and Physiology of the Human Body

CHAPTER 9

Anatomic Descriptors and Fundamental Body Structure

Words to Know Challenge

Spelling: Each line contains three spellings of a word. Underline the correctly spelled word.

1.	antonomy	anotomy	anatomy
2.	anterior	aunterior	antieror
3.	cavitie	cavity	cavety
4.	conective	connective	connecktive
5.	cephalic	sephalic	cefalic
6.	doorsal	dursal	dorsal
7.	edama	edema	edemma
8.	epigastric	epagastric	epaghastric
9.	epatheleal	epathelial	epithelial
10.	jean	geen	gene
11.	illiac	iliac	illac
12.	lateral	latarel	laterel
13.	lumbar	lumber	lambar
14.	midlane	mildline	midline
15.	muscelle	muscel	muscle
16.	orgen	organ	organne
17.	posterior	posteror	posterear
18.	smoothe	smooth	smouth
19.	vantral	ventril	ventral

Matching: Match the term in column I to its description in column II. (Note: Not all descriptions will be used.)

COLUMN I	COLUMN II
____ 1. Cardiac	A. Groin area
____ 2. Cranial	B. A nerve cell
____ 3. Cytoplasm	C. A covering on a nerve
____ 4. Diaphragm	D. Heart tissue
____ 5. Dorsal	E. Toward the midline
____ 6. Epigastric	F. Change in the genetic code
____ 7. Homeostasis	G. Part of extremity nearest the body
____ 8. Hypochondriac	H. Pertaining to the cranium or skull
____ 9. Inguinal	I. Midline
____ 10. Lateral	J. Muscle tissue in organs
____ 11. Medial	K. Abdominal area around navel
____ 12. Myelin	L. Stores hereditary material of the cell
____ 13. Neuron	M. Consists of like cells
____ 14. Proximal	N. Skeletal muscle tissue
____ 15. Smooth	O. Below the body's transverse line
____ 16. Striated	P. Cellular fluid
____ 17. Thoracic	Q. Part of extremity farthest away from body
____ 18. Tissue	R. State of normal functioning
____ 19. Umbilical	S. Muscle that divides anterior cavity
____ 20. Ventral	T. Away from the midline
____ 21. Mutation	U. Carried by X chromosome
____ 22. Chromosome	V. The anterior section
____ 23. X-linked gene	W. Pertaining to the abdominal area above umbilical
____ 24. Midsagittal	X. Chest area
____ 25. Caudal	Y. Of or pertaining to the posterior section
	Z. The abdominal area below the umbilical
	AA. The cell nucleus
	BB. Swelling in the tissues
	CC. Abdominal area below ribs

Chapter Review

Short Answer

1. Describe the meaning of the phrase "anatomical position." _____
   _____
   _____

2. List the organs within each body cavity.
   a. Thoracic: _____
   b. Abdominal: _____
   c. Pelvic: _____
   d. Cranial: _____
   e. Spinal: _____

3. The abdomen can be divided into four sections for reference purposes. Name the sections.
   a. _____
   b. _____
   c. _____
   d. _____

4. List the structures of a cell.
   a. _____
   b. _____
   c. _____
   d. _____
   e. _____
   f. _____
   g. _____
   h. _____
   i. _____
   j. _____

5. List three things that may cause a mutation to occur.
   a. _____
   b. _____
   c. _____

6. Name three types of inheritance patterns and explain how they affect an individual's inherited traits.
   a. _____
   b. _____
   c. _____

7. List the six processes by which materials pass through cell membranes.
   a. _____
   b. _____
   c. _____
   d. _____
   e. _____
   f. _____

8. What is the name of the project that sequenced genes? _____

9. Explain the term "DNA fingerprinting" and how it can be used. _____

_____

_____

10. List the four types of tissues. Identify three places in the body where the tissue can be found.

a. _____

1. _____

2. _____

3. _____

b. _____

1. _____

2. _____

3. _____

c. _____

1. _____

2. _____

3. _____

d. _____

1. _____

2. _____

3. _____

11. List the 10 systems of the body.

a. _____

b. _____

c. _____

d. _____

e. _____

f. _____

g. _____

h. _____

i. _____

j. _____

Fill in the Blank: Use information from the chapter to complete the sentence.

1. In anatomical position, the patient's right side is across from your _____ side.

2. Something toward the midline is said to be _____ ; if it is away from the midline it is

_____ .

3. Arms and legs are known as _____ .

4. The front of the body is called the _____ or _____ section.

5. The back section is called the _____ or _____ side.

6. The body has two main cavities. The anterior cavity is further divided into an upper _____ and
a lower _____ cavity.

7. The posterior body section has a(n) _____ cavity and a(n) _____ cavity.

Labeling

1. Label the nine anatomical divisions and one reference point of the abdomen on the following illustration. Refer to Figure 9–7 in the textbook.

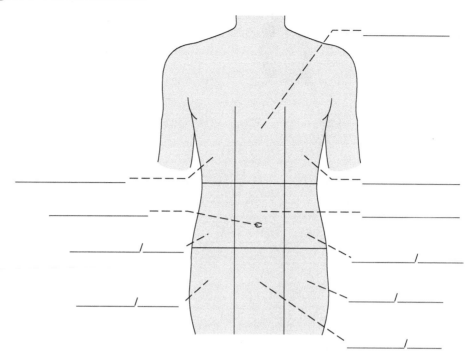

2. Label the directional reference terms on the illustrations of anatomical position. Refer to Figure 9–1 in the textbook.

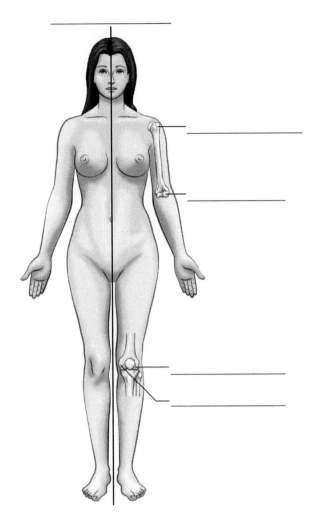

3. Label the directional reference terms on the illustration of anatomical position. Refer to Figure 9–3 in the textbook.

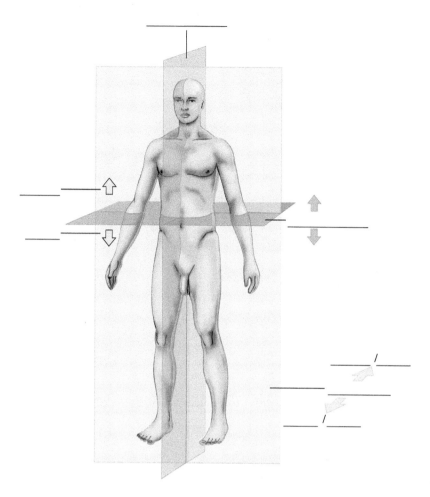

4. Label the eight body cavities on the following illustration. Refer to Figure 9–4 in the textbook.

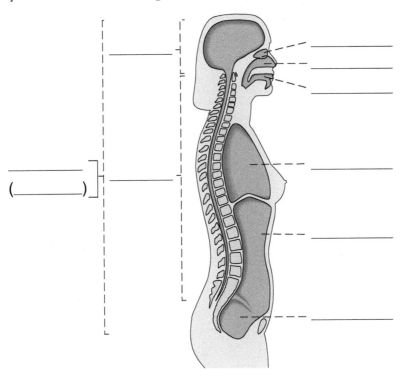

5. Label the thoracic and abdominal organs. Refer to Figure 9–5 in the textbook.

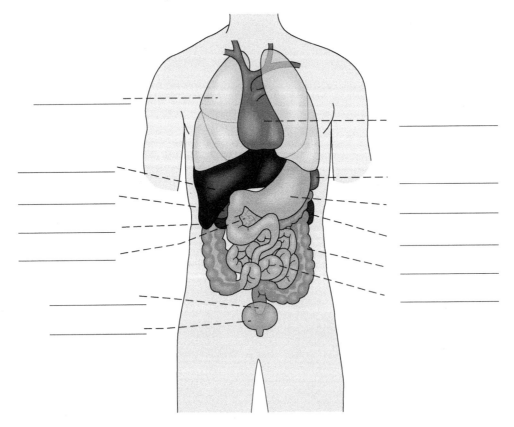

Matching

1. Match the acid or base in column I with its possible material in column II.

COLUMN I	COLUMN II
____ 1. Acetic acid	A. Batteries
____ 2. Boric acid	B. Household liquid cleaners
____ 3. Hydrochloric acid	C. Lye
____ 4. Sulfuric acid	D. Vinegar
____ 5. Ammonium hydroxide	E. The stomach
____ 6. Magnesium hydroxide	F. Weak eyewash
____ 7. Sodium hydroxide	G. Milk of magnesia

2. The following genetic conditions have visible abnormal characteristics that make them readily recognized. Match the condition in column I to its visible sign in column II.

COLUMN I	COLUMN II
____ 1. Cleft lip	A. Male with long legs and short, obese trunk
____ 2. Cleft palate	B. Malformation of one or both feet
____ 3. Down syndrome	C. Vertical split in upper lip
____ 4. Spina bifida	D. Female with webbing of the neck
____ 5. Klinefelter's syndrome	E. Opening in the top of mouth
____ 6. Talipes	F. Small head and slanting eyes
____ 7. Turner's syndrome	G. A malformation of the back

Chapter Application

Case Studies with Critical Thinking Questions

Scenario 1

Your best friend shares with you that she is trying to become pregnant. You know that she is 39 years old and has a younger brother with Down syndrome. She tells you she has not talked to a physician about pregnancy.

1. What type of physician does she need to see? _____
_____
_____

2. How do you feel about asking her if she considered the risks of this pregnancy? _____
_____
_____

3. How would you determine if it might be appropriate to talk with her about how she would deal with it if she learned she was having a Down child? _____
_____
_____
_____
_____

Scenario 2

A neighbor confides in you that her 15-year-old son has not shown any signs of sexual maturity, even though he is in high school and almost six feet tall. You know from previous discussions that he has had some difficulty in school. She has asked you what you think.

1. What kind of questions do you need to ask to determine what she means by sexual maturity? _____

    _____

    _____

    _____

    _____

2. What could you tell her if it sounds like he might have a hormone deficiency? _____

    _____

    _____

    _____

    _____

3. How can you help her to identify a physician for her to consult? _____

    _____

    _____

    _____

Research Activity

Select one of the congenital disorders discussed in the text. Do an Internet search to learn more about the condition. Find out about the causes and treatment. Is there a support group for people and families dealing with the condition? Is there a national, state, or local association supporting the disorder? (You may need to refer to your phone directory for local information.) Prepare a short written report of your findings.

As an alternative to a disorder search, find out more about gene therapy, genetic engineering, or genetic counseling. Look for new techniques or options for genetic conditions.

Role-Play Activity

Working in a group of three, one is the model, one is the medical assistant, and one asks the questions. Using the textbook Figures 9–1, 9–2, 9–3, 9–4, 9–6, and 9–7, the questioner asks the medical assistant to show on the model 10 of the directional terms, body cavities, or abdominal regions. Then, the group changes roles and continues the identification. Repeat as long as desired.

CHAPTER 10

The Nervous System

Words to Know Challenge

Spelling: Each line contains three spellings of a word. Underline the correctly spelled word.

1. angiography   angiografie   angeography
2. aracknoid   arachnoid   arachenoid
3. autonomech   autanomic   autonomic
4. cerebellam   ceribellum   cerebellum
5. hypothalamous   hypothalamus   hypathalmus
6. meninges   menegies   maninges
7. periferal   peripherel   peripheral
8. sciatika   sciatica   siaticka
9. sympathetic   synpethetic   synpathitic
10. ventrickle   ventricle   ventracle

Matching: Match each word in column I with its definition in column II.

COLUMN I	COLUMN II
____ 1. Meninges	A. The skull
____ 2. Midbrain	B. Nerve that causes action or movement
____ 3. Occipital	C. Small brain part at top of brain stem
____ 4. Cranium	D. Contains sensory nerve cell bodies
____ 5. Autonomic	E. Membranes covering the central nervous system
____ 6. Frontal	F. Nerve of vision
____ 7. Motor	G. Part of the peripheral nervous system
____ 8. Ganglion	H. Posterior lobe of cerebrum
____ 9. Optic	I. Cavity within the brain
____ 10. Ventricle	J. Portion of cerebrum behind forehead

Chapter Review

Short Answer

1. List the two main divisions of the nervous system.

   a. _____

   b. _____

2. What is a synapse? _____

   _____

   _____

3. Identify two types of peripheral nerves.

   a. _____

   b. _____

4. List the two types of spinal nerves and describe their functions.

   a. _____

   b. _____

5. What is the purpose or function of the autonomic nervous system? _____

   _____

   _____

6. Name the two divisions of the autonomic nervous system, explaining their actions.

   a. _____

   b. _____

7. List the five divisions of the brain and identify what function each division provides.

   a. _____

   _____

   b. _____

   c. _____

   d. _____

   e. _____

8. List the lobes of the cerebrum and their associated functions.

   a. _____

   _____

   b. _____

   c. _____

   _____

   d. _____

9. List the two structures between the cerebrum and the midbrain, describing their functions.

   1. _____

   2. _____

   _____

   _____

   _____

10. List the three meninges, describing their characteristics as given in the text.

    a. _____

    b. _____

    c. _____

11. What are the spaces called between the (a) dura mater and the arachnoid and (b) the arachnoid and the pia mater?

    _____

12. Name the fluid within the cavities of the CNS and describe its function. _____

    _____

    _____

Matching: For each symptom, write the letter of the appropriate disease or disorder.

____ 1. Sudden, acute onset of fever, headache, and vomiting, which progresses to a stiff neck and back, drowsiness, and eventual coma

____ 2. Blurred or double vision with sensations of tingling or numbness; periods of attacks and remission characterized by tremor, muscular weakness, and paralysis

____ 3. Severe muscle rigidity, drooling, tremor, and a bent-forward position when walking

____ 4. Temporary double vision, slurred speech, dizziness, staggering, and falling

____ 5. Loss of sensation with paralysis of one side of the body

____ 6. Sharp, piercing pain in the back of the thigh extending down the side of the leg

____ 7. Weakness and paralysis on one side of the face causing drooping mouth, drooling, and inability to close the affected eye

____ 8. Fluid-filled vesicles on the skin associated with fever, severe pain, itching, and abnormal skin sensations

____ 9. Seizures of varying duration, possible loss of consciousness, loss of body function control, and convulsions

____ 10. Abnormally large head, distended scalp veins, shiny scalp skin, irritability, vomiting

____ 11. Hyperactive tendon reflexes, underdeveloped affected extremities, muscular contractions; may also have seizures, mental retardation, and impaired speech

____ 12. High fever, chills, headache, positive Brudzinski's and Kernig's signs

____ 13. Severe pain along the course of a nerve anywhere in the body

____ 14. Excruciating facial pain upon stimulation of a trigger zone

_____ 15. Paralysis with loss of sensation and reflexes in lower extremities

_____ 16. Muscular weakness and atrophy; problems with speech, chewing, and swallowing; respirations may be affected; choking and drooling

_____ 17. Prodromal symptoms of fatigue, visual disturbances, tingling of face and lips, sensitivity to light, nausea, and vomiting

_____ 18. Incomplete closure of one or more vertebra, bladder and bowel control problems, hydrocephalus, weakness or paralysis of legs, often includes mental retardation

_____ 19. Vomiting, lethargy, liver dysfunction, hyperventilation, delirium and coma, with eventual respiratory arrest

A. Amyotrophic lateral sclerosis
B. Bell's palsy
C. Cerebral palsy
D. Encephalitis
E. Epilepsy
F. Herpes zoster
G. Hemiplegia
H. Hydrocephalus
I. Meningitis
J. Migraine headache

K. Multiple sclerosis
L. Neuralgia
M. Paraplegia
N. Parkinson's disease
O. Reye's syndrome
P. Sciatica
Q. Spina bifida
R. Transient ischemic attack
S. Trigeminal neuralgia

Matching: Match the diagnostic tests in column I with their purposes in column II.

COLUMN I	COLUMN II
_____ 1. Arteriography	A. Detects abnormal electrical impulses in the brain
_____ 2. Brain scan	B. Detects tumors, bleeding, clots, brain size, and edema
_____ 3. Glasgow Coma Scale	C. Measures cerebrospinal fluid pressure or obtains a sample of fluid
_____ 4. CAT scan	D. Images enhanced with color
_____ 5. EEG	E. Detects cranial fractures or dense cerebral areas
_____ 6. Electromyography	F. Instills a dye or air to show irregularities in the CNS
_____ 7. Lumbar puncture	G. Detects cerebral hemorrhage, aneurysm, or CVA
_____ 8. Myelography	H. Detects neuromuscular disorders or nerve damage
_____ 9. Skull X-ray	I. Radioisotopes are measured to detect abnormal masses or blood vessel lesions
_____ 10. Position emission tomography	J. Describes the level of consciousness

Fill in the Blank: Use information from the chapter to fill in the blank space in the sentence.

1. Simple reflex actions involve an impulse traveling along a nerve to the _____ and _____.

2. A common test used to illustrate this action is called the _____.

3. Complex reflex actions involve an impulse traveling from its source through _____ to the _____ and up to the _____. The message is interpreted and the _____ _____ carry the response message back to the _____ and out the appropriate nerve.

Labeling

Label the illustration of the lateral view of the brain using the following terms. Refer to Figure 10–10A in the textbook.

Brain stem   Medulla   Sulci
Cerebellum   Midbrain   Temporal lobe
Cerebrum   Occipital lobe
Convolutions   Parietal lobe
Frontal lobe   Pons

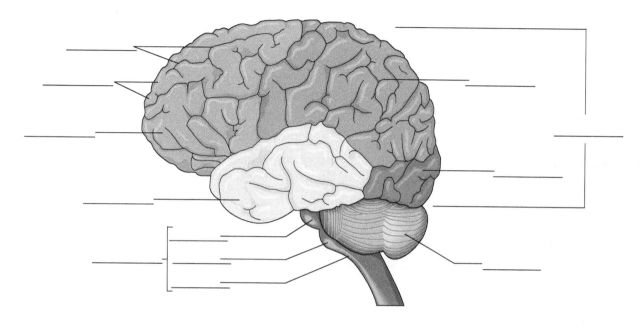

Chapter Application

Case Studies with Critical Thinking Questions

Scenario 1

Yesterday your nephew was severely injured in a motorcycle accident. The provider believes there is a fracture in the thoracic spine but needs to have a radiological workup to determine the extent of the injury. Your brother is very concerned because his son has no sensations or control of his body from the waist down. He has asked you what you think of his condition.

1. Is it important to ask what the nephew's physician has told your brother? _____

_____

_____

_____

2. How would you answer your brother if he asks if the paralysis may be permanent? _____

_____

_____

_____

_____

3. How much encouragement for recovery should you give him? _____

_____

_____

Scenario 2

A male patient phoned the office to request the provider to call the pharmacy to order some cream to apply on a rash on the right side of his chest. He said it started a couple days ago and is getting worse.

1. What do you need to know about the appearance of the rash? _____

_____

_____

2. What subjective symptoms would you want to ask the patient about? _____

_____

_____

3. Does this patient need to be seen? _____

_____

_____

Role-Play Activities

Choose a partner to participate in some nerve testing and to experience some neurological responses.

1. Following instruction from your teacher, use a percussion hammer to perform the knee-jerk test on your partner. Do it on both legs. Is the reaction equal? Does it seem too reactive or under-responsive?

2. With your partner lying on an exam table with his or her legs relaxed and shoes off, stroke the bottom of each foot, from the heel to the toes, with the hammer handle. What happened?

3. Try to perform the Brudzinski and Kernig tests.

4. Experience hemiplegia: For 15 minutes, refrain from using your dominant hand and arm. Try to not use your dominant leg except to support you; you cannot make it move. Try to get up from a sitting position without the use of your dominant hand or leg.

5. If possible, spend at least one hour in a wheelchair during lab time when you should be moving about. Can you express your feelings about not being able to perform routine tasks?

CHAPTER 11

The Senses

Words to Know Challenge

Spelling: Each line contains three spellings of a word. Underline the correctly spelled word.

1. acqueous   acquous   aqueous
2. tinnitus   tinitis   tinnitis
3. staples   stappes   stapes
4. chorhoid   choroid   chorid
5. cochlea   choclea   cocklea
6. cataraxt   cattaract   cataract
7. lacramal   lacrimal   lacramil
8. vittreous   vitreous   vitrious

Fill in the Blank: Complete the following sentences with Words to Know from this chapter.

1. _____, commonly called nearsightedness, is a defect in vision so that objects can only be seen when very near. The opposite of this is _____, or farsightedness.

2. _____ is a condition known commonly as "lazy eye."

3. Within the middle ear, sound waves vibrate the membrane and the _____ (hammer) attached to its inner surface. This in turn "strikes" the _____ (anvil), which moves the _____ (stirrups).

4. The middle ear is connected to the throat via the _____.

5. The gradual loss of hearing that occurs normally as part of the aging process is known as _____.

6. _____ causes pain and hearing loss; two types include externa and media.

7. The most common cause of conductive deafness is _____.

Chapter Review

Short Answer

1. List the five senses of the human body and identify the organ(s) responsible for the perception.

   a. _____

   b. _____

   c. _____

   d. _____

   e. _____

2. Name the structures of the eye through which light passes in the process of sight.

   a. _____

   b. _____

   c. _____

   d. _____

   e. _____

   f. _____

3. Explain the function of the lens and the process of accommodation. _____

   _____

   _____

4. How does the cornea affect vision? _____

   _____

   _____

5. Name the two humors and describe their purpose.

   a. _____

      1. _____

      2. _____

   b. _____

      1. _____

      2. _____

6. Explain how sounds are heard. _____

   _____

   _____

   _____

   _____

7. How is equilibrium maintained? _____

   _____

   _____

   _____

8. Describe the structure of the olfactory organ and explain how an odor can be detected. _____

   _____

   _____

9. Define the following terms:

   a. Epistaxis _____

   b. Allergic rhinitis _____

   c. Nasal polyp _____

10. Identify the sensations that are perceivable by the skin.

a. _____

b. _____

c. _____

d. _____

e. _____

f. _____

g. _____

Matching

1. Match the disease or disorder of the eye in column II with the major symptoms in column I.

COLUMN I	COLUMN II
_____ 1. Scratch from foreign body or injury to the cornea	A. Age-related macular degeneration
_____ 2. Red-rimmed, crusted eyelids with scales, itching, and burning	B. Amblyopia
_____ 3. Aching, loss of peripheral vision, visual halos around lights	C. Arcus senilis
_____ 4. Visual deviation of the eyeball; blurred or double vision	D. Blepharitis
_____ 5. Drooping of the upper eyelid	E. Cataract
_____ 6. Inward turning of one eye with blurred vision	F. Conjunctivitis
_____ 7. Redness, pain, and occasional discharge caused by an infectious microbe	G. Corneal abrasion
_____ 8. Painless, gradual visual blurring, and loss of vision	H. Corneal ulcers
_____ 9. Pain, especially on blinking; excessive tearing; exudate; irregular cornea; blurred vision	I. Diabetic retinopathy
_____ 10. Red, painful swelling of gland of the eyelid	J. Glaucoma
_____ 11. Inability to accommodate for near vision	K. Hordeolum
_____ 12. Visual floating spots, light flashes, and gradual vision loss	L. Myopia
_____ 13. Glare, blurred vision, reduced visual acuity, eventual blindness	M. Presbyopia
_____ 14. A thin, grayish-white circle at edge of cornea	N. Ptosis
_____ 15. Gradual loss of central vision	O. Detached retina
_____ 16. Vision is blurred except close objects due to misshapen eyeball	P. Strabismus

2. Match the major symptoms in column II with the diseases and disorders of the ear in column I.

COLUMN I

_____ 1. Auditory canal obstruction

_____ 2. Ménière's disease

_____ 3. Motion sickness

_____ 4. Otitis externa

_____ 5. Otitis media

_____ 6. Otosclerosis

_____ 7. Presbycusis

COLUMN II

A. Loss of equilibrium, headache, nausea, and vomiting due to movement

B. Severe, deep, throbbing pain; fever; hearing loss; nausea; vomiting; dizziness; bulging eardrum

C. Slow, progressive conduction hearing loss

D. A degree of hearing loss; possible discomfort; may be a foreign body

E. Severe vertigo, tinnitus, nerve hearing loss, nausea, and vomiting

F. Infection in auditory canal, pain, fever, conduction hearing loss

G. Loss of ability to hear high-frequency sounds, tinnitus, possible depression

Labeling

1. Add labels to each part of the eye. Refer to Figure 11–1 in the textbook.
   Anterior chamber
   Choroid coat
   Ciliary body
   Conjunctiva
   Cornea
   Fovea centralis
   Iris
   Lens
   Optic nerve
   Path of light
   Posterior chamber
   Pupil
   Retina
   Sclera
   Vitreous body

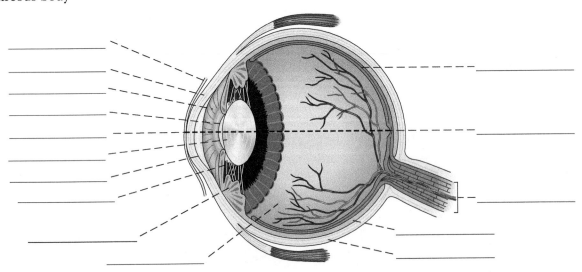

2. Label the illustrations of the outer, middle, and inner ear using the following terms. Refer to Figures 11–11 and 11–12 in the textbook.

Outer and Middle Ear

Auricle
Cochlea
Eustachian tube
External auditory canal
Incus
Malleus
Semicircular canals
Stapes
Tympanic membrane
Vestibulocochlear nerve

Inner Ear

Cochlea
Cochlear nerve
Lateral semicircular canal
Oval window
Posterior semicircular canal
Superior semicircular canal
Vestibular nerve
Vestibule

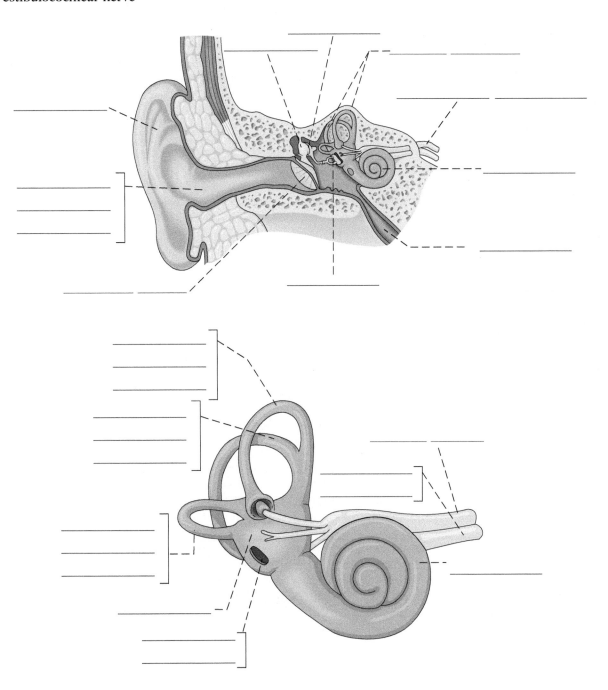

Chapter Application

Case Studies with Critical Thinking Questions

Scenario 1

You notice that a little girl in your daughter's preschool class has one eye that turns inward. You have never seen the child with glasses. You have a chance to talk with the mother at a preschool program. She says she is not worried about it because she thinks her daughter will outgrow it and they don't have any insurance coverage.

1. How far should you go to impress on the mother that the child needs to be evaluated by a pediatric ophthalmologist? _____

_____

_____

2. What could you say to the mother to impress on her that her daughter's vision might be lost if the eye is not treated? _____

_____

_____

3. How can you find out if treatment is available without a lot of cost to the parents? _____

_____

_____

_____

_____

Scenario 2

A 24-year-old male patient is being seen in the office for treatment of an upper respiratory infection. During your interview he proudly announces that he has quit smoking. In the process of your assessment you notice his teeth are quite stained, especially on one side. He explains to you that he is using a little smokeless tobacco to satisfy his need for nicotine.

1. What should you tell him about his new habit? _____

_____

_____

2. Where can you obtain some written materials for him? _____

_____

3. What should you question about his dental care? _____

_____

_____

Research Activity

There are four rather common conditions that may lead to blindness, sometimes unnecessarily. Make a chart that divides a piece of paper horizontally into four sections after saving the top inch for headings. You will need five vertical columns, one small and four of equal size. In the first, smaller column, enter: Age-related macular degeneration, Diabetic retinopathy, Glaucoma, and Retinal detachment, one in each of the horizontal sections. Across the top row enter for titles: Description, Signs/symptoms, Etiology, and Treatment. Referring to the text, enter the information on each condition. When completed, look at the descriptors in each column. Which disorders occur slowly and which are sudden? Which ones require immediate treatment? Which ones can be "cured"? Are there any that could be avoided with good health practices? Which ones cause pain? Which ones are most likely to go unnoticed until some damage has occurred? Your knowledge of these conditions may someday help save someone's vision.

CHAPTER 12

The Integumentary System

Words to Know Challenge

Spelling: Each line contains three spellings of a word. Underline the correctly spelled word.

1. dermatitus   <u>dermatitis</u>   dermitius
2. <u>epidermis</u>   epedermis   epidermus
3. erathema   erithema   <u>erythema</u>
4. intagumantary   integumentory   <u>integumentary</u>
5. <u>psoriasis</u>   psariasis   spsorisis
6. sabeceous   <u>sebaceous</u>   sebaceus
7. subcutanous   <u>subcutaneous</u>   subcuteneous
8. <u>urticaria</u>   urtecaria   urticarea
9. varrucai   <u>verrucae</u>   varrucae
10. <u>alopecia</u>   alopechia   alepecia
11. egsema   egzema   <u>eczema</u>
12. mellonoma   <u>melanoma</u>   mellenoma
13. leshion   <u>lesion</u>   leishon

Matching: Match the terms in column I to their definitions in column II.

COLUMN I	COLUMN II
_____ 1. Erythema	A. Color
_____ 2. Melanin	B. Skin with little or no color
_____ 3. Pustule	C. Provides lubrication
_____ 4. Pigment	D. A chronic condition
_____ 5. Sebaceous	E. Sunburn
_____ 6. Subcutaneous	F. A lesion with exudates
_____ 7. Dermis	G. A skin layer
_____ 8. Vesicle	H. True skin
_____ 9. Albino	I. Round elevations of skin
_____ 10. Wheals	J. A pigment
_____ 11. Psoriasis	M. A blister-like lesion

Chapter Review

Short Answer

1. List the five functions of the skin.

   a. _____

   b. _____

   c. _____

   d. _____

   e. _____

2. How does the skin regulate body temperature? _____
   _____
   _____

3. How does the body cool its surface? _____
   _____
   _____

4. List the three layers of skin tissue; identify the characteristic structure of each layer.
   _____
   _____
   _____
   _____
   _____

5. What causes wrinkles? _____
   _____
   _____

6. Why does exposure to the sun cause the skin to darken? _____
   _____
   _____

7. Why does the skin become red when a person blushes? _____
_____
_____

8. What causes birthmarks? _____
_____
_____

9. What is a mole? _____
_____
_____

10. Define "albinism" and describe the main characteristics of the condition. _____
_____
_____

11. Define the lesion in column I by placing the number of its correct definition from column II in the space.

COLUMN I	COLUMN II
____ 1. Macule	1. A small, circumscribed lesion filled with exudate and lymph
____ 2. Papule	2. A round lesion with a white center and a red periphery that usually itches
____ 3. Pustule	3. A variously colored spot that is neither elevated nor depressed
____ 4. Vesicle	4. A solid, elevated circular red mass about a pinhead to a pea in size
____ 5. Wheal	5. A blister-like, elevated mass containing serous fluid

12. Identify the ABCD and E rules of melanoma.
_____
_____
_____
_____
_____
_____
_____
_____
_____

13. What two words describe the skin in the following age groups?
a. Infant and child _____
b. Teenager _____
c. Aging _____
d. Aged _____

14. Identify the body systems involved in Lyme disease.
_____
_____
_____
_____

Matching

1. Match the primary disease characteristics in column I with the disease or disorder in column II.

COLUMN I

COLUMN II

____ 1. Dry skin, redness, itching, edema, scaling

A. Scabies

____ 2. A small red macule becomes a vesicle and then changes into a pustule with yellow crust and outer rim

B. Psoriasis

____ 3. A thickened scar

C. Urticaria

____ 4. Itching red papules covered with silvery scales

D. Dermatitis

____ 5. Flat lesion that can be dry and scaly or moist and crusty: has characteristic outer ring with clear center

E. Verrucae

____ 6. Threadlike red nodules at the inner wrists, elbows, between fingers, and in axilla

F. Ringworm

____ 7. Distinct raised wheals surrounded by reddened areas; usually itches

G. Impetigo

____ 8. Rough, elevated, rounded surface, especially on the hands and fingers: some forms appear on soles of feet and on genitalia

H. Keloid

____ 9. A loss of hair, usually on the scalp

I. Lyme disease

____ 10. A lesion exhibiting some of the ABCD characteristics

J. Herpes simplex

____ 11. Red, dry, itching, and scaly skin; occurs in both acute and chronic forms, often producing watery discharge

K. Pediculosis capitis

____ 12. Cold sores or blisters on the mouth or face

L. Hirsutism

____ 13. A deep abscess involving several follicles with multiple drainage points

M. Melanoma

____ 14. A bull's-eye rash and a bite site

N. Eczema

____ 15. Oval, grayish, dandruff-appearing flecks, itching scalp, matted hair

O. Alopecia

____ 16. Excessive body hair on females and children, in an adult male growth pattern

P. Carbuncle

2. Match the definition in column II with the correct term in column I.

	COLUMN I		COLUMN II
___	1. Dermis	A.	Reddened, flat area with definite edge
___	2. Epidermis	B.	Bottom layer of skin
___	3. Keloid	C.	Hives
___	4. Macule	D.	The middle layer of skin
___	5. Melanin	E.	Raised areas surrounded by reddened area
___	6. Pustule	F.	Raised lesion containing serous fluid
___	7. Subcutaneous	G.	Lesion with purulent material
___	8. Urticaria	H.	The top layer of skin
___	9. Vesicle	I.	Pigment in the skin
___	10. Wheals	J.	An overgrowth of scar tissue
___	11. Whorl	K.	The lack of skin pigment
		L.	An oil gland
		M.	Fingerprints

Chapter Application

Case Studies with Critical Thinking Questions

Scenario 1

Johnny's mother called the office almost hysterical because he brought home a note from school saying one of his classmates has head lice. She is sure the entire family has lice because they've all started to itch.

1. How can you help her to determine if they actually have lice? _____
   _____
   _____

2. If a family member does have lice, what steps should be taken besides treating the hair? _____
   _____
   _____
   _____

Scenario 2

You are following a coworker up a flight of stairs when you notice a very unusually colored mole on the calf of her leg. When you ask her about it, she says it's been there for a while and it doesn't bother her. She thinks it's just a mole because she has several on her back and chest area.

1. What could you say to express your concern? _____
   _____
   _____

2. When would it be appropriate to schedule an appointment for her with a dermatologist? _____
   _____
   _____
   _____

Research Activity

Look in your local phone directory. How many providers specialize in dermatology? Make a list of the different services or treatments they provide. You will notice they range from cosmetic to serious conditions.

Role-Play

Choose a partner to explore the skin.

1. Use a magnifying glass to identify the few places on the body where there is no hair.

2. Using finger paint or an ink stamp pad, make a page of right thumbprints of all classmates. Look at the differences in the lines and patterns.

3. See how the skin surface reacts to hot or cold. Apply a hot, wet cloth to your partner's forearm for two minutes. Remove it and record what you observe. Now apply a cold, wet cloth wrapped around ice for two minutes. Remove and record your findings. What is the skin trying to do in each situation?

4. Blindfold your partner and see if his or her skin can perceive different stimuli. Have your partner tell you what you are doing; be considerate and do not cause harm.

   a. Touch the skin on the forearm lightly with your fingertip.

   b. Gently pinch the skin.

   c. Press a pencil or pen into the skin.

   d. Press an object that you've held under hot water against the skin.

   e. Press an item that is cold against the skin.

   f. Try to tickle the surface with the edge of a tissue, barely touching the skin.

CHAPTER 13

The Skeletal System

Words to Know Challenge

Spelling: Each line contains three spellings of a word. Underline the correctly spelled word.

1. axeal   axyal   <u>axial</u>

2. carpelle   carpel   <u>carpal</u>

3. <u>epiphysis</u>   ephiphysis   epyphysis

4. cocyx   <u>coccyx</u>   coscix

5. <u>ischium</u>   ishium   ishiem

6. kyfosis   kiphosis   <u>kyphosis</u>

7. osteopersis   <u>osteoporosis</u>   osteoperosis

8. phalancks   <u>phalanx</u>   phalenx

9. prosthesys   prothesis   <u>prosthesis</u>

10. <u>synovial</u>   sinovial   sinoval

Matching: Match the terms in column I with their definitions in column II.

COLUMN I	COLUMN II
____ 1. Fracture	A. Sensation after amputation
____ 2. Femur	B. Floating mass in blood vessel
____ 3. Alignment	C. Incomplete fracture
____ 4. Callus	D. To stretch a ligament
____ 5. Greenstick	E. To straighten a fracture
____ 6. Phantom limb	F. Break
____ 7. Ligament	G. Fills long bones
____ 8. Vertebrae	H. Bones of the hands and feet
____ 9. Ulna	I. Bone in the rib cage
____ 10. Humerus	J. Pelvic bone
____ 11. Marrow	K. Attaches bone to bone at joints
____ 12. Embolus	L. Thigh bone
____ 13. Ilium	M. Upper arm bone
____ 14. Phalanges	N. Bones of the spine
____ 15. Sternum	O. Bone of forearm
____ 16. Sprain	P. Bulgy deposit around a new fracture

Chapter Review

Short Answer

1. What is bone composed of? _____

_____

2. List six functions of the skeletal system.

   a. _____

   b. _____

   c. _____

   d. _____

   e. _____

   f. _____

3. Describe the spinal column. _____

_____

4. How is a long bone constructed? _____

_____

_____

5. How do long bones grow? _____

_____

6. Identify three kinds of synovial joints, giving examples of each.

   a. _____

   b. _____

   c. _____

7. List the seven types of fractures, describing the characteristics of each type.

   a. _____

   b. _____

   c. _____

   d. _____

   e. _____

   f. _____

   g. _____

8. Identify each type of fracture illustrated below. Refer to Figure 13–11 in the textbook.

Transverse

Oblique

(A) _____   (B) _____   (C) _____   (D) _____   (E) _____   (F) _____

(G) _____   (H) _____

9. Describe the initial and follow-up treatment of fractures. _____
_____
_____
_____
_____
_____

10. How does bone heal? _____
_____
_____
_____

11. What is a fat embolus and how does it occur? _____
_____
_____

12. What conditions might result in the need for an amputation?
    a. _____
    b. _____
    c. _____
    d. _____

13. Explain the condition known as phantom limb. _____
_____
_____

Fill in the Blank: Use information from the chapter to fill in the blank space in the sentence.

1. The skeletal system is divided into sections. The axial skeleton is made up of the _____ , _____ , and _____ . The appendicular skeleton is made up of the _____ , _____ , _____ , _____ , _____ , and _____ .

2. The rib cage consists of ____ pairs of ribs that attach by _____ to the _____ anteriorly and to the _____ posteriorly. The top ____ pairs are attached both anteriorly and posteriorly. The bottom ____ pairs are attached only to the _____ and are therefore called _____ .

3. The rib cage is also classified as having _____ and _____ ribs. This division considers the first ___ pairs to be _____ ribs because _____ . The last ___ pairs are called _____ ribs because _____ .

4. The primary function of the rib cage is to protect the _____ and _____ .

Labeling

1. Label the skeletal system with these terms. Refer to Figure 13–1 in the textbook.

Carpals
Clavicle
Coccyx
Cranium
Facial bones
Femur
Fibula
Greater trochanter
Humerus

Ilium
Ischium
Metacarpals
Metatarsals
Patella
Phalanges (used twice)
Pubis
Radius
Ribs

Sacrum
Scapula
Sternum
Tarsals
Tibia
Ulna
Vertebral column

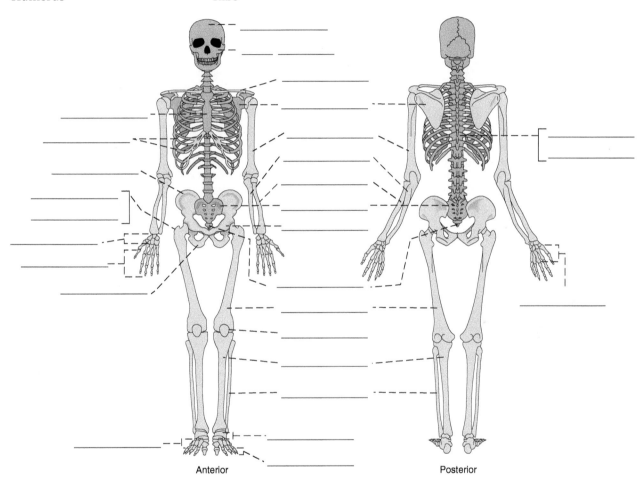

Anterior   Posterior

2. Label the illustration of the vertebral column using the following terms. Refer to Figure 13–5 in the textbook.
   Cervical vertebrae
   Coccyx
   Intervertebral disc
   Lumbar vertebrae
   Sacrum
   Thoracic vertebrae
   Vertebral body

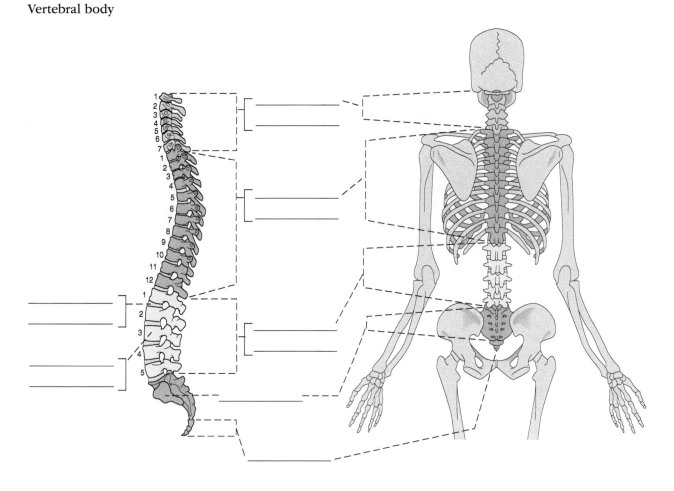

3. Label the illustration of the rib cage with the following terms. Refer to Figure 13–7 in the textbook.
   Clavicle
   Costal cartilage
   False ribs
   Floating ribs
   Manubrium
   Spinal column
   Sternum
   True ribs
   Xiphoid process

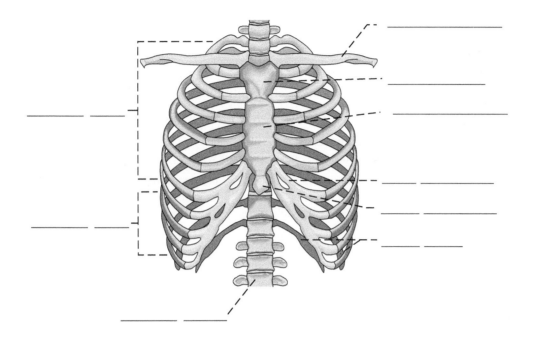

Matching: Match the disease or disorder in column I with the appropriate symptoms in column II.

	COLUMN I		COLUMN II
____	1. Osteoarthritis	A.	Painful displacement of the bones of the joint, usually fingers, shoulders, knees, often resulting in joint fracture
____	2. Rheumatoid arthritis	B.	A metabolic disease resulting in severe joint pain due to deposits of urates
____	3. Bursitis	C.	A lateral spinal curvature, usually thoracic, resulting from spinal column rotation
____	4. Congenital hip dysplasia	D.	Porous, brittle bones, prone to fracture; caused by metabolic disorder; found primarily in postmenopausal women
____	5. Dislocation	E.	Progressive deterioration of joint cartilage, usually hip and knee; joint pain; stiffness; grating; and joint fluid
____	6. Epicondylitis	F.	The dislocation of a child's hip joint at birth
____	7. Gout	G.	A bowing of the back, usually at the thoracic level
____	8. Hallux valgus	H.	Inflammation of forearm extensor tendon at its attachment on the humerus; more painful with twisting of forearm
____	9. Herniated disc	I.	Chronic inflammatory disease occurring intermittently; damages synovial membrane, causing edema and congestion, bone atrophy, deformities
____	10. Kyphosis	J.	Causes severe low back pain, radiating deep into buttocks and down back of the leg
____	11. Osteoporosis	K.	A tear of the ligaments of a joint resulting in pain, swelling, and local bleeding
____	12. Scoliosis	L.	Painful inflammation of the joint sac, usually at the knee, elbow, or shoulder
____	13. Sprain	M.	Lateral deviation of the great toe with enlarged first metatarsal and the formation of a bunion
____	14. Carpal tunnel syndrome	N.	Partial or incomplete dislocation of the articulating surfaces of bones at a joint, causing deformity, pain, and extremity length change
____	15. Bunion	O.	An inflamed bursa of the great toe filled with fluid and covered with a callus
____	16. Lordosis	P.	Decreased sensitivity in the first two fingers and thumb, often with atrophy of the thumb muscle on the palm side
____	17. Subluxation	Q.	Abnormal anterior convex curvature of the lumbar spine

Chapter Application

Case Studies with Critical Thinking Questions

Scenario 1

You are alone in the office when the wife of a patient calls to find out what she should do. Her husband suffered a leg fracture at work yesterday, but in the last hour he started perspiring and looks pale. He also seems to be breathing faster, and his pulse is above normal. She wonders if this is normal.

1. What should you initially tell the patient's wife? _____

_____

_____

_____

_____

2. When is it appropriate for you try to reach the provider? _____

_____

_____

_____

3. Why might this be a real emergency? _____

_____

_____

Scenario 2

Your neighbor calls to tell you he sprained his ankle the night before, but it is a lot more swollen and painful today. He tells you he has been keeping the heating pad on it like his friend told him, but it just seems to be getting worse.

1. What advice should you give him first? _____

_____

_____

_____

_____

2. How can you be certain it's just a sprain? _____

_____

_____

_____

3. When should you recommend medical evaluation? _____

_____

_____

Role-Play: Bone Identification and Spelling

1. Practice identifying the bones of the body. With a partner, use a model of a skeleton or a chart without labels and try to identify all the bones of the body. Your partner can say whether you are right or wrong.

2. Choose a partner and play hangman using the Words to Know. Each person makes a list of 10 words and then tries to win against his or her partner.

The Muscular System

Words to Know Challenge

Spelling: Each line contains three spellings of a word. Underline the correctly spelled word.

1.	distrophy	dystrophy	dystraphy
2.	pecktoralis	pectoralles	pectoralis
3.	extensor	extenser	egtensor
4.	gastructnemius	gastrocnemius	gastrocnemious
5.	hiccupp	hiccough	hicough
6.	intercostal	intracostal	intercoastal
7.	spincter	sphinctor	sphincter
8.	tortacollis	torticollis	torticolis
9.	fibramyositis	fibromyositis	fibromyasitis

Matching: Match the term in column I with its description in column II. (*Note*: Not all descriptions will be used.)

COLUMN I	COLUMN II
___ 1. Abduction	A. Spasmodic contractions of the diaphragm
___ 2. Adduction	B. Excessive stress on a skeletal muscle
___ 3. Anchor	C. A doughnut-shaped muscle
___ 4. Atrophy	D. A progressive wasting of muscle tissue from lack of use
___ 5. Contracture	E. A tough membrane sheath attachment
___ 6. Dystrophy	F. To move an extremity away from the body's center
___ 7. Fascia	G. The origin of a muscle
___ 8. Hiccough	H. Permanent shortening of flexor muscles with bent joints
___ 9. Spasm	I. Congenital progressive skeletal muscle wasting
___ 10. Strain	J. A state of partial muscle contraction
	K. To move an extremity toward the body's center
	L. A painful contracted muscle that will not relax

Chapter Review

Short Answer

1. What is a motor unit? _____

_____

2. Why does muscular activity produce heat in the body? _____

_____

_____

_____

3. List six functions of skeletal muscles.

a. _____

b. _____

c. _____

d. _____

e. _____

f. _____

4. What is the purpose of a muscle team? Give one example. _____

_____

_____

5. What does the term *muscle tone* mean? _____

_____

6. Describe the structure and function of a tendon, locating the body's strongest example. _____

_____

_____

_____

7. Explain the meaning of the terms *origin* and *insertion*. _____
   _____
   _____
   _____

8. Describe a muscle sheath and bursa; explain their functions. _____
   _____
   _____
   _____

9. Identify the muscles of respiration and explain their actions. _____
   _____
   _____
   _____

10. Explain peristaltic action. _____
    _____
    _____

11. Describe the structure and function of a sphincter. _____
    _____
    _____
    _____

Labeling

1. Label the six illustrations below to indicate direction of movement in the muscle teams. Refer to Figures 14–3 and 14–4 in the textbook.

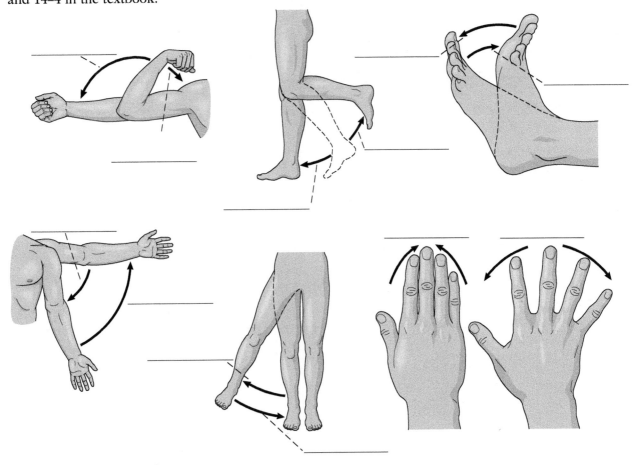

2. Label the illustration with the following major anterior body muscles. Refer to Figure 14–6 in the textbook.
   Bicep brachii
   Deltoid
   External oblique
   Intercostals
   Masseter
   Orbicularis oculi
   Orbicularis oris
   Pectoralis major
   Quadriceps femoris
   Rectus abdominis
   Sartorius
   Soleus
   Tibialis anterior
   Vastus lateralis

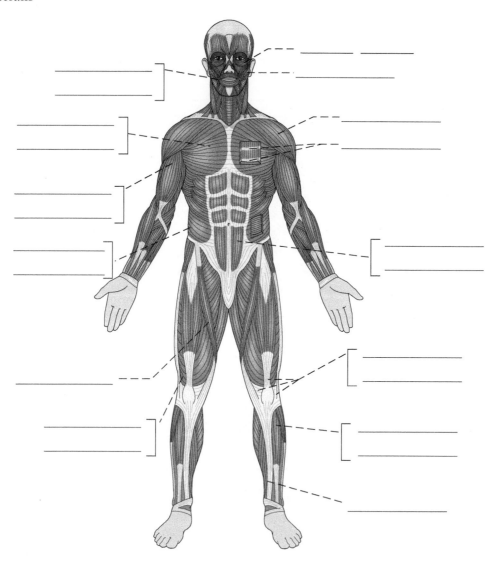

3. Label the illustration with the following major posterior body muscles. Refer to Figure 14–7 in the textbook.

Achilles tendon
Biceps femoris
Deltoid
Gastrocnemius
Gluteus maximus
Gluteus medius
Hamstring group
Latissimus dorsi
Occipitalis
Semimembranosus
Semitendinosus
Sternocleidomastoid
Trapezius
Triceps brachii

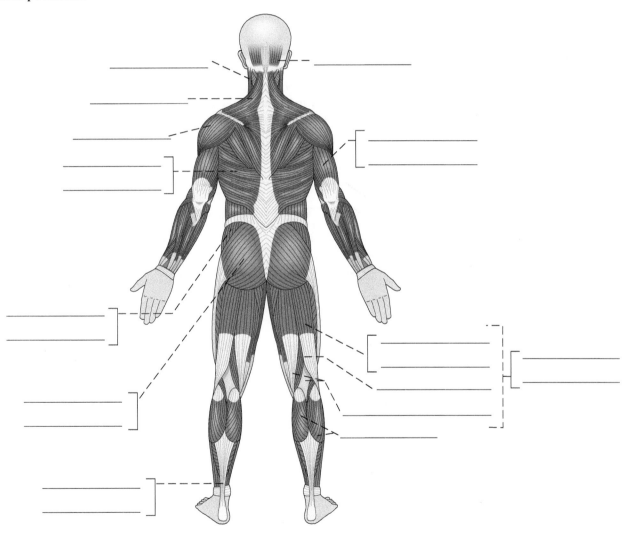

Design a table: List the three types of muscular tissue, describe the characteristics of each type, the location in the body, and the function performed.

TYPE	CHARACTERISTICS	LOCATION	FUNCTION
a. _____ _____	_____ _____	_____ _____	_____ _____
b. _____ _____ _____	_____ _____ _____	_____ _____ _____	_____ _____ _____
c. _____ _____ _____	_____ _____ _____	_____ _____ _____	_____ _____ _____

Chapter Application

Case Studies with Critical Thinking Questions

Scenario 1

A male patient has been treated for tendonitis of the elbow. He calls the office to complain that for the past two days he has experienced an increase of pain and feels he is worse than when he was first diagnosed. He has been applying heat like he was advised. He wants to know what to do.

1. What additional information should you get? _____
   _____
   _____

2. What advice will the provider likely give him? _____
   _____
   _____

3. Do you think the provider needs to see him again? _____
   _____
   _____

Scenario 2

One of your best friends calls you and is very upset. She tells you the provider thinks she may have fibromyalgia. She has never heard of the condition and is asking you for information. You realize she needs help and support.

1. Why should you question her about her symptoms? _____
   _____

2. Why should you determine what the provider has already told her? _____
   _____
   _____
   _____

3. Where else can she go for help? _____

_____

_____

_____

_____

Role-Play: Muscle identification and spelling

1. Practice identifying the muscles of the body. With a partner, use a model of the muscular system or a chart without labels and try to identify the principal muscles of the body. Your partner can say whether you are right or wrong.

2. Choose a partner and play hangman using the Words to Know. Each person makes a list of 10 words and then tries to win against his or her partner.

CHAPTER 15

The Respiratory System

Words to Know Challenge

Spelling: Each line contains three spellings of a word. Underline the correctly spelled word.

1. alveala   alveola   <u>alveoli</u>
2. <u>cyanosis</u>   cyaniosis   cyinosis
3. emphasema   empfazema   <u>emphysema</u>
4. hickcoughs   <u>hiccoughs</u>   hiccoufs
5. <u>influenza</u>   enfluenza   influensa
6. larengitis   <u>laryngitis</u>   laringitis
7. pnewmonia   <u>pneumonia</u>   pneumonea
8. spontaneus   <u>spontaneous</u>   spauntaneous
9. ventalation   ventelation   <u>ventilation</u>

Matching: Match the disorders or diseases in column I with their major symptoms in column II.

	COLUMN I		COLUMN II
_____	1. Allergic rhinitis	A.	A progressive, complex disease with marked dyspnea, productive cough, frequent respiratory infections, barrel chest, respiratory failure
_____	2. Asthma	B.	A nosebleed
_____	3. Atelectasis	C.	Coldlike symptoms initially, progressing to involve liver, spleen, and lymph glands; productive cough, dyspnea, weakness
_____	4. Bronchitis	D.	Acute, contagious disease with chills, fever, headache, muscular aches, nonproductive cough
_____	5. COPD	E.	Sharp, stabbing pain with lung respirations, some dyspnea, usually one-sided
_____	6. Emphysema	F.	Surgical removal of the larynx
_____	7. Epistaxis	G.	Fluid collection within lung tissue associated with heart disease; causes dyspnea, orthopnea, frothy bloody sputum
_____	8. Histoplasmosis	H.	Dyspnea, chest pain, rapid heart, productive cough, low-grade fever; caused by blood vessel obstruction
_____	9. Respiratory distress syndrome	I.	Reaction to airborne allergens causing sneezing, profuse watery nasal discharge, and nasal congestion
_____	10. Influenza	J.	Prolonged apnea in infants, irregular heart rate, severe lack of oxygen
_____	11. Laryngectomy	K.	Nodular lesions and patchy infiltration of lung tissue causing fatigue, weakness, lack of appetite, weight loss, night sweats
_____	12. Legionnaires' disease	L.	An infectious, acute, or chronically developed disease causing wheezing, dyspnea, productive cough
_____	13. Paroxysmal nocturnal dyspnea	M.	Sore throat, nasal congestion, headache, burning, watery eyes, fever, nonproductive cough
_____	14. Pleural effusion	N.	Diarrhea, lack of appetite, headache, chills, fever that persists, weakness, grayish sputum
_____	15. Pleurisy	O.	Bronchospasms; an allergic disorder causing wheezing, dyspnea, sputum production
_____	16. Pneumonoconiosis	P.	Affects infants, causing respiratory distress, rapid and shallow breathing, retracted sternum, flared nostrils, grunting
_____	17. Pneumonia	Q.	Acute infection causing coughing, sputum, chills, fever, pleural chest pain; impairs exchange of oxygen and carbon dioxide
_____	18. Pneumothorax	R.	Inability to exchange oxygen and carbon dioxide, causing chronic cough, pursed-lips breathing, cyanosis, weight loss
_____	19. Pulmonary edema	S.	Sudden sharp pain, unequal chest wall expansion, may be chest wound; weak rapid pulse, dyspnea, lung collapse
_____	20. Pulmonary embolism	T.	Environmental disease causing dyspnea, lack of oxygen, bronchial congestion
_____	21. SIDS	U.	Dyspnea due to collapse of the alveoli
_____	22. Tuberculosis	V.	Awaken from sleep with feeling of suffocation
_____	23. URI	W.	Hypoxia due to the presence of excess fluid in the pleural space

Chapter Review

Short Answer

1. Where is oxygen produced, and how important is it to the human body? _____
   _____
   _____

2. What causes a breath to be taken? _____
   _____
   _____

3. Trace the pathway of oxygen to an internal cell. _____
   _____
   _____
   _____
   _____

4. How is voice sound produced? _____
   _____
   _____

5. Explain the difference between external and internal respiration. _____
   _____
   _____
   _____

6. What is surfactant and how does it affect inflation of the lungs? _____
   _____
   _____

7. List five instances when a breathing pattern is altered normally.
   a. _____
   b. _____
   c. _____
   d. _____
   e. _____

8. Describe the pleural coverings of the lungs and explain their purpose. _____
   _____
   _____
   _____

Matching: Match the diagnostic examination from column I with its purpose in column II.

	COLUMN I		COLUMN II
____	1. Bronchoscopy	A.	To evaluate pulmonary emboli
____	2. Chest X-ray	B.	To withdraw fluid from the pleural space
____	3. Lung scan	C.	To determine basic condition of the lungs or identify a disease process
____	4. Sputum analysis	D.	To observe the trachea and bronchial tree, obtain a sample, or remove a foreign body
____	5. Thoracentesis	E.	To diagnose infectious organisms or cancer cells
____	6. Arterial blood gases	F.	Aid in diagnosing pulmonary emboli and evaluating pulmonary circulation in certain heart conditions before surgery
____	7. Lung perfusion scan	G.	To measure the partial pressures of O_2 and CO_2 in the lungs by determining the pH of the blood
____	8. Lung ventilation scan	H.	To provide a visual image of pulmonary blood flow to diagnose blood vessel obstruction
____	9. Pulmonary angiography	I.	To determine the distribution pattern of an inhaled gas to identify obstructed airways

Design a Table: Enter the structure and function of each of the following parts of the respiratory system.

PART	STRUCTURE	FUNCTION
a. Nose		
b. Pharynx		
c. Epiglottis		
d. Larynx		
e. Trachea		
f. Bronchi		
g. Bronchioles		
h. Alveoli		

Labeling

Label the illustration of the lungs. Refer to Figure 15–6 in the textbook.

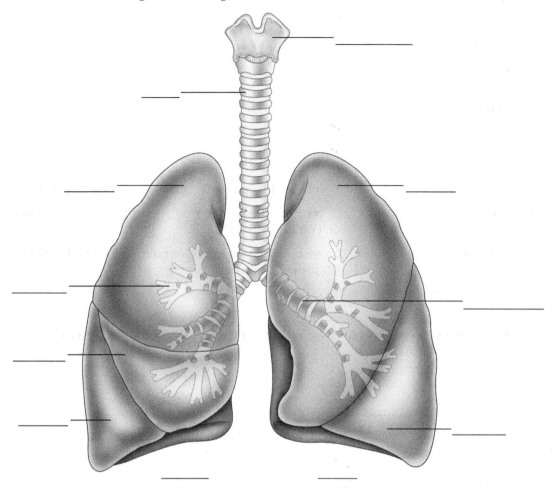

Chapter Application

Case Studies with Critical Thinking Questions

Scenario 1

You are employed in a pediatrician's office. A young, first-time mother calls the office crying because her toddler is having a temper tantrum and is holding his breath until he gets red and then gasps for air. She is afraid he is going to quit breathing and die. She wants to know what to do.

1. What should you ask the mother before responding? _____

   _____

   _____

   _____

2. Is this common for toddlers? _____

   _____

   _____

3. Should you check with the provider about referring her to a behavior specialist or child psychiatrist? _____

   _____

   _____

   _____

Scenario 2

An elderly patient calls to complain of a high fever, muscle aches, a headache, and chills. He thinks he is getting the flu. He stated he had a flu shot about nine months ago, even though he didn't want it, and he is not supposed to get sick.

1. Should you take his self-appraisal of his condition without further question? _____
   _____
   _____

2. How would you explain to him the nature of the flu vaccine and its effectiveness? _____
   _____
   _____
   _____
   _____

Research Activity

There are four lung diseases or disorders that are very interesting and quite serious that should be further researched. The four conditions are pulmonary fibrosis, respiratory distress syndrome (RDS), sudden infant death syndrome (SIDS), and tuberculosis (TB). Select one and prepare a report to share with the class. Perhaps the instructor could divide the class and each group could work on the assigned report. In your research, determine the cause, the rate of incidence within the population, the age group affected, symptoms, treatment, prognosis, and any other aspect of the disease. RDS and SIDS, for example, each have a profound impact on parents. Discuss this situation. Can you identify any support groups? Tuberculosis was thought to be a thing of the past, but it has returned. Why? Pulmonary fibrosis is probably unknown to most people, yet it is not that uncommon.

CHAPTER 18

The Digestive System

Words to Know Challenge

Spelling: Each line contains three spellings of a word. Underline the correctly spelled word.

1. apendix	appendix	appenddix
2. cirrhosis	cirhosis	cirrosis
3. collitis	colytis	colitis
4. diahrrea	diarhea	diarrhea
5. digestion	digestation	digeshion
6. dudenum	duodenum	duodunem
7. esofagus	esophagus	esophegus
8. hepattitis	hepetitis	hepatitis
9. ileocecal	illucecal	illuocecal
10. insalen	insilun	insulin
11. jaundice	jawndice	jaundace
12. nasea	nausea	nausae
13. pancrase	pancrease	pancreas
14. sigmiod	sigmoid	sigmyod
15. stenosis	stenasis	stenesis
16. stomack	stomach	stomache
17. tong	tungue	tongue
18. varies	varices	verices

Matching: Match the term in column I with its description in column II.

COLUMN I	COLUMN II
____ 1. Alimentary canal	A. Inability to control bowel elimination
____ 2. Bile	B. A backup of stomach contents
____ 3. Cholelithiasis	C. The organ between the mouth and stomach
____ 4. Cystic duct	D. Smooth muscle action that moves material
____ 5. Duodenum	E. Engorged veins
____ 6. Esophagus	F. Protrusion of an organ through an opening
____ 7. Flatus	G. The chain of organs of the GI system
____ 8. Gastric	H. The yellowish discoloration caused by bile in the tissues
____ 9. Gastroscopy	I. An instrument to visualize the rectum
____ 10. Hernia	J. Stored by the gallbladder
____ 11. Incontinent	K. The first section of the small intestine
____ 12. Jaundice	L. Intestinal gas
____ 13. Peristalsis	M. Refers to the stomach
____ 14. Proctoscope	N. An instrument to view the stomach
____ 15. Reflux	O. Gallstones
____ 16. Varices	P. The drainage tube for the gallbladder

Chapter Review

Short Answer

1. Define *digestion*. _____

_____

_____

2. List the raw materials the body requires to promote good health.

a. _____

b. _____

c. _____

d. _____

e. _____

f. _____

g. _____

3. List, in order, the organs of the alimentary tract through which food passes.

a. _____

b. _____

c. _____

d. _____

e. _____

f. _____

4. List the accessory digestive organs of the mouth; explain their function in the digestive process.

 a. _____

 b. _____

 _____

 c. _____

 _____

 _____

5. a. What are the initial teeth called? _____

 b. When do they appear? _____

 c. Initial teeth are lost beginning about age ___ and are replaced by _____ .

 d. Identify the four types of "secondary" teeth and their specific duties.

 a) _____

 b) _____

 c) _____

 d) _____

6. How is swallowing accomplished? _____

 _____

 _____

 _____

7. How is food moved through the esophagus? _____

 _____

 _____

8. Describe the structure of the stomach and explain its function. _____

 _____

 _____

 _____

 _____

 _____

 _____

 _____

9. Describe the structure of the small intestine, naming its sections and explaining its function. _____

 _____

 _____

 _____

 _____

10. What functions does the liver perform, including the relationship with the portal circulation?

 a. _____

 b. _____

 c. _____

 d. _____

 e. _____

 f. _____

 g. _____

 h. _____

 i. _____

 _____

 _____

11. What role does the gallblader play and how is it related to the liver? _____
_____
_____

12. Explain why the duodenum is vital to digestion. _____
_____

13. Describe the location and function of the pancreas. _____
_____
_____
_____

14. Where in the body are nutrients absorbed, and how is absorption accomplished? _____
_____
_____
_____
_____

15. Explain the function of the colon and name its five sections. _____
_____

   a. _____
   b. _____
   c. _____
   d. _____
   e. _____

16. What function does the rectum perform? _____
_____

17. Describe the structure and function of the anal canal. _____
_____
_____

Labeling

1. Label the illustration of the structures involved in swallowing using the following terms. Refer to Figure 18–4 in the textbook.

(windpipe)　　　　　(food tube)

1. Epiglottis	5. Pharynx
2. Food	6. Soft palate
3. Hard palate	7. Tongue
4. Jawbone	

2. Label the organs of digestion on the illustration using the following terms. Refer to Figure 18–1 in the textbook.

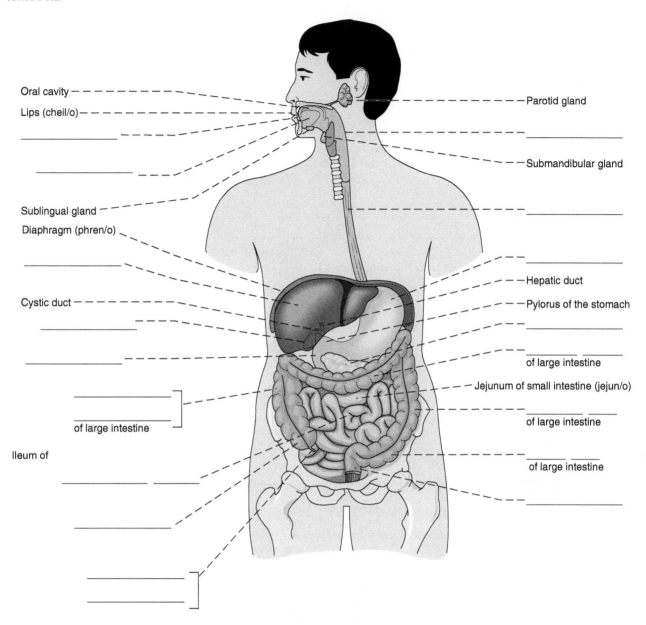

Oral cavity

Lips (cheil/o)

_____

_____

Sublingual gland

Diaphragm (phren/o)

_____

Cystic duct

_____

_____

_____

of large intestine

Ileum of

_____

_____

Parotid gland

_____

Submandibular gland

_____

_____

Hepatic duct

Pylorus of the stomach

_____

_____ _____

of large intestine

Jejunum of small intestine (jejun/o)

_____ _____

of large intestine

_____ _____

of large intestine

_____

1. Ascending colon
2. Cecum
3. Descending colon
4. Duodenum
5. Esophagus
6. Gallbladder
7. Liver
8. Pancreas
9. Pharynx

10. Rectum
11. Sigmoid colon
12. Small intestine
13. Stomach
14. Teeth
15. Tongue
16. Transverse colon
17. Vermiform appendix

3. Label the illustration using the following terms. Refer to Figure 18–7 in the textbook.

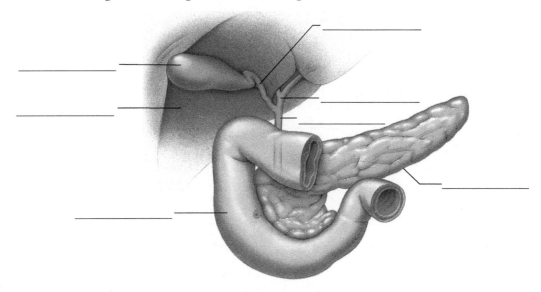

1. Common bile duct
2. Cystic duct
3. Duodenum
4. Gallbladder
5. Hepatic duct
6. Liver
7. Pancreas

Matching: Match the disease or conditions in column I with the appropriate symptoms or description in column II.

COLUMN I	COLUMN II
___ 1. Anorectal abscess or fistula	A. Frequent, liquid stools
___ 2. Cirrhosis	B. Enlarged spleen, ascites, bloody emesis and stools, reduced platelets
___ 3. Colitis	C. Dilated anal veins, painful defecation, bleeding
___ 4. Colostomy	D. Protruding mass at inguinal area or loop of intestine in scrotum
___ 5. Diarrhea	E. Tenderness and discomfort of the colon
___ 6. Diverticulitis	F. Jaundice, hepatomegaly, loss of appetite, fatigue, clay-colored stools, weight loss
___ 7. Esophageal varices	G. Absence of peristalsis, abdominal distention, distress, vomiting
___ 8. Anal fissure	H. Severe epigastric pain, not relieved by vomiting; a rigid abdomen, rales, tachycardia, fever, cold, perspiring extremities
___ 9. Gastroenteritis	I. Asymptomatic growths protruding from the intestinal lining
___ 10. Hemorrhoids	J. Painful, throbbing lump near the anus, with or without drainage

____	11. Hepatitis	K.	Fever, nausea and vomiting, abdominal cramps, traveler's diarrhea
____	12. Hiatal hernia	L.	Forceful vomiting, dilation of stomach, difficulty emptying contents of stomach into duodenum
____	13. Inguinal hernia	M.	Recurrent bloody diarrhea with mucus and exudate, weight loss, weakness, anorexia, nausea, vomiting, abdominal pain
____	14. Ileostomy	N.	Itching of anal area, especially following bowel movement, reddened skin, weeping and thickened skin, darkening of tissue
____	15. Pancreatitis	O.	Lack of appetite, indigestion, nausea, vomiting, nosebleeds, bleeding gums, enlarged and firm liver, jaundice, ascites
____	16. Paralytic ileus	P.	Alternating periods of constipation and diarrhea, lower abdominal pain, daytime diarrhea, mucous stools
____	17. Peptic ulcer	Q.	A single or double opening on the abdomen through which solid fecal material passes
____	18. Polyps	R.	Heartburn, epigastric pain relieved by food, weight gain, bubbling hot water sensation
____	19. Pruritus ani	S.	Opening of small intestine into the abdomen through which liquid stool is expelled
____	20. Pyloric stenosis	T.	Bulging pouches in the intestine that cause abdominal pain, nausea, flatus, irregular bowel movements, high white blood cell count
____	21. Spastic colon	U.	Burning rectal pain with a few drops of blood with passing of stool, sentinel pile
____	22. Ulcerative colitis	V.	Heartburn, regurgitation, vomiting, fullness, stomach spasms, difficulty swallowing, gastric reflux

Chapter Application

Case Studies with Critical Thinking Questions

Scenario 1

A male patient called to schedule an appointment. He is complaining about what he thinks is an ulcer. Almost every time he eats he gets a feeling of indigestion and discomfort. He usually has heartburn and sometimes brings food up into his throat. The provider is away on vacation for the next 10 days, and you cannot schedule an appointment.

1. How would you decide if this situation is an emergency? _____

_____

_____

2. Should he be offered an alternative provider since his current physician is away? _____

_____

_____

Scenario 2

Your neighbor tells you her 14-year-old daughter has not felt well for the past couple of days. The neighbor explains that her daughter first had a general discomfort in her abdomen, but then it became more severe and seemed to be located just below her umbilicus on her right side. She was nauseated and couldn't eat. She also had a slight fever. However, she had a good night's sleep, and the pain has gone away; she is feeling better today. The mother thinks she probably ate something that didn't agree with her.

1. Why do you think she should be advised to have the daughter examined? _____
   _____
   _____

2. What else could be causing her symptoms? _____
   _____
   _____

3. What are the possible complications that could develop if nothing is done? _____
   _____
   _____

Research Activity

The incidence of GERD is very common. Go online to http://digestive.niddk.nih.gov/ddiseases/pubs/gerd to read the information and find the answers to the following questions.

1. What is GERD?

2. What are the symptoms?

3. What causes GERD?

4. How is GERD treated?

5. What if GERD symptoms persist?

6. What are the long-term complications of GERD?

7. What is Barrett's esophagus?

CHAPTER 19

The Urinary System

Words to Know Challenge

Spelling: Each line contains three spellings of a word. Underline the correctly spelled word.

1. noturia   nocturea   <u>nocturia</u>

2. <u>oliguria</u>   oligurea   olliguria

3. pollyurea   polyurea   <u>polyuria</u>

4. <u>calyces</u>   calcyces   callcyces

5. <u>ptosis</u>   tosis   phtosis

6. dialasis   <u>dialysis</u>   dilyasis

7. sectretion   secreton   <u>secretion</u>

8. <u>lithotripsy</u>   lithatripsy   lithotrypsy

9. unuria   auria   <u>anuria</u>

10. glommerulus   <u>glomerulus</u>   glomurelus

Matching: Match the term in column I with its signs and symptoms in column II.

COLUMN I	COLUMN II
____ 1. Cystitis	A. Urgency, dysuria, nocturia, hematuria, ammoniac or fishy odor to urine, high fever, chills, flank pain, fatigue
____ 2. Glomerulonephritis	B. Small stream of urine, prolonged urination time
____ 3. Nephrotic syndrome	C. Oliguria, azotemia, severe electrolyte imbalance, acidosis, uremia, other body system involvement
____ 4. Polycystic kidney disease	D. Frequency, dysuria, bladder spasms, sharp stabbing pain on urination
____ 5. Pyelonephritis	E. Severe pain beginning in kidney, moving to groin area, nausea, vomiting, chills, and fever
____ 6. Renal failure	F. Generalized dependent edema, pleural effusion, ascites, lethargy, fatigue, pallor, swollen external sexual organs
____ 7. Stricture	G. Urine products in the blood, coma, toxic waste levels in blood, eventual death
____ 8. Calculi	H. Moderate edema, proteinuria, hematuria, oliguria, fatigue, urinary casts, hypertension
____ 9. Uremia	I. Pointed nose, small chin, floppy low-set ears, inner eyelid folds, eventually widened body, swollen, tender abdomen, life-threatening bleeding, ureteral spasms

Chapter Review

Short Answer

1. List the three main functions of the urinary system, explaining the meaning of each.

   a. _____

   b. _____

   c. _____

2. Identify the organs of the urinary system; describe their physical characteristics.

   a. _____
   _____
   _____

   b. _____
   _____
   _____

   c. _____
   _____
   _____

   d. _____
   _____
   _____

3. How does the urinary system work with the other body systems to accomplish its job? _____

_____
_____
_____
_____
_____
_____

4. How is the interior of the kidney constructed? _____

_____
_____
_____

5. List the parts of the nephron and describe the function of each part.
   a. Bowman's _____
   b. Glomerulus _____
   _____
   c. Proximal _____
   _____
   d. Distal _____

6. Describe kidney dialysis, and identify two major methods. _____

_____
_____
_____
_____
_____
_____

7. What are the two main categories of diagnostic examinations? Give one example of each type. _____

_____
_____
_____

8. Name the three types of incontinence.
   a. _____
   b. _____
   c. _____

9. Name four methods for connecting a patient to hemodialysis.
   a. _____
   b. _____
   c. _____
   d. _____

10. Identify the types of peritoneal dialysis.
   a. _____
   b. _____
   c. _____

Labeling

1. Label the illustration of the urinary system using the following terms. Refer to Figure 19–1 in the textbook.
   Abdominal aorta
   Adrenal gland
   Inferior vena cava
   Left kidney
   Left renal artery
   Prostate gland (in males)
   Renal cortex
   Renal medulla
   Renal pelvis
   Right and left ureters
   Right kidney
   Ureteral orifices
   Urethra
   Urethral meatus
   Urinary bladder

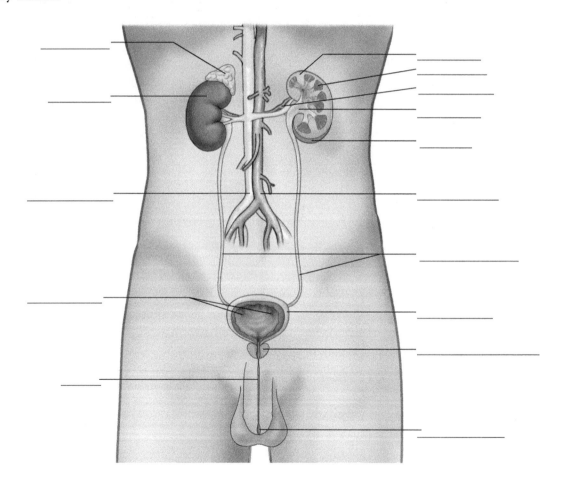

2. Label the illustration of the interior of the kidney and the nephron with the following terms. Refer to Figure 19–2 in the textbook.

Afferent arteriole
Bowman's capsule
Collecting duct
Efferent arteriole
Glomerulus
Medulla
Peritubular capillaries
Renal artery X 2
Renal cortex
Renal pelvis
Renal tubules
Renal vein X 2
Ureter

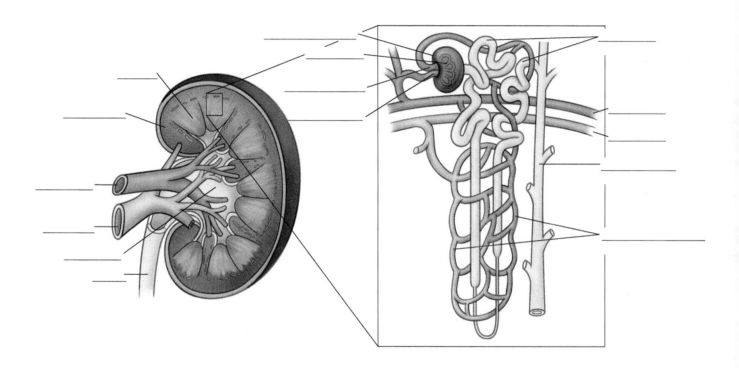

Chapter Application

Case Study with Critical Thinking Questions

A female patient calls to find out whether she is experiencing a reaction to a cystoscopic examination three days ago. She has started going to the bathroom frequently, and now it is beginning to be painful. She thinks it looks like there might be a little blood in her urine. She wonders if this is common.

1. What other symptoms would you ask her if she is experiencing? _____

_____

2. Why should you ask if she has done anything to treat herself? _____

_____

_____

Research Activity

Select one of the urinary system disorders discussed in the text. Do an Internet search to learn more about the condition. Find out about the causes and treatment. Is there a support group for people and families dealing with the condition? Is there a national, state, or local association supporting the disorder? (You may need to refer to your phone directory for local information.) Prepare a short written report of your findings.

CHAPTER 21

The Reproductive System

Words to Know Challenge

Spelling: Each line contains three spellings of a word. Underline the correctly spelled word.

1. circumcision   circumsision   circumcisun
2. dysmenorrhea   dismenorehea   dysmenorrea
3. epididimus   epididymis   epididymus
4. genetalia   genitalea   genitalia
5. menapause   menopause   menoplaus
6. menorrhagia   menarrhagia   menorrhagea
7. prostratectomy   prostatectemy   prostatectomy
8. syfhillis   syphillis   syphilis

Define the Terms: Define the following diseases or disorders of the female reproductive system.

1. Abortion _____
2. Cervical erosion _____
3. Cervicitis _____
4. Cystic breast disease _____
5. Cystocele _____
6. Dysmenorrhea _____
7. Endometriosis _____
8. Fibroids _____
9. Hysterectomy _____
10. Malignancy of the breast _____

11. Ovarian cyst _____

12. PMS _____

13. Polyp _____

14. Rectocele _____

Chapter Review

Short Answer

1. What is the difference between asexual and sexual reproduction? _____
   _____
   _____

2. Explain the process of differentiation of the reproductive organs; compare the male organ to the female
   organ. _____
   _____
   _____
   _____
   _____
   _____
   _____

3. How is sperm able to fertilize an egg? _____
   _____
   _____

4. List the nine male sex organs or structures and describe their function.
   a. _____
   b. _____
   c. _____
   d. _____
   _____
   e. _____
   f. _____
   _____
   g. _____
   _____
   h. _____
   i. _____

5. How do pituitary hormones affect the function of the testes? _____
   _____
   _____

6. List the secondary male sex characteristics.
   a. _____
   b. _____
   c. _____
   d. _____
   e. _____
   f. _____
   g. _____

7. List, in order, the structures through which sperm pass.

    a. _____

    b. _____

    c. _____

    d. _____

    e. _____

8. What is the composition of semen?

    a. _____

    b. _____

    c. _____

    d. _____

9. List the four diseases and disorders of the male reproductive system; define the condition and identify the main symptoms and/or cause of the condition.

    a. _____
    _____

    b. _____
    _____
    _____

    c. _____
    _____
    _____

    d. _____
    _____
    _____

10. List the eight female sexual structures and describe their function.

    a. _____

    b. _____

    c. _____

    d. _____

    e. _____

    f. _____

    g. _____

    h. _____

11. How do hormones from the pituitary gland affect the development of the female reproductive organs?

    _____
    _____
    _____

12. List the female secondary sex characteristics.

    a. _____

    b. _____

    c. _____

    d. _____

    e. _____

    f. _____

    g. _____

    h. _____

    i. _____

13. List the four phases of the menstrual cycle.

    a. _____

    b. _____

    c. _____

    d. _____

14. Describe the fertilization of an ovum. _____

    _____

    _____

    _____

    _____

15. List the usual signs and symptoms of early pregnancy.

    a. _____

    b. _____

    c. _____

    d. _____

    e. _____

    f. _____

16. List symptoms that occur later in pregnancy.

    a. _____

    b. _____

    c. _____

    d. _____

    e. _____

    f. _____

    g. _____

    h. _____

17. Describe the characteristics of the three stages of labor.

    First   a. _____

             b. _____

    Second   a. _____

             b. _____

             c. _____

             d. _____

    Third   a. _____

             b. _____

18. List eight reasons to use contraceptives.

    a. _____

    b. _____

    c. _____

    d. _____

    e. _____

    f. _____

    g. _____

    h. _____

19. List seven routine screening and diagnostic pregnancy tests. _____
_____
_____

20. Name 14 methods of contraception.

a. _____ h. _____
b. _____ i. _____
c. _____ j. _____
d. _____ k. _____
e. _____ l. _____
f. _____ m. _____
g. _____ n. _____

21. Identify the main characteristics of each of the following disease conditions.

a. Chlamydia _____
_____
_____

b. Gonorrhea _____
_____
_____

c. Herpes _____
_____

d. NGU _____

e. PID _____
_____
_____

f. Syphilis (four stages) (1) _____
_____

(2) _____
_____
_____

(3) _____

(4) _____

g. Trichomoniasis _____

Matching: Match the test or procedure in column I with its description in column II.

COLUMN I

_____ 1. Alpha-fetoprotein screening
_____ 2. Mammograph
_____ 3. Maturation index
_____ 4. Papanicolaou test
_____ 5. Pregnancy test
_____ 6. Ultrasonography
_____ 7. Colposcopy
_____ 8. Hysteroscopy

COLUMN II

A. Examination with an instrument connected to a monitor to view the endometrium

B. Determines hormonal level from cells scraped from vaginal walls

C. High-frequency sound waves that detect and aid in the diagnosis of breast irregularities

D. A urine specimen test to detect the presence of HCG

E. A blood test to detect birth defects

F. Examination of cervical secretions for cancer cells

G. An X-ray of the breast

H. An examination of the cervix following a questionable Pap smear

Labeling

1. Label the male reproductive system illustration using these terms. Refer to textbook Figure 21–7.

Anal opening
Bulbourethral gland or Cowper's gland
Ejaculatory duct
Epididymis
Membranous urethra
Penis
Prepuce
Prostate gland
Rectum

Scrotum
Seminal vesicle
Spermatic cord
Symphysis pubis
Testis
Vas deferens (two times)
Urethra
Urinary bladder

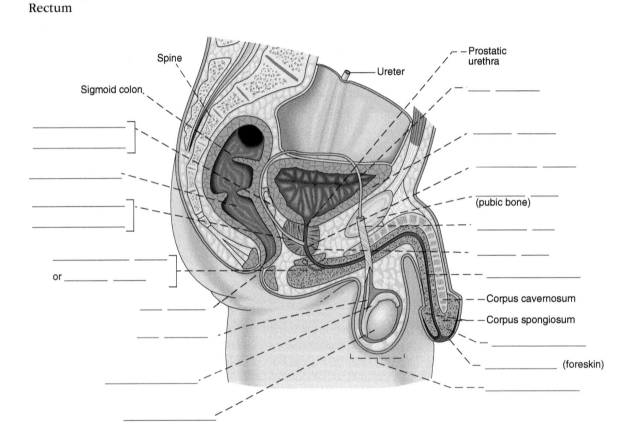

2. Label the female reproductive system illustration using the following terms. Refer to Figure 21–15 in the textbook.

Anus
Cervix
Corpus of uterus
Crus of clitoris
Fallopian tube
Fundus of uterus

Ovary
Symphysis pubis
Ureter
Urethra
Urinary bladder
Vagina

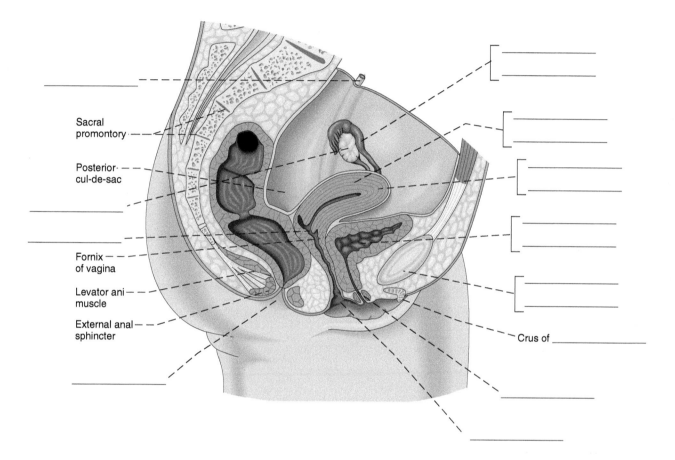

Sacral
promontory

Posterior
cul-de-sac

Fornix
of vagina

Levator ani
muscle

External anal
sphincter

Crus of _____

3. Label the external female structures on the illustration using the following terms. Refer to Figure 21–16 in the textbook.

Anus   Mons pubis
Clitoris   Perineum
Hymen   Urethral orifice
Labia majora   Vaginal orifice
Labia minora   Vestibule

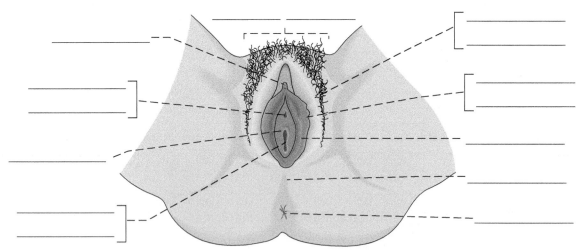

Fill in the Blank: Use information from the chapter to fill in the blank space in the sentence.

1. A male infant develops if the zygote contains a _____ chromosome.

2. At about the seventh or eighth week, the _____ begin to develop within the _____.

3. During the eighth or ninth month, the _____ move from the _____ through the _____ into the _____.

Chapter Application

Case Studies with Critical Thinking Questions

Scenario 1

A 65-year-old male patient calls the office asking if the provider would call in a prescription for his kidney infection. He is complaining of frequent urination, getting up at night, and even some dribbling in between. He says about a year ago his younger brother had the same problem.

1. What additional information about symptoms do you need before you talk to the doctor? _____

_____

_____

_____

_____

_____

2. Why do you need to tell him the provider will probably want to see him before he prescribes something?

_____

_____

_____

Scenario 2

Your 16-year-old daughter tells you that some of the girls at school have been talking about having sex. One of the girls said that she didn't worry about getting any diseases or getting pregnant because she always uses a vinegar douche directly afterward. Your daughter wonders if that really works.

1. Why is it important for you to explain to your daughter the physiology of conception? _____

_____

_____

_____

_____

2. Why would you discuss your opinions toward sexual behavior? _____

_____

_____

_____

_____

_____

_____

Application Activity

This application deals with pregnancy, something many women experience and share with their friends. Suppose this is your sister's first pregnancy, and she is very excited about the development of the baby. She is constantly asking you questions. She wants to know:

1. When is the formation of the embryo complete? _____

2. What is the baby called when it is two months old? _____

3. When can the baby's sex be determined? _____

4. When will she feel movement? _____

5. How big is the baby at the end of five months? _____

6. When can you hear its heartbeat? _____

She is amazed when you tell her that at _____ the fetus will open its eyes and by _____ it can hear sounds inside the uterus.

SECTION 3

The Front Office

Business Communications

CHAPTER 22

Telephone Communications

X Words to Know Challenge

Spelling: Each line contains three spellings of a word. Underline the correctly spelled word.

1. <u>confirmed</u>   confired   confirmd
2. <u>confidential</u>   confadential   confedential
3. <u>communication</u>   comunication   communacation
4. <u>preference</u>   perference   preferance
5. emputhy   empathie   <u>empathy</u>
6. ettiquete   <u>ettiquette</u>   <u>etiquette</u>
7. ecspress   <u>express</u>   escpress
8. <u>fax</u>   facs   facts
9. <u>patient portal</u>   patience portal   patience portle
10. pirsonallity   personallity   <u>personality</u>
11. <u>screening</u>   screaning   skreaning
12. treage   <u>triage</u>   treaje
13. <u>teleconferencing</u>   teleconfrencing   telaconfrencing
14. antissipate   <u>anticipate</u>   antisipate

Fill in the Blank: Complete the following sentences with correctly spelled words from the Spelling section.

1. Because the phone call is often the first contact a patient has with the office, your manner of speaking and the _____ you convey are a part of establishing an appropriate image of the practice.

2. An established phone _____ manual (sometimes called a _____ manual) should be kept near each phone for reference so that each assistant who answers the phone will ask standard questions and give the standard response that has been preauthorized by the provider.

3. You must _____ the needs of the patient and provider by asking the proper questions to route accurate information to the appropriate person with the level of urgency required.

4. Appointments should be _____ by reading the scheduled time back to the patient after it has been recorded in the appointment book or scheduling system.

5. The general rule is that a medical assistant does not give out information or call in a prescription without the _____ direction of the physician.

6. Professional _____ dictates that the provider will not keep a colleague waiting unless he or she is involved with an emergency or surgical procedure.

7. Your voice is part of your _____, but over the phone, your voice is you.

8. Messages from the answering service need to be returned in the order of importance within an appropriate and reasonable time period. Remember to check the _____ machine and _____ for other patient-related messages.

9. Before you telephone a patient regarding PHI, review (the) _____ form for what number to call and if it is okay to leave a message. _____ is a way to include people at a remote location in a meeting discussion.

Chapter Review

Short Answer

1. Explain the proper protocol (steps) for answering the telephone in the medical office, including an example.
   Answer phone with smile and greeting "Good morning, Central Medical Office, Ellen speaking, How may I help you?"

2. What does *screening* mean?
   A logical set of questions that reveal callers conditions, help determine when patient should be seen by provider.

3. For each type of call in the following list, identify who it should be routed to: provider; take a message for provider; clinical medical assistant; or administrative medical assistant.
   a. Critical lab results: *Take message for provider, clinical medical assistant*
   b. A patient with a question about insurance: *administrative medical assistant*
   c. A patient calling for a routine prescription refill: *Message for provider*
   d. A patient wanting some medical advice: *clinical medical assistant*

   e. Another physician: *Provider*
   f. A patient needing to schedule an appointment: *Administrative medical assistant*
   g. A patient upset about his last visit: *Administrative medical assistant, clinical Medical Assistant.*
   h. A patient with a question about a statement received by mail: *Administrative Med. As.*
   i. A patient having a heart attack: *Clinical Medical Assistant*

4. List at least six pieces of information that should be included in all telephone messages.

Full Name, date, time, M/F, Phone Number, Nature of call

X 5. Fill in the following chart, identifying four types of telephone calls a medical assistant might have to answer in the medical office; explain how each should be handled. The first one has been filled in for you as an example.

Type of Phone Call	How It Should Be Handled
Appointments	Positively identify the patient (with two identifiers) and confirm the last appointment date. Assess the type of appointment needed and note in the schedule.
Referrals Test Results	Confirm with provider, observe office policy, give test results after verifying patient identity.
Emergency Calls	Get all details, remain calm, notify EMS if urgent.
Providers, Hospitals	Ask for name and inform the provider, ask if call is regarding a patient.
Personal calls	Provider will inform you on how to handle calls from family members.

6. List at least four types of community resources for patients' health care needs and four types of emergency services and how to research current information.

X Matching: Match the tone of voice in column I to the translation in column II.

COLUMN I

C 1. Monotone flat voice

E 2. Slow speed and low pitch

D 3. High-pitched and empathic voice

B 4. Abrupt speed and loud tone

A 5. High-pitch combined with drawn-out speed

COLUMN II

A. "I don't believe what I'm hearing."

B. "I'm angry and not open to input."

C. "I'm bored and have absolutely no interest in what you're talking about."

D. "I'm enthusiastic about this subject."

E. "I'm depressed and want to be left alone."

Chapter Application

Case Studies with Critical Thinking Questions

Scenario 1

Jennifer, the clinical medical assistant, answers the telephone for the receptionist, who is busy, and encounters a patient who is very upset and anxious. The patient quickly informs Jennifer that her three-year-old daughter has fallen and is bleeding badly. The patient tells Jennifer her name and phone number but hangs up before Jennifer can find anything to write with or record the message on.

1. How should Jennifer handle this situation? _____
_____
_____

2. How can she ensure that this will not happen again? _____
_____
_____

3. What should Jennifer do before answering the phone the next time? _____
_____
_____

Scenario 2

Several of the telephone lines are ringing at once, and Sarah is already on the line with one patient who needs to have an important question answered immediately.

1. What should Sarah do about answering the other lines? _____
_____
_____

2. Should she continue to talk with the first caller and let the other lines ring? _____
_____
_____

3. What device could help in this situation? _____
_____
_____

Competency Practice

1. **Perform a Telephone Screening Demonstrating Professional Telephone Techniques**

    Using Procedure 22–1 as a guideline, with a partner read the situations in A and B out loud in class and role-play how you would handle them using the information in the textbook to properly screen a call demonstrating professional telephone techniques.

    A. "I Have to See the Physician—Today!"

Physician's Identity:	(Use names of local providers or make up)
Solo or Group:	Two-provider partnership
Specialty:	Family practice
Time:	8:30 a.m.
Situation:	Both providers are on hospital rounds and are not expected until 10:00 a.m. The appointment book is full.
Patient:	(Insert name of student or fictitious name), a patient since infancy

"I need an appointment today—right away. I'm leaving for college tomorrow, and the physician just has to see me. Just for a minute. I need a quick physical and a form filled out. It's nothing really. I can't register for class unless the physician sees me. I just have to have an appointment. I know this is last-minute—but just this once, please. Certainly, you understand; you have to."

B. Call to Notify Patient

Physician's Identity:	(Use names of local providers or make up)
Solo or Group:	Two-provider partnership
Specialty:	OB/GYN
Time:	1:00 p.m.
Situation:	Both providers have called to say that they will be late in returning to the office. It seems all the babies in town decided to be born today. Dr. ___, anticipating a cesarean section, says he might not be in at all. Dr. ____ says he will be at least one hour late and maybe longer. Office protocol is to notify patients, who have not yet arrived, of the delay.
Patient:	(Insert fictitious name)

You call Mrs. ____ and tell her of the delay. She has an appointment for 3:00 p.m., which she made about three weeks ago. You can tell from the tone of her voice that she is upset. The medical assistant knows from past experience that the best thing to do is cancel Mrs. ____'s appointment and reschedule her. This cannot be done. The earliest time that Dr. ____ can see Mrs. ____ will be 5:00 to 5:30 p.m. Mrs. ____ is not enthusiastic about either alternative.

2. **Document Telephone Messages Accurately**

   Using Procedure 22–2 as a guideline, obtain messages from a phone recording device (or answering service) as noted in the following scenario. Record the messages, noting the date and time of call, patient/caller name, and the reason for the call. After documenting the messages, prioritize and route/respond appropriately.

   Scenario: Upon arriving at the office Monday morning, you check for messages, retrieving them from the answering device (or answering service) and fax machine. There are five messages from the answering service and no fax messages.

   a. Ms. Emily Riley called at 2:30 p.m. on Saturday to say her son Ryan has been running a fever (101°F) and seems to be very congested. She would like to bring him to the office first thing Monday morning. Her callback number is 555-0125.

   b. Jorge Monroy called at 6:18 p.m. on Friday to say he needed a work release form from Dr. ___ as soon as possible so he can return to work. His callback number is 555-0183.

   c. Sheniqua Jackson called at 7:26 a.m. Monday. She was discharged from the same-day surgery center on Friday, and she is feeling very short of breath and would like to see Dr. ___ this morning. No number provided.

   d. James Brosnovich called at 5:08 p.m. on Friday to say he would like to set up an appointment with Dr. ___ to review a new drug sample available. His callback number is 555-0102.

   e. Mrs. Millie Garza called at 6:46 p.m. on Saturday to cancel her appointment Monday morning at 9:45 a.m. due to a family emergency. No number provided.

3. **Telephone a Patient with Test Results**

Using Procedure 22–3 as a guideline, with a partner read the read the following situation out loud in class and role-play how you would handle it using the information and techniques described in the textbook to telephone a patient with test results.

Physician's Identity:	(Use names of local providers or make up)
Solo or Group:	Two-provider partnership
Specialty:	Internal Medicine
Time:	3:00 p.m.
Situation:	Your provider has forwarded a message to you to call a patient with her lab results.
Patient:	(Insert fictitious name)

Call Mrs. _____ and tell her the results of her cholesterol test has been received. Per the message from the provider, her LDL is 118 mg/dL, her HDL is 59 mg/dL, and her triglycerides are 148 mg/dL. Dr. ___ is very happy with the levels and recommends that she stay on Atorvastatin 20 mg qd, and he has sent in a new 90-day prescription with three refills to her mail-away prescription carrier, CareTrackerRx. He wants Mrs. ___ to return for repeat lab work in six months. When finished with the call, enter a recall for the repeat lab work into the patient's chart.

4. **Develop a Current List of Community Resources Related to Patient Health Care Needs**

Using Procedure 22–4 as a guideline, create a list of resources for senior services available in your community. (Create additional resource lists for nutritional services or smoking cessation.)

5. **Facilitate Referrals to Community Resources in the Role of Patient Navigator**

Using Procedure 22–5 as a guideline, access the Internet (or alternatively access the Federal Emergency Management Agency [FEMA] website to create a list of resources for emergency services available in your community). Using at least two topics in Competency Practice 22–4 (Senior Services, Nutritional Services, or Smoking Cessation), facilitate referral(s) to community resources in the role of patient navigator.

The Office Environment, Computers, and Equipment

Words to Know Challenge

Spelling: Each line contains three spellings of a word. Underline the correctly spelled word.

1. dicktation   dictation   diktation
2. incoder   encorder   encoder
3. faximilie   faxsimilie   facsimile
4. periferral   peripheral   peripherral
5. interface   intraface   interfface
6. erganomic   ergonomic   eargonomic
7. hazzard   hazard   hazerd
8. atmostphere   atmosfere   atmosphere
9. biohazzardous   biohazardour   biohazardous
10. continuity of care   conintious of care   continuty of care
11. environment   enviroment   enviramenet
12. HT7 Protocol   HL7 Protocol   HLZ Protocol
13. invantore   invantory   inventory
14. reception   recepshun   resepction
15. threchold   thrashold   threshold
16. trascription   transcription   transkription
17. volatile   volotile   vollatile
18. hardwhere   hardware   hardwere
19. softwhere   software   softwere
20. assoult   asault   assault
21. electronic helth record   electronic helth recerd   electronic health record

Matching: Now, using the correctly spelled terms from the Words to Know section, write each word next to the correct definition.

	COLUMN I	COLUMN II
____	1. Atmosphere	A. Any material that has been in contact with body fluid and is potentially capable of transmitting disease
____	2. Inventory	B. The delivery of services provided to a person that proceeds without a lapse or interruption, with the intended purpose of maintaining a level of health and treatment
____	3. HL7 Protocol	C. An itemized list of goods in stock
____	4. Hazard	D. Any surrounding influence
____	5. Biohazardous	E. Writing over from one book or medium into another; typing in full ordinary letters
____	6. Continuity of Care	F. Danger; risk
____	7. Environment	G. The fact or manner of being received; a social gathering
____	8. Threshold	H. Easily changed into a gas or tending to change into a vapor; usually considered potentially dangerous
____	9. Reception	I. The standard for exchanging information between medical applications
____	10. Transcription	J. A minimum amount of supplies to be maintained; also known as par level
____	11. Volatile	K. Surroundings

Chapter Review

Short Answer

1. List five things to check in the reception area at the beginning of the day.

_____

_____

_____

2. List five tasks to perform when preparing the front desk at the beginning of the day.

_____

_____

_____

3. List five tasks to perform when preparing an examination room for use.

_____

_____

_____

4. Describe the difference between computer hardware and software.

_____

_____

_____

_____

5. Give two examples of hardware and two examples of software.

_____

_____

_____

_____

6. Define application software and application suites. Include examples in your answer.

_____
_____
_____
_____
_____

7. Explain why caution should be taken when gathering information from the Internet.

_____
_____
_____
_____

8. Describe four guidelines for finding credible information on the Internet.

_____
_____
_____
_____
_____

9. Explain the computer term *downtime* and describe when it would be used.

_____
_____
_____

10. Fill in the following chart, describing common software applications used in medical offices.

Software Application	Description/Capabilities
Practice management	
Electronic health records	
Encoder software	

Matching: Match the office equipment in column I with the appropriate function in column II.

COLUMN I

COLUMN II

_____ 1. Most machines can be set to use either letter- or legal-sized paper and duplicate a document.

A. Fax machine

_____ 2. A small electronic device that is activated by a telephone signal.

B. Copy machine

_____ 3. An electronic device, operating under the control of instructions stored in its own memory unit, which can accept and store data, perform mathematical and logical operations on that data without human intervention, and produce output from the processing.

C. Transcriber

_____ 4. The machine scans a document and converts the image to electronic impulses that are transmitted over the telephone lines.

D. Computer

_____ 5. Providers dictate their notes following patients' appointments, and the medical assistant uses this machine for the chart notes.

E. Pager

_____ 6. The machine produces hard copies from computer files.

F. Printer

Chapter Application

Case Studies with Critical Thinking Questions

Scenario 1

As Mary Ramirez, the medical assistant, escorts the first patient into the exam room, she notices that the room is disorganized and that there is evidence of the last patient from the day before. Mary needs to take the patient's vitals and notices that the blood pressure cuff is missing, so she leaves the room to find it.

1. What might the patient's impression of the office be? _____

_____

2. What should the medical assistant have done before bringing the patient to the exam room? _____

_____

3. How can this situation be prevented in the future? _____

_____

Competency Practice

1. **Open the Office and Evaluate the Work Environment to Identify Unsafe Working Conditions**

   Using Procedure 24–1 and the information in your textbook as a guideline, create a typed checklist to use when opening the medical office. In the checklist, be sure to include items to be observed for safety as well as any environmental considerations and other precautions that should be taken. Using the checklist you created, evaluate a work environment (or personal living space—your apartment, your home, your parents' home, and so on) for safe and unsafe conditions and complete the checklist. Write down five safe conditions and five unsafe conditions present.

   Place of evaluation:

   Evaluate the work environment to identify unsafe working conditions.

	Safe Conditions Present	Unsafe Conditions Present
1.		
2.		
3.		
4.		
5.		

2. **Perform an Inventory of Equipment and Supplies with Documentation**

   Using Procedure 24–2 and the information from the textbook as a guideline, perform an inventory of the school laboratory supplies listed on the following inventory sheet. Accurately count and record the number and amount of each item. Indicate if reordering is necessary, following the protocol for the exact inventory that should be available.

Item	Amount on Hand	Minimum Needed	Place Order?	Date
Urine reagent strips		2 bottles		
Urine specimen cups		25		
Microhematocrit tubes		2 bottles		
Sealing clay		2		
ESR kits		1		
Rapid strep kits		2		
Glass slides		10 boxes		
Cover slips		3 boxes		
Pregnancy test kits		2		
Lens paper		5 tablets		

3. **Close the Office and Evaluate the Work Environment to Identify Unsafe Working Conditions**

   Using Procedure 24–3 and the information in your textbook as a guideline, create a typed checklist to use when closing the medical office. In the checklist, include items to be observed for safety as well as any environmental considerations and other precautions that should be taken. Using the checklist you created, role-play closing the office.

4. **Use Proper Ergonomics**

   Using Procedure 24–4 and the information in your textbook as a guideline, log on to the OSHA Website, locate eTools and select the Nursing Home eTool. Then click on the ergonomics-related topics. Review the ergonomic topics and suggestions (programs). Write a summary of or role-play at least two topics.

5. **Perform Routine Maintenance of Administrative or Clinical Equipment**

   Using Procedure 24–5 and the information in your textbook as a guideline, create a typed checklist to use when performing routine maintenance of administrative and clinical equipment. In the checklist, include items to be observed for cleanliness, safety, and operability. Provide a column where you can note and report any equipment requiring repair.

   Using the checklist you created, perform routine maintenance of any three of the following examples of administrative and clinical equipment.

   Examples:

   a. Fax machine

   b. Printer

   c. Scanner

   d. Computer (or tablet)

   e. Autoclave

   f. Refrigerator

   g. Freezer

   h. Microscope

Beginning the Patient's Record

Scheduling Appointments and Receiving Patients

Words to Know Challenge

Spelling: Each line contains three spellings of a word. Underline the correctly spelled word.

1.	matricks	mattrix	matrix
2.	unstructured	unstrictured	unstructered
3.	waive	wave	weave
4.	cloustering	clustering	clustaring
5.	modified wave	modified waive	modifide wave
6.	streeming	streming	streaming
7.	oblitarate	obliterrate	obliterate
8.	single-booking	singel-booking	signel-booking
9.	open ours	open hours	opin hours
10.	double-bookking	double-booking	dubble-bookking
11.	utilization	utilisation	Utilazition
12.	reel time adjustment	real time adjudication	real time adjustment

Matching: Using the correct spellings from the spelling activity, enter the correct terms next to the following appropriate description.

_____ 1. Patients scheduled during first half hour, last half hour left open for same-day appointments

_____ 2. Patient booked for a specific amount of time

_____ 3. Appointments time allocated based on need

_____ 4. Scheduling patients for a specific type of visit (physical, new patient, and so on)

_____ 5. Scheduled time as a wave, except in the last half hour, when appointments are spaced at 10- to 20-minute intervals

_____ 6. Same appointment is given to more than one patient

_____ 7. No appointment is needed; patients seen in order of arrival

_____ 8. Open block of time

Chapter Review

Short Answer

1. Name three criteria or pieces of information the medical assistant needs to obtain when making appointments. _____

_____

_____

2. When scheduling an inpatient admission, name at least five items that should be provided to the hospital representative.

_____

_____

_____

3. Describe how the medical assistant should handle a patient who arrives without an appointment.

_____

_____

_____

4. Why should entries in the records or appointment books never be obliterated?

_____

5. Describe how the administrative medical assistant should greet and receive patients.

_____

_____

_____

6. List the information that should be obtained for every new patient.

_____

_____

_____

7. Explain the importance of discussing general office policies to patients.

_____

_____

_____

8. What benefits can be obtained through assisting patients with payment planning?

_____

_____

_____

Fill in the blank

1. A _____ scheduling system has increased functionality and flexibility over the handwritten or paper schedule.

2. When scheduling a hospital admission, a _____ is required.

3. A _____ is the person who will be responsible for the medical services rendered.

4. A HIPAA release of information does not authorize the release of all information. _____

Chapter Application

Case Studies with Critical Thinking Questions

Scenario 1

A mother arrives in the office around 11:00 a.m., demanding an appointment immediately for her child, who is quiet but alert. The child has been seen before. The mother states that the child has a temperature but denies nausea, vomiting, diarrhea, or other signs or symptoms. The office has been busy all day, with several interruptions calling the physician away. The provider will be seeing patients in the afternoon, and there are a couple of same-day appointments available on your schedule. You offer her an appointment for later that day, but she insists that it must be NOW.

1. How do you handle this situation?

_____
_____
_____
_____
_____
_____
_____
_____

2. What ramifications are possible if you are unable to handle the situation successfully?

_____
_____
_____

For Scenarios 2 and 3, review the following appointment scheduling guidelines:
- New patients: 50 minutes
- Established patients: 20 minutes
- Physical examinations: 30 minutes
- Immunizations and prescription refills: 10 minutes

Scenario 2

Elizabeth Jones, age 76, is an established patient in your family practice office. She calls to report that she is out of two of her regular medications, has been running a fever for two days, and has a cough.

1. What type of appointment is needed? _____
_____
_____

2. How much time is required to see this patient? _____

Scenario 3

Johnny Rodriguez is a five-year-old who is about to start kindergarten. His mother called to ask for an appointment for a school physical. The family has been without insurance due to a loss of jobs, and it is unclear when Johnny was last seen by a medical provider.

1. What type of appointment is most appropriate for this patient?

   _____

   _____

   _____

2. What information should Ms. Rodriguez be asked to bring to the appointment?

   _____

   _____

   _____

Competency Practice

1. **Manage the Appointment Schedule Using Established Priorities**

   Using Procedure 25–1 as a guideline, manage the appointment schedule using the criteria outlined below (if using an EHR, perform basic keyboarding skills to manage the appointment schedule):

   - Office hours are from 8:00 a.m. to 5:30 p.m.
   - Lunch for staff and personal appointments at noon for 1½ hours
   - Mornings: Schedule Monday, Wednesday, and Friday mornings for 20-minute appointments to see follow-ups and well-person physicals.
   - Tuesday afternoons: Childhood immunizations in 20-minute visits
   - Thursday afternoons: 40-minute new-patient appointments
   - Tuesday and Thursday mornings: Surgeries or special procedures

   SCENARIO A: Manage the appointment schedule using the modified wave system.

   SCENARIO B: Manage the appointment schedule using the streaming method.

2. **Schedule a Patient Procedure**

   Inpatient Admission: Katherine Jameson is 45 years old and has a history of endometriosis. Her OB/GYN physician has determined that she needs to have a total abdominal hysterectomy. Ms. Jameson needs her laboratory work and a KUB done prior to admission. She will need to be in the hospital approximately five days following her procedure. A medical-surgical unit will be appropriate following surgery unless complications arise. Postoperative laboratory, abdominal X-ray, and pain medications should be anticipated. What kind of paperwork must be completed, and what information will the hospital require prior to admission?

   _____

   _____

   _____

3. **Apply HIPAA Rules in Regard to Patient Privacy and Release of Information When Scheduling a Patient Procedure**

   Using Procedure 25–3 as a guideline, schedule the following patient procedures and apply HIPAA rules in regard to patient privacy and release of information. Also apply the Patient's Bill of Rights as it relates to choice of treatment, consent for treatment, or refusal of treatment.

   Outpatient Procedure: Kenneth Jones, age 50, has had a positive treadmill test that suggests an underlying cardiac condition. The cardiologist has asked you to schedule him for a cardiac catheterization with planned stent placement, which will require an overnight stay. He also needs a CBC, electrolyte panel, and an echocardiogram done prior to the catheterization. What information will need to be provided when scheduling the procedure? How will you access and/or transmit this information complying with HIPAA rules? How will you apply the Patient's Bill of Rights when you schedule the procedure?

   _____

4. **Explain General Office Policies to the Patient**

Using Procedure 25–4 as a guideline, explain to the following patients both the practice's expectations for the patient as well as what legal and ethical rights the patient can expect, including HIPAA Privacy and Release guidelines and the Bill of Rights as it relates to choice or treatment, consent for treatment, and refusal of treatment. Remember that new patients must complete and sign all patient registration forms, consent, HIE, NPP, and financial responsibility documents.

a. New Patient: Jason Carlton, age 56, Type 2 diabetes

b. New Patient: Bwembya Roza el, age 22

c. Established Patient: Lillian Epstein, age 44, Type 2 diabetes, rheumatoid arthritis, hypertensive. Ms. Epstein has missed her last two appointments.

CHAPTER 26

The Medical Record, Documentation, and Filing

Words to Know Challenge

Spelling: Each line contains three spellings of a word. Underline the correctly spelled word.

1. awdit   audet   audit

2. ubjective   objective   objetive

3. progress notes   progras notes   progriss notes

4. subjective   sobjective   subjetave

5. docyumentation   documintation   documentation

6. ethnicity   ethincity   ethnicaty

7. privacy   prevasy   prevacy

8. chronalogic   chronologic   kronologic

Fill in the Blank: Complete the following sentences with Words to Know from this chapter.

1. EHR is an acronym for _____ .

2. Per HIPAA, each office is required to have a designated _____ . This person must keep track of who has access to protected health information within a facility.

3. Progress notes are entered in the chart in _____ order.

4. Three types of charting styles discussed in this chapter include _____ _____ and _____ .

5. In the early 1970s, Lawrence L. Weed, M.D., originated a system of recordkeeping for patients called the _____ . Progress notes are organized and entered based on where they come from, whether from a provider, laboratory, or other source.

6. The _____ is the presenting problem and should be recorded in the medical record in the patient's own words.

7. A _____ can be an expanding file, a card file, or even a portion of a file drawer. It consists of dividers with the names of all the months and dividers numbered from 1 to 31 for the days of the month.

8. _____ means to clean out.

Chapter Review

Short Answer

1. What is meant by "meaningful use of EHRs"?

_____
_____
_____
_____
_____

2. What types of *non*medical information is kept as part of the medical record?

_____
_____
_____

3. Why is it important to obtain records about new patients from other providers?

_____
_____
_____

4. What is an OUTguide used for in filing?

_____
_____
_____

5. Describe the necessary steps for pulling a file.

_____
_____
_____

6. Name the steps for filing a record.

_____

7. What is a tickler file?

_____
_____
_____

8. What is meant by indexing files?

_____
_____
_____

9. Fill in the blanks in the following chart, telling what each initial of SOAP represents and what the meaning is.

	Initial Represents	Meaning	Activity That Takes Place in This Phase
S	_____	_____	Patient account of symptoms, sensations, timing, or associated events
O	_____	_____	Physical exam, vital signs, laboratory testing, radiologic examinations, other diagnostics
A	_____	_____	Assimilates subjective and objective data into most likely diagnosis along with other considerations to rule out
P	_____	_____	Prescriptions, additional laboratory or radiologic assessment, admissions, therapy, referrals

Matching: Tell what each initial of CHEDDAR represents and then match each initial (letter) with its description.

Initial:	Initial Represents:	Description:
____	_____	A. Medications and amounts
____	_____	B. Follow-up
____	_____	C. Test results, additional findings
____	_____	D. Diagnosis and plan
____	_____	E. Presenting problem
____	_____	F. Past medical events and problems
____	_____	G. Objective findings

Matching: For each of the following statements, identify whether the statement is subjective or objective.

_____ 1. I have a burning pain in my chest.

_____ 2. My daughter has a fever.

_____ 3. The baby is lethargic and has no tears when she cries.

4. She looks queasy.

5. His skin is pale and diaphoretic.

6. The child's temperature is 38.1°C/100.5°F orally.

_ing Questions

nt information in the chart, it is noticed that an error was made.

ure for making the correction.

_____

_____

_____

note entry, use the preceding procedure you described and correct the entry: Ms.
_ts of right-upper quadrant abdominal pain.

_es called regarding complaints of left upper quadrant abdominal pain that gets worse with eat-
_re has been using TUMS for relief and feels better when sitting up. Will make appointment with
_nderson for tomorrow. Kelly Taylor, MA

4:1-_

Credit Card
XXXXXXXXX7464
XX/XX
464710

$ 5.00

Card Type:
Card No.:
Expires:
Appr Code:

Purchases:

Tip:

Total:

REGENSBURGER/RACHEL B

I agree to pay the above total amount
according to the card issuer agreement.

Competency Practice

1. **Create and Organize a Patient's Medical Record.**

   Using Procedure 26–1 as a guideline, create and organize a patient's medical record.

   Gather patient records, privacy forms, chart or folder, and tabs. The following documents are suggested to use to create a patient's chart (but you are not limited to those detailed below). If using an EHR, set up and create an electronic chart for a patient (use yourself or a dummy patient as directed by your instructor). Forms will be provided by your instructor or can be obtained from a variety of websites. *Hint:* Think about forms you have created and/or completed in earlier chapters and those you will complete in later chapters. Continue adding them to the newly created patient medical record if suggested by your instructor. Forms to include (but are not limited to):

   a. Patient registration form

   b. NPP

   c. Referral form

   d. Lab results

   e. Eligibility results

   f. Medical history forms

   g. Patient telephone message (ToDo)

   h. Receipt for co-pay

   i. Prescription

   j. Immunization record

   k. Progress note

   l. Assessment and Plan

   m. Consult letter

   n. Explanation of Benefits

   o. Claim Status Detail

   p. Patient Statement

   q. Collections letter

2. **Use an Alphabetic Filing System.**

   Using Procedure 26–2 as a guideline, alphabetically organize the 14 patient charts that were seen by the providers as noted in the following table.

Chart Number	Name
42405371	Lyndsey, Jordyn
42405377	Ramirez, Sonia S.
42557605	Smith, Cosima
42445211	Smith, Craig W.
54778201	Morgan, Jane W.
17887482	Mcginniss, Jim
88774680	Jeorge, Larry T.
44575850	Barret, Thomas
44511357	Watson, Barbara
42507342	Hernandez, Julia

55478885	Thompson, Adam
42383755	Douglas, Spencer M.
42405367	Smith, James M.
45518700	Smith, Craig X.

List out the correct alphabetic order of these patient charts using the blank table below.

Order	Name
1	
2	
3	
4	
5	
6	
7	
8	
9	
10	
11	
12	
13	
14	

3. **Use a Numeric Filing System.**

Using Procedure 26–3 as a guideline, numerically organize the charts for the 14 patients that were seen by the providers as noted in the previous table. List out the correct numerical order of the patient charts using the blank table below.

Order	Chart Number	Name
1		
2		
3		
4		
5		
6		
7		
8		

9	_____	_____
10	_____	_____
11	_____	_____
12	_____	_____
13	_____	_____
14	_____	_____

Medical Insurance and Coding

Health Insurance

Words to Know Challenge

Spelling: Each line contains three spellings of a word. Underline the correctly spelled word.

1. <u>capitation</u>   capitiation   capitition
2. preauthorisation   preauthoriziation   <u>preauthorization</u>
3. indemity plan   <u>indemnity plan</u>   indenmity plan
4. diductable   <u>deductible</u>   deducteble
5. <u>precertification</u>   precertafication   precertefication
6. quality insurance   quality asurance   <u>quality assurance</u>
7. coassurance   <u>coinsurance</u>   coinsurence
8. <u>dependent</u>   dependant   deependent
9. subscibor   subscribir   <u>subscriber</u>
10. <u>beneficiary</u>   benefichary   benefichairy
11. gate keeper   gatkeeper   <u>gatekeeper</u>
12. feeschedule   free schedule   <u>fee schedule</u>
13. <u>co-payment</u>   copyment   copaymnt

Fill in the Blank: Complete the following sentences with Words to Know from this chapter.

1. The _____ is the amount a patient must pay before his or her insurance begins to pay for services.

2. Payment made to providers by insurance carriers on a per-member, per-month basis is known as _____ .

3. _____ _____ is approval obtained from an insurer before services are rendered; additionally relates to whether the services are medically necessary.

4. This determines the primary insurance when the patient is a child who has health care coverage through both parents; it is called the _____ .

5. When a provider contracts with an insurer and agrees that payment made is payment in full for the services, the provider is said to _____ .

6. This form, the _____ , is provided to Medicare patients when services might not be covered.

7. Reviewing services prior to their provision to determine appropriateness and medical necessity is known as a _____ .

8. When a patient agrees to allow the provider to submit charges on his or her behalf and for the insurer to send payment directly to the provider, this is known as _____ .

9. _____ refers to procedures used when a patient has more than one insurance to make sure that the responsible insurer pays for the claim.

10. After services are provided and the insurer has been billed, a patient receives a(n) _____ , a written description of benefits provided to the member by the insurer.

11. A commercial plan in which the company (insurance) or group reimburses providers or beneficiaries for services and allows subscribers more flexibility in obtaining services is known as a(n) _____ plan.

12. _____ is defined as inclusive of policies, procedures, and practices as standards for reliable results that include documentation.

Chapter Review

Short Answer

1. What is the purpose of health insurance? _____

_____

_____

2. What was the initial purpose of an HMO? _____

_____

_____

3. Identify and define the different types of managed care. _____

_____

_____

_____

_____

_____

_____

_____

_____

_____

_____

4. Define consumer-driven health care and list three types of plans. _____
   _____
   _____
   _____

5. Describe the concept of primary and secondary coverage and what impact it has on health care coverage.
   _____
   _____
   _____
   _____
   _____
   _____
   _____
   _____

6. Why is it necessary for a provider to obtain preauthorization and precertification for some services?
   _____
   _____
   _____

7. What is a diagnostic-related group (DRG) and in what type of health facility is it used? _____
   _____
   _____
   _____

Matching: Identify the types of insurance plans and models from the following list. (*Hint*: Not all words in the list will be used.)

HMO	flexible spending arrangement	Medicare Advantage
health savings account	indemnity	Medigap
TRICARE	CHAMPVA	Medicaid
point-of-service plan	workers' compensation	Fee for service
preferred provider organization	Medicare	

_____	1.	Government program established by the federal government and administered by each individual state.
_____	2.	Government insurance program for individuals 65 years of age and older or disabled.
_____	3.	Coverage for military personnel and their dependents.
_____	4.	Plan that employee contributes to with pretax dollars; employee must use the funds in the benefit year or lose them.
_____	5.	Type of account in which employees deposit pretax money, and any balance can be used the next year.
_____	6.	A managed care plan that requires all members to have a primary care physician who is responsible for all that patient's care.
_____	7.	Insurance coverage that allows subscribers more flexibility in seeking care. This type of plan has the least amount of structural guidelines for patients to follow.
_____	8.	Coverage individuals purchase to cover the out-of-pocket expenses of Medicare.

Chapter Application

Case Studies with Critical Thinking Questions

Scenario 1

Josephine Robinson is a 65-year-old patient new to Medicare, and she also has a Medigap plan. She was seen in the office recently for her annual physical. She asks for an explanation of what she will be charged for the visit.

1. What preventive care services will Medicare beneficiaries receive as a result of the ACA? _____

   _____

   _____

2. She asks if her Medigap plan will cover any of the visit and if she has a deductible that needs to be paid. How would you explain this to her? _____

   _____

   _____

   _____

Scenario 2

Robert Olson was seen two months ago for an ear infection. Robert's mother is on the phone asking why she is receiving a bill for this visit. She indicates during the conversation that Robert is covered by both her insurance and her ex-husband's, so there shouldn't be any balances due.

1. What could have caused her to receive a bill for this service? _____

   _____

   _____

2. What kind of proactive action can you take to avoid such issues in the future with the Olsons and with other patients? _____

   _____

   _____

   _____

Competency Practice

1. **Verify Insurance Coverage and Eligibility for Services**

   Using the detailed instructions and rationales outlined in Procedure 27–1 as a guideline, interpret information on an insurance card and verify a patient's insurance coverage prior to rendering services, by accessing the website for the patient's insurance carrier (or the EHR application with electronic eligibility features). Select a different patient, different insurance card, and different insurance company than indicated in the textbook. Include documentation.

2. **Obtain Precertification or Preauthorization (Predetermination) and Inform a Patient of Financial Obligations for Services Rendered**

   Using Procedure 27–2 as a guideline, complete the "Managed Care Out-of-Network Request Form." Using the detailed instructions noted in Procedure 27–2 of the textbook, access the BCBSMA website. Scroll down to the "Administrative" section and select the "Managed Care Out-of-Network Request Form." Complete the referral form and obtain precertification.

CHAPTER 28

Procedural and Diagnostic Coding

Words to Know Challenge

Spelling: Each line contains three spellings of a word. Underline the correctly spelled word.

1. specifisity   specificity   spesificity

2. primary diangosis   primary dignosis   primary diagnosis

3. comordibities   comobititys   comorbidities

4. contributory factors   contributary factors   contributery factors

5. key components   key componnents   key componends

6. bundelled   bundled   bundeled

7. medical nessecity   medial necessity   medical necessity

8. modifyer   modifier   modifire

9. sequenced   sequinced   sequeenced

10. reimbersement   reimbursment   reimbursement

Fill in the Blank: Complete the following sentences with correctly spelled words from the Spelling section.

1. Each E/M code description identifies the _____ as well as _____ that must be met to report that code.

2. Codes are _____ in relation to the intensity and level of service provided; this involves listing the primary reason for the office visit first and other reasons next in order of their importance.

3. It is important to remember the reason rule, which says that the reason for the patient visit (the _____) is coded *first*; any other issues the patient presents with (_____) are coded next in order of importance.

4. _____ are used with HCPCS codes to indicate that something is different about the way the service or procedure was performed.

5. Use of ICD-9-CM codes establishes the _____ for the services or procedures provided to the patient.

6. One of the reasons for the move to ICD-10-CM is that ICD-9-CM lacks sufficient _____ and detail to report morbidity adequately in the twenty-first century.

7. _____ means it is included in another procedure or service code.

8. It is critical for any codes submitted to an insurance carrier to be accurate; the provider's _____ is based upon the codes that are submitted.

Chapter Review

Short Answer

1. What are the two main coding systems? Describe what each reports and how the two differ.

_____

_____

_____

2. List the sections of the CPT manual.

_____

_____

_____

3. List six of the general CPT coding rules. **Students should list any six of these:**

_____

_____

_____

_____

_____

_____

4. Why are modifiers used? What codes are they appended to?

_____

_____

_____

5. What is the significance of the reason rule and sequencing?

_____

_____

_____

6. List the four general rules for diagnostic coding.

   (1) _____

   _____

   (2) _____

   (3) _____

   (4) _____

   _____

7. Describe the impact of ICD-10-CM on the health care delivery system.

_____
_____
_____
_____
_____
_____

8. Identify four types of insurance fraud and why they should be avoided.

_____
_____
_____
_____
_____
_____
_____
_____

Matching: Identify the key components and contributory factors in E/M code descriptions.

_____ 1. Amount of time physician spent   A. Key component

_____ 2. Nature of the presenting problem   B. Contributory factor

_____ 3. Level of history obtained

_____ 4. Coordination of care

_____ 5. Degree of medical decision making involved

_____ 6. Counseling

_____ 7. Level examination performed

Labeling: Use the following list to identify each symbol found in the CPT book.

Modifier 51 exempt   FDA approval pending   Add-on code

Revised guidelines   Reinstated code   New code

Revised code description   Code includes moderate sedation

Symbol	Meaning
+	_____
▲	_____
•	_____
►◄	_____
⃠	_____
⊙	_____
⚡	_____
○	_____

Chapter Application

Case Study with Critical Thinking Questions

Scenario

Ins Plan	Allowed	Payment	Transfers	Variance
Blue Cross	$50.00	($0.00)	($50.00)	$50.00

Payment variance scenario:

The lack of payment by the insurance company indicates that the insurance company may have denied payment, and the Transfers amount of $50.00 indicates that the amount may have been transferred to a coinsurance.

Step 1: Determine the cause of the payment variance and the steps you should take.

Step 2: Work the payment

If the insurance company denied the claim, then you need to further process the payment. For example, you may need to bill the patient, override the variance, or resubmit the claim to the insurance company.

Referring to the scenario above:

1. Brainstorm about reasons the insurance company denied the claim.

   _____

   _____

   _____

2. Come up with ideas to solve the problem for this claim and prevent denials of future claims.

   _____

   _____

   _____

3. Further analyze and debate findings and discuss how you reached your conclusions.

   _____

   _____

   _____

Coding Practice

1. **ICD-9-CM Coding: Underline the main term in the following diagnostic statements and then find the appropriate ICD-9-CM code.**

   1. Macular _____ (senile), unspecified   _____
   2. Congenital heart _____   _____
   3. Corpus luteum cyst or _____   _____
   4. Genital tract-skin _____ female   _____
   5. Onchocerca volvulus _____   _____
   6. Shoulder joint _____   _____
   7. Cauda equina _____ with neurogenic bladder   _____
   8. Idiopathic fibrosing _____   _____
   9. _____ of skull fracture   _____
   10. Congenital choledochal ___   _____

2. **CPT Coding: Identify the main term you would use to find the following procedures.**

1. Darrach procedure _____

2. Placement of shunt _____

3. New-patient office visit _____

4. ECG, 12-lead w/interpretation and report _____

5. Removal of mass, right breast _____

6. Laparoscopic removal of gallbladder _____

7. Suture open wound to left cheek _____

8. Annual physical _____

9. Hernia repair _____

10. Dead tissue removal _____

Competency Practice

1. **Perform Procedural Coding**

Using the detailed instructions and rationales outlined in Procedure 28–1 as a guideline, complete the encounter form with proper procedure codes for a new-patient office visit. Patient received an ECG, urinalysis, and HEP B vaccine.

_____

_____

_____

2. **Utilize Medical Necessity Guidelines**

Using the detailed instructions and rationales outlined in Procedure 28–2 as a guideline, complete the Medical Necessity form.

_____

_____

_____

_____

3. **Perform Diagnostic Coding**

a. Using the detailed instructions and rationales outlined in Procedure 28–3 as a guideline, complete the encounter form with proper diagnostic codes for a new-patient exam; assessment of COPD, HTN, overweight, and dysuria.

_____

_____

b. Now using the detailed instructions and rationales outline in Procedure 28–3 as a guideline, complete the encounter form with proper ICD-10-CM diagnostic codes for a new-patient exam; assessment of COPD, HTN, overweight, and dysuria.

_____

_____

_____

Billing and Payment for Medical Services

CHAPTER 29

Patient Accounts

Words to Know Challenge

Spelling: Each line contains three spellings of a word. Underline the correctly spelled word.

1. debbit	debt	debit
2. bookkeeper	bookeeper	bookkeepper
3. jurnalizing	journalizing	journelizing
4. ledger	leger	legger
5. ascets	assets	asets
6. ajustment	adjusment	adjustment
7. posting	posteing	poasting
8. creddit	credit	credibt

Matching: Match each term in column I to its meaning in column II.

	COLUMN I	COLUMN II
____	1. Accountant	A. Reflects that amount paid is less than total due
____	2. Accounts receivable	B. Each transaction is recorded in two accounts
____	3. Business associate agreement	C. All the outstanding accounts, amounts due to the office
____	4. Trial balance	D. Reflects that the amount paid is greater than was due, or the account is being paid in advance of service provided
____	5. Credit balance	E. Analyzes financial transactions and prepares reports
____	6. Debit balance	F. Signed by an outside company that provides bookkeeping services to a medical office
____	7. Single-entry bookkeeping system	G. Bookkeeping strategy to confirm accuracy in debits and credits in ledger
____	8. Double-entry bookkeeping system	H. Similar to a checkbook register

Chapter Review

Short Answer

1. Explain the cost estimate sheet.

   _____

   _____

2. What should be recorded on a cash control sheet?

   _____

   _____

3. List at least four advantages of computerized accounting.

   _____

   _____

4. List three disadvantages of computerized accounting.

   _____

   _____

5. Describe how the patient encounter form is used in the office.

   _____

   _____

6. What is the role of a bookkeeper?

   _____

7. Why would you use a Business Associate Agreement (BAA)?

   _____

   _____

   _____

8. What are day sheets and patient ledgers?

   _____

   _____

   _____

Matching: Identify whether the statements describe a single-entry bookkeeping system or a double-entry bookkeeping system.

_____ 1. Only the revenues and expenses are totaled, not individual values of each one.

_____ 2. For each debit there is an equal and opposite credit, and the total of all debits must equal the total of all credits.

_____ 3. Undetected errors can occur and might only be discovered through bank statement reconciliation.

_____ 4. Two entries are made for each transaction.

_____ 5. There is no direct link between income and the balance sheet.

_____ 6. Ability to prepare financial statements directly from the accounts

_____ 7. The bookkeeping system most often used in the large and busy medical setting

A. Single-entry bookkeeping system

B. Double-entry bookkeeping system

Chapter Application

Case Study with Critical Thinking Questions

A young mother checks in at the front desk and is asked to fill out a new-patient form. Her husband recently left her with two children to raise and no income. She is enrolled in a job-training program, but she will be on a state aid program until she can finish her training. The young mother is embarrassed about the fact that she must be on a welfare program, even for a short time. After reviewing the form, the administrative medical assistant calls to the patient across the waiting area and announces to everyone that she will need a copy of her Medicaid card.

1. How could the administrative medical assistant have handled this situation in a more professional manner?

   _____

   _____

2. How do you think the patient felt?

   _____

   _____

Competency Practice

1. **Perform Accounts Receivable Procedures to Patient Accounts, Including Posting Charges, Payments, and Adjustments.**

   Using the detailed instructions and rationales outlined in Procedure 29–1 as a guideline, complete the following scenario and perform accounts receivable procedures to patient accounts, including posting charges, payments, and adjustments.

   Scenario: Record the following charges and credits on the Patient Ledger form (Workbook Form 29–1); note that some entries already exist on the form. Use yourself as the patient and your provider's name as the physician. Use today's date.

   - Insurance information: Insurance Company – Health Care One; Insurance ID – 123-45-6789-A; Coverage Code A – Group II; office visit co-payment ($20); this is your own health insurance through your job. You pay with a credit card.

   - Description: You are an established patient requiring a problem-focused exam (99212, $75), throat culture (87060, $60), antibiotic injection (90788, $40), ECG (93000TB, $40), spirometry (94010TB, $40), and chest X-ray review (76140-26, $25).

   - Diagnoses: Acute bronchitis (493.9), pneumonia (486). The physician wants to see you in two weeks.

   - Insurance payments: On 06/01/20XX, your insurance company made a $50 payment for the problem-focused exam and, on 07/01/20XX, your insurance company made a $200 payment for the office procedures performed on the limited exam date.

WORKBOOK FORM 29–1

PATIENT LEDGER

Date:

MR#:   **Address:**   **Provider:**

Name: **City/State/Zip:**   **Date of Birth:**   **Sex:**

Charges

Date of Service:	Procedure:	Description:	Diagnosis Codes:	Amount
2/1/20XX	70373	X-Ray	052.9 354.0 503 847.2	$75.00
2/1/20XX	29130	App. of Finger Splint	052.9 354.0 503 847.2	$30.00
2/1/20XX	99204	Office Visit New	052.9 354.0 503 847.2	$75.00
3/1/20XX	J1820	Inj, Insulin, Up to 100 Units	052.9 354.0 503 847.2	$20.00

Total: **$_____**

Insurance Payments

Date of Payment:	Payment Code:	Line Description:	Transaction Description:	Amount
2/1/20XX	XP	XYZ Insurance Payment	XYZ	($40.00)
2/1/20XX	XP	XYZ Insurance Payment	XYZ	($20.00)

Total: **($_____)**

Insurance Adjustments

Date of Payment:	Payment Code:	Line Description:	Transaction Description:	Amount
5/1/20XX	MED ADJ	Medicare Writeoff	Adjustment	($10.00)
5/1/20XX	MED ADJ	Medicare Writeoff	Adjustment	($10.00)

Total: ($20.00)

Patient Payments

Date of Payment:	Payment Code:	Payment Description:	Transaction Description:	Amount
2/1/20XX	COCHECK	Co-pay Check Payment		($20.00)
3/1/20XX	CCARDCOP	Credit Card Co-pay		($20.00)

Total: **($_____)**

Total Payments **($_____)**

Amount Due: **$_____**

PATIENT LEDGER

Date:

MR#:   **Address:**   **Provider:**

Name: **City/State/Zip:**   **Date of Birth:**   **Sex:**

Charges

Date of Service:	*Procedure:*	*Description:*	*Diagnosis Codes:*	*Amount*
2/1/20XX	70373	X-Ray	052.9 354.0 503 847.2	$75.00
2/1/20XX	29130	App. of Finger Splint	052.9 354.0 503 847.2	$30.00
2/1/20XX	99204	Office Visit New	052.9 354.0 503 847.2	$75.00
3/1/20XX	J1820	Inj, Insulin, Up to 100 Units	052.9 354.0 503 847.2	$20.00

Total:

Insurance Payments

Date of Payment:	*Payment Code:*	*Line Description:*	*Transaction Description:*	*Amount*
2/1/20XX	XP	XYZ Insurance Payment	XYZ	($40.00)
2/1/20XX	XP	XYZ Insurance Payment	XYZ	($20.00)

Total: _____

Insurance Adjustments

Date of Payment:	*Payment Code:*	*Line Description:*	*Transaction Description:*	*Amount*
5/1/20XX	MED ADJ	Medicare Writeoff	Adjustment	($10.00)
5/1/20XX	MED ADJ	Medicare Writeoff	Adjustment	($10.00)

Total: ($20.00)

Patient Payments

Date of Payment:	*Payment Code:*	*Payment Description:*	*Transaction Description:*	*Amount*
2/1/20XX	COCHECK	Co-pay Check Payment		($20.00)
3/1/20XX	CCARDCOP	Credit Card Co-pay		($20.00)

Total: _____

Total Payments _____

Amount Due: _____

Research Activity

Search the Internet to find *two* company websites that provide information on their computerized medical office accounting software systems. Print out the basic information the companies offer regarding computerized accounting systems. Contrast and compare the systems, and prepare an analysis of the system most applicable to the medical practice. List pros and cons of each system.

Preparing Insurance Claims and Posting Insurance Payments

Words to Know Challenge

Spelling: Each line contains three spellings of a word. Underline the correctly spelled word.

1. reimbursement	rembursement	rembursment
2. cleeringhouse	clearinghose	clearinghouse
3. career	carrier	carrere
4. secondery	secondary	secondarry
5. scrub	skrub	scruub

Matching: Match the abbreviations in column I to their meanings in column II.

	COLUMN I	COLUMN II
____	1. NPI	A. Centers for Medicare and Medicaid Services
____	2. CMS	B. Electronic claims sent to CMS
____	3. EOB	C. Specifies reasons a provider may submit paper claims
____	4. EDI	D. Standard claim form filed by provider's office for reimbursement
____	5. ECT	E. Unique 10-digit identifier for covered health care providers
____	6. ASCA	F. Electronic system required for filing electronic claims to CMS
____	7. EMC	G. Document explaining payments made by the insurance company
____	8. CMS-1500	H. Method for monitoring the status and payment of insurance claims

Fill in the Blank: Complete the following sentences with Words to Know from this chapter.

1. _____ is the most common way to monitor insurance claims today.

2. The _____ may be filed electronically for provider Medicare and Medicaid reimbursement and is the standard claim form used in provider offices.

3. An _____ is received by the patient and shows what the insurance company has paid.

4. A _____ is a company that provides a service between providers and payers, running a claims scrub on all claims to check for missing or invalid data.

5. In many instances, a(n) _____ will pay most, if not all, of the balance left over from the primary insurance to the provider.

6. Use of _____ transactions allow a medical facility or a provider's office to submit transactions faster and therefore be paid for claims faster.

7. When you _____ a claim, it ensures that claims are correctly coded before being sent to the insurance company, which reduces denials and increase payments to the practice.

8. A unique 10-digit number identification for covered health care providers is known as the _____

_____.

9. The _____ standard electronic data interchange (EDI) enrollment form must be completed prior to submitting _____ or other EDI transactions to Medicare.

10. There are limited situations when paper claim forms may be submitted for payment in lieu of electronic claims, and there are specific conditions the provider must meet to do this and receive payment from Medicare. These conditions are set forth by the _____

Chapter Review

Short Answer

1. What two things should the office claims processor have before processing a patient's claim?

_____

_____

_____

2. Explain the differences between manual and electronic tracking systems.

_____

_____

_____

_____

3. List five pieces of information found on an EOB.

_____

_____

_____

4. Explain the history of claim forms.

_____

_____

_____

5. List four pieces of information to have before calling to follow up on a delinquent insurance claim.

_____

_____

_____

Matching: Look at a copy of a CMS-1500 form and match the following information in column I with the claim form's numbered sections listed in column II.

COLUMN I	COLUMN II
____ 1. Health care coverage being billed	A. Section 4
____ 2. Patient's name	B. Section 10a
____ 3. Insured's name	C. Section 11d
____ 4. Patient's condition is result of employment	D. Section 21
____ 5. Indicate there is another health plan	E. Section 1
____ 6. Diagnosis code	F. Section 24d
____ 7. Insured's policy group or FECA number	G. Section 2
____ 8. Procedure code	H. section 11
____ 9. Name of referring provider	I. section 25
____ 10. Federal tax ID number	J. section 17

Chapter Application

Case Study with Critical Thinking Questions

You are working in a medical practice that sends out billing electronically, but the software does not include a claim scrubber program.

1. What are some of the effects of not having a claim scrubbed prior to submission?

_____

_____

_____

_____

2. What can you, as an administrative medical assistant, do?

_____

_____

_____

_____

Competency Practice

1. **Complete an Insurance Claim Form.** Use the detailed instructions and rationales outlined in Procedure 30–1 as a guideline and complete the insurance claim form CMS-1500. Complete two CMS-1500 claim forms, including correct code selection, using the following practice information. (Additional blank CMS-1500 clam forms can be downloaded from the Student Companion website.)

Practice Information: Angela Dickinson, MD; 890 Medical Center Road, Suite A7, Moontown, US 09876-5432. EIN #11-3456780, Phone (222) 555-0000, NPI #0011223344.

Case 1:

- Austin C. Henderson, 7 Penney Lane, Moontown, US 09876, Telephone (222) 555-1111, DOB 9/4/1978. Single.
- Insurance: One Health Plan, ID #239457669. Group Number 887. Employer: Jacobson Paint Supply. Patient is subscriber. Signature on file.
- Office visit for acute bronchitis: ICD-9-CM Code: 466.0 (IDC-10-CM Code: J20.9) Date of service: 3/19/XX
  - Level 4 established patient visit (CPT Code: 99214)   Amount: 105.00
  - Chest x-ray, complete (CPT Code: 71020)   Amount: 135.00

Case 2:

- Octavia DeFillipo, 90 Elm Street, Moontown, US 09876, Telephone (222) 555-9988, DOB 3/25/1954. Married and employed full time.
- Insurance: Blue Cross Blue Shield US, ID #445590871. Group Number 112. Employer: Applied Jet Technology. Patient is spouse of subscriber: Ernesto P. DeFillipo, DOB 01/18/1952. Signature on file.
- Office visit for annual physical: ICD-9-CM Code: V70.0
- Date of service: 04/05/XX
  - Level 5 Established Patient (CPT Code: 99215)   Amount: 236.00
  - Pap smear (CPT Code: Q0091)   Amount: 49.00

Complete the following five insurance forms, using the following information:

Code 11, office, for places of service (24B). The provider is Samuel E. Matthews, MD, Suite 120, 100 E. Main Street, Yourtown, US 98765-4321. His SS# is 987-65-4321. Phone number (222) 789-0123. NPI 7654321. The patients all live in Yourtown, US 98765.

Case 3:

Juan Gomez, 293 West High Street 98765

Medicare, ID# 29116696A. Phone (222) 263-5538. DOB 2/17/31. Male, single. Patient is insured person. Signature on file. Abdominal pain and diabetes mellitus. (Consult code book for code numbers needed for procedures.) Seen in office.

5/18/XX	Office visit, Est. Pt., Level 2	65.00
	Test stool for blood	30.00
	Automated hemogram	30.00
	Venipuncture	30.00

Case 4:

LaChar Holley, 4567 Charcoal Lane 98765

Travelers Insurance, ID# 505209821. Phone (222) 122-7768. DOB 10/7/60. Female. Patient is insured person. No other insurance. Not related to employment or accident. Signature on file. Arthritis, acute back pain. Seen in office.

6/15/XX	Office visit, Est. Pt., Level 2	65.00
	X-ray lumbar spine, AP & lat.	200.00
	Venipuncture	30.00
	Automated hemogram	30.00

Case 5:

Tina Schmidt, daughter. DOB 12/27/11. Phone (222) 891-7145. Insured George Schmidt, 1249 E. Remington Road 98769. Self-employed. BC and BS Insurance, ID# 888207777. DOB 10/6/87. No other insurance. Phone (222) 441-0050. Signature on file. Impetigo. Seen in office.

6/20/XX	Office visit, Est. Pt., Level 1	40.00

Case 6:

Joan Moriarty, wife. DOB 12/19/62. Insured Patrick Moriarty, 397 North Tony Road 98768. Self-employed. Metropolitan-Insurance, ID# 887105566. DOB 11/14/60. Phone (222) 431-6943. No other insurance. Signature on file. Cervicitis, cystitis, acute edema. Patient seen in office.

9/20/XX	Office visit, Est. Pt., Level 3	80.00
	Catheterization, urethra	120.00
	Endometrial biopsy	300.00
	Urinalysis	25.00

Case 7:

Boris Kostrevski 1493 S. James Road 98765. Aetna Insurance, ID# 505208800-A.

DOB 7/14/52. Phone (222) 298-6483. Signature on file. Diabetes mellitus, coronary atherosclerosis. Seen in office.

9/24/XX	Office visit, Est. Pt., Level 2	65.00
	Glucose screen	25.00
	Venipuncture	30.00

2. **Process Insurance Claims.** Use the detailed instructions and rationales outlined in Procedure 30–2 as a guideline and process insurance claims. Students can download the Patient Ledger Card from the Student Companion website to complete this activity and use as work product for this procedure. (*Note:* Some entries may already be completed. Students must add entries and perform calculations.) Use the following information to complete the insurance payment processing and insurance adjustment for scoring of the competency checklist:

   • Use yourself as the patient and your provider as the physician. Use today's date as date of payment.

   • Insurance company is XYZ Insurance Company.

   • The insurance payment check is for $75.00 (check number 1234).

   • The insurance adjustment check is for $5 (check number 1235) for a procedure.

HEALTH INSURANCE CLAIM FORM

APPROVED BY NATIONAL UNIFORM CLAIM COMMITTEE (NUCC) 02/12

CARRIER

| | PICA | | | | | PICA | |

1. MEDICARE (Medicare#)   MEDICAID (Medicaid#)   TRICARE (ID#/DoD#)   CHAMPVA (Member ID#)   GROUP HEALTH PLAN (ID#)   FECA BLK LUNG (ID#)   OTHER (ID#)

1a. INSURED'S I.D. NUMBER   (For Program in Item 1)

2. PATIENT'S NAME (Last Name, First Name, Middle Initial)

3. PATIENT'S BIRTH DATE MM DD YY   SEX   M ☐ F ☐

4. INSURED'S NAME (Last Name, First Name, Middle Initial)

5. PATIENT'S ADDRESS (No., Street)

6. PATIENT RELATIONSHIP TO INSURED   Self ☐ Spouse ☐ Child ☐ Other ☐

7. INSURED'S ADDRESS (No., Street)

CITY   STATE

8. RESERVED FOR NUCC USE

CITY   STATE

ZIP CODE   TELEPHONE (Include Area Code) ( )

ZIP CODE   TELEPHONE (Include Area Code) ( )

9. OTHER INSURED'S NAME (Last Name, First Name, Middle Initial)

10. IS PATIENT'S CONDITION RELATED TO:

11. INSURED'S POLICY GROUP OR FECA NUMBER

a. OTHER INSURED'S POLICY OR GROUP NUMBER

a. EMPLOYMENT? (Current or Previous)   ☐ YES ☐ NO

a. INSURED'S DATE OF BIRTH MM DD YY   SEX M ☐ F ☐

b. RESERVED FOR NUCC USE

b. AUTO ACCIDENT?   ☐ YES ☐ NO   PLACE (State)

b. OTHER CLAIM ID (Designated by NUCC)

c. RESERVED FOR NUCC USE

c. OTHER ACCIDENT?   ☐ YES ☐ NO

c. INSURANCE PLAN NAME OR PROGRAM NAME

d. INSURANCE PLAN NAME OR PROGRAM NAME

10d. CLAIM CODES (Designated by NUCC)

d. IS THERE ANOTHER HEALTH BENEFIT PLAN?   ☐ YES ☐ NO   *If yes*, complete items 9, 9a, and 9d.

READ BACK OF FORM BEFORE COMPLETING & SIGNING THIS FORM.

12. PATIENT'S OR AUTHORIZED PERSON'S SIGNATURE I authorize the release of any medical or other information necessary to process this claim. I also request payment of government benefits either to myself or to the party who accepts assignment below.

SIGNED _____   DATE _____

13. INSURED'S OR AUTHORIZED PERSON'S SIGNATURE I authorize payment of medical benefits to the undersigned physician or supplier for services described below.

SIGNED _____

PATIENT AND INSURED INFORMATION

14. DATE OF CURRENT ILLNESS, INJURY, or PREGNANCY (LMP) MM DD YY   QUAL.

15. OTHER DATE QUAL.   MM DD YY

16. DATES PATIENT UNABLE TO WORK IN CURRENT OCCUPATION   FROM MM DD YY   TO MM DD YY

17. NAME OF REFERRING PROVIDER OR OTHER SOURCE   **17a.**   **17b.** NPI

18. HOSPITALIZATION DATES RELATED TO CURRENT SERVICES   FROM MM DD YY   TO MM DD YY

19. ADDITIONAL CLAIM INFORMATION (Designated by NUCC)

20. OUTSIDE LAB?   ☐ YES ☐ NO $ CHARGES

21. DIAGNOSIS OR NATURE OF ILLNESS OR INJURY Relate A-L to service line below (24E)   ICD Ind.

A. _____ B. _____ C. _____ D. _____
E. _____ F. _____ G. _____ H. _____
I. _____ J. _____ K. _____ L. _____

22. RESUBMISSION CODE   ORIGINAL REF. NO.

23. PRIOR AUTHORIZATION NUMBER

24. A. DATE(S) OF SERVICE From MM DD YY To MM DD YY	B. PLACE OF SERVICE	C. EMG	D. PROCEDURES, SERVICES, OR SUPPLIES (Explain Unusual Circumstances) CPT/HCPCS MODIFIER	E. DIAGNOSIS POINTER	F. $ CHARGES	G. DAYS OR UNITS	H. EPSDT Family Plan	I. ID. QUAL.	J. RENDERING PROVIDER ID. #
1									NPI
2									NPI
3									NPI
4									NPI
5									NPI
6									NPI

25. FEDERAL TAX I.D. NUMBER   SSN ☐ EIN ☐

26. PATIENT'S ACCOUNT NO.

27. ACCEPT ASSIGNMENT? (For govt. claims, see back)   ☐ YES ☐ NO

28. TOTAL CHARGE $

29. AMOUNT PAID $

30. Rsvd for NUCC Use

31. SIGNATURE OF PHYSICIAN OR SUPPLIER INCLUDING DEGREES OR CREDENTIALS (I certify that the statements on the reverse apply to this bill and are made a part thereof.)

SIGNED _____   DATE _____

32. SERVICE FACILITY LOCATION INFORMATION

a. **NPI**   b.

33. BILLING PROVIDER INFO & PH # ( )

a. **NPI**   b.

PHYSICIAN OR SUPPLIER INFORMATION

NUCC Instruction Manual available at: www.nucc.org   *PLEASE PRINT OR TYPE*

© *Courtesy of the Centers for Medicare and Medicaid Services, www.cms.gov.*

HEALTH INSURANCE CLAIM FORM

APPROVED BY NATIONAL UNIFORM CLAIM COMMITTEE (NUCC) 02/12

◄── CARRIER

| | PICA | | | | | | | PICA | |

1. MEDICARE *(Medicare#)* MEDICAID *(Medicaid#)* TRICARE *(ID#/DoD#)* CHAMPVA *(Member ID#)* GROUP HEALTH PLAN *(ID#)* FECA BLK LUNG *(ID#)* OTHER *(ID#)*

1a. INSURED'S I.D. NUMBER (For Program in Item 1)

2. PATIENT'S NAME (Last Name, First Name, Middle Initial)

3. PATIENT'S BIRTH DATE MM DD YY **SEX** M☐ F☐

4. INSURED'S NAME (Last Name, First Name, Middle Initial)

5. PATIENT'S ADDRESS (No., Street)

6. PATIENT RELATIONSHIP TO INSURED Self☐ Spouse☐ Child☐ Other☐

7. INSURED'S ADDRESS (No., Street)

CITY / STATE

8. RESERVED FOR NUCC USE

CITY / STATE

ZIP CODE / TELEPHONE (Include Area Code) ( )

ZIP CODE / TELEPHONE (Include Area Code) ( )

9. OTHER INSURED'S NAME (Last Name, First Name, Middle Initial)

10. IS PATIENT'S CONDITION RELATED TO:

11. INSURED'S POLICY GROUP OR FECA NUMBER

a. OTHER INSURED'S POLICY OR GROUP NUMBER

a. EMPLOYMENT? (Current or Previous) ☐YES ☐NO

a. INSURED'S DATE OF BIRTH MM DD YY **SEX** M☐ F☐

b. RESERVED FOR NUCC USE

b. AUTO ACCIDENT? PLACE (State) ☐YES ☐NO

b. OTHER CLAIM ID (Designated by NUCC)

c. RESERVED FOR NUCC USE

c. OTHER ACCIDENT? ☐YES ☐NO

c. INSURANCE PLAN NAME OR PROGRAM NAME

d. INSURANCE PLAN NAME OR PROGRAM NAME

10d. CLAIM CODES (Designated by NUCC)

d. IS THERE ANOTHER HEALTH BENEFIT PLAN? ☐YES ☐NO **If yes,** complete items 9, 9a, and 9d.

READ BACK OF FORM BEFORE COMPLETING & SIGNING THIS FORM.
12. PATIENT'S OR AUTHORIZED PERSON'S SIGNATURE I authorize the release of any medical or other information necessary to process this claim. I also request payment of government benefits either to myself or to the party who accepts assignment below.

SIGNED _____ DATE _____

13. INSURED'S OR AUTHORIZED PERSON'S SIGNATURE I authorize payment of medical benefits to the undersigned physician or supplier for services described below.

SIGNED _____

◄── PATIENT AND INSURED INFORMATION

14. DATE OF CURRENT ILLNESS, INJURY, or PREGNANCY (LMP) MM DD YY QUAL.

15. OTHER DATE QUAL. MM DD YY

16. DATES PATIENT UNABLE TO WORK IN CURRENT OCCUPATION FROM MM DD YY TO MM DD YY

17. NAME OF REFERRING PROVIDER OR OTHER SOURCE

17a. 17b. NPI

18. HOSPITALIZATION DATES RELATED TO CURRENT SERVICES FROM MM DD YY TO MM DD YY

19. ADDITIONAL CLAIM INFORMATION (Designated by NUCC)

20. OUTSIDE LAB? ☐YES ☐NO **$ CHARGES**

21. DIAGNOSIS OR NATURE OF ILLNESS OR INJURY Relate A-L to service line below (24E) ICD Ind.

A. ___ B. ___ C. ___ D. ___
E. ___ F. ___ G. ___ H. ___
I. ___ J. ___ K. ___ L. ___

22. RESUBMISSION CODE ORIGINAL REF. NO.

23. PRIOR AUTHORIZATION NUMBER

24. A. DATE(S) OF SERVICE From MM DD YY To MM DD YY	B. PLACE OF SERVICE	C. EMG	D. PROCEDURES, SERVICES, OR SUPPLIES (Explain Unusual Circumstances) CPT/HCPCS | MODIFIER	E. DIAGNOSIS POINTER	F. $ CHARGES	G. DAYS OR UNITS	H. EPSDT Family Plan	I. ID. QUAL.	J. RENDERING PROVIDER ID. #
1									NPI
2									NPI
3									NPI
4									NPI
5									NPI
6									NPI

25. FEDERAL TAX I.D. NUMBER SSN☐ EIN☐

26. PATIENT'S ACCOUNT NO.

27. ACCEPT ASSIGNMENT? (For govt. claims, see back) ☐YES ☐NO

28. TOTAL CHARGE $

29. AMOUNT PAID $

30. Rsvd for NUCC Use

31. SIGNATURE OF PHYSICIAN OR SUPPLIER INCLUDING DEGREES OR CREDENTIALS (I certify that the statements on the reverse apply to this bill and are made a part thereof.)

SIGNED _____ DATE _____

32. SERVICE FACILITY LOCATION INFORMATION

a. **NPI** b.

33. BILLING PROVIDER INFO & PH # ( )

a. **NPI** b.

◄── PHYSICIAN OR SUPPLIER INFORMATION

NUCC Instruction Manual available at: www.nucc.org   **PLEASE PRINT OR TYPE**

© Courtesy of the Centers for Medicare and Medicaid Services, www.cms.gov.

HEALTH INSURANCE CLAIM FORM

APPROVED BY NATIONAL UNIFORM CLAIM COMMITTEE (NUCC) 02/12

☐☐ PICA   PICA ☐☐

CARRIER →

| 1. MEDICARE ☐ (Medicare#) MEDICAID ☐ (Medicaid#) TRICARE ☐ (ID#/DoD#) CHAMPVA ☐ (Member ID#) GROUP HEALTH PLAN ☐ (ID#) FECA BLK LUNG ☐ (ID#) OTHER ☐ (ID#) | 1a. INSURED'S I.D. NUMBER   (For Program in Item 1) |

| 2. PATIENT'S NAME (Last Name, First Name, Middle Initial) | 3. PATIENT'S BIRTH DATE MM DD YY   SEX M ☐ F ☐ | 4. INSURED'S NAME (Last Name, First Name, Middle Initial) |

| 5. PATIENT'S ADDRESS (No., Street) | 6. PATIENT RELATIONSHIP TO INSURED Self ☐ Spouse ☐ Child ☐ Other ☐ | 7. INSURED'S ADDRESS (No., Street) |

| CITY | STATE | 8. RESERVED FOR NUCC USE | CITY | STATE |

| ZIP CODE | TELEPHONE (Include Area Code) ( ) | | ZIP CODE | TELEPHONE (Include Area Code) ( ) |

| 9. OTHER INSURED'S NAME (Last Name, First Name, Middle Initial) | 10. IS PATIENT'S CONDITION RELATED TO: | 11. INSURED'S POLICY GROUP OR FECA NUMBER |

| a. OTHER INSURED'S POLICY OR GROUP NUMBER | a. EMPLOYMENT? (Current or Previous) YES ☐ NO ☐ | a. INSURED'S DATE OF BIRTH MM DD YY   SEX M ☐ F ☐ |

| b. RESERVED FOR NUCC USE | b. AUTO ACCIDENT? PLACE (State) YES ☐ NO ☐ | b. OTHER CLAIM ID (Designated by NUCC) |

| c. RESERVED FOR NUCC USE | c. OTHER ACCIDENT? YES ☐ NO ☐ | c. INSURANCE PLAN NAME OR PROGRAM NAME |

| d. INSURANCE PLAN NAME OR PROGRAM NAME | 10d. CLAIM CODES (Designated by NUCC) | d. IS THERE ANOTHER HEALTH BENEFIT PLAN? YES ☐ NO ☐ *If yes*, complete items 9, 9a, and 9d. |

READ BACK OF FORM BEFORE COMPLETING & SIGNING THIS FORM.

12. PATIENT'S OR AUTHORIZED PERSON'S SIGNATURE I authorize the release of any medical or other information necessary to process this claim. I also request payment of government benefits either to myself or to the party who accepts assignment below.

SIGNED _____ DATE _____

13. INSURED'S OR AUTHORIZED PERSON'S SIGNATURE I authorize payment of medical benefits to the undersigned physician or supplier for services described below.

SIGNED _____

PATIENT AND INSURED INFORMATION →

| 14. DATE OF CURRENT ILLNESS, INJURY, or PREGNANCY (LMP) MM DD YY QUAL. | 15. OTHER DATE QUAL.   MM DD YY | 16. DATES PATIENT UNABLE TO WORK IN CURRENT OCCUPATION MM DD YY FROM   TO MM DD YY |

| 17. NAME OF REFERRING PROVIDER OR OTHER SOURCE | 17a. | | 18. HOSPITALIZATION DATES RELATED TO CURRENT SERVICES MM DD YY FROM   TO MM DD YY |
| | 17b. NPI | | |

| 19. ADDITIONAL CLAIM INFORMATION (Designated by NUCC) | 20. OUTSIDE LAB? YES ☐ NO ☐ $ CHARGES |

21. DIAGNOSIS OR NATURE OF ILLNESS OR INJURY Relate A-L to service line below (24E) ICD Ind.	22. RESUBMISSION CODE ORIGINAL REF. NO.
A. ____ B. ____ C. ____ D. ____	
E. ____ F. ____ G. ____ H. ____	23. PRIOR AUTHORIZATION NUMBER
I. ____ J. ____ K. ____ L. ____	

24. A. DATE(S) OF SERVICE			B. PLACE OF SERVICE	C. EMG	D. PROCEDURES, SERVICES, OR SUPPLIES (Explain Unusual Circumstances)		E. DIAGNOSIS POINTER	F. $ CHARGES	G. DAYS OR UNITS	H. EPSDT Family Plan	I. ID. QUAL.	J. RENDERING PROVIDER ID. #
From MM DD YY	To MM DD YY				CPT/HCPCS	MODIFIER						
1												NPI
2												NPI
3												NPI
4												NPI
5												NPI
6												NPI

| 25. FEDERAL TAX I.D. NUMBER SSN ☐ EIN ☐ | 26. PATIENT'S ACCOUNT NO. | 27. ACCEPT ASSIGNMENT? (For govt. claims, see back) YES ☐ NO ☐ | 28. TOTAL CHARGE $ | 29. AMOUNT PAID $ | 30. Rsvd for NUCC Use |

| 31. SIGNATURE OF PHYSICIAN OR SUPPLIER INCLUDING DEGREES OR CREDENTIALS (I certify that the statements on the reverse apply to this bill and are made a part thereof.) SIGNED _____ DATE _____ | 32. SERVICE FACILITY LOCATION INFORMATION a. **NPI** b. | 33. BILLING PROVIDER INFO & PH # ( ) a. **NPI** b. |

PHYSICIAN OR SUPPLIER INFORMATION →

NUCC Instruction Manual available at: www.nucc.org   *PLEASE PRINT OR TYPE*

© *Courtesy of the Centers for Medicare and Medicaid Services, www.cms.gov.*

HEALTH INSURANCE CLAIM FORM

APPROVED BY NATIONAL UNIFORM CLAIM COMMITTEE (NUCC) 02/12

		PICA								PICA	

1. MEDICARE	MEDICAID	TRICARE	CHAMPVA	GROUP HEALTH PLAN	FECA BLK LUNG	OTHER	1a. INSURED'S I.D. NUMBER	(For Program in Item 1)
(Medicare#)	(Medicaid#)	(ID#/DoD#)	(Member ID#)	(ID#)	(ID#)	(ID#)		

2. PATIENT'S NAME (Last Name, First Name, Middle Initial)

3. PATIENT'S BIRTH DATE MM DD YY — SEX M☐ F☐

4. INSURED'S NAME (Last Name, First Name, Middle Initial)

5. PATIENT'S ADDRESS (No., Street)

6. PATIENT RELATIONSHIP TO INSURED Self☐ Spouse☐ Child☐ Other☐

7. INSURED'S ADDRESS (No., Street)

CITY — STATE

8. RESERVED FOR NUCC USE

CITY — STATE

ZIP CODE — TELEPHONE (Include Area Code) ( )

ZIP CODE — TELEPHONE (Include Area Code) ( )

9. OTHER INSURED'S NAME (Last Name, First Name, Middle Initial)

10. IS PATIENT'S CONDITION RELATED TO:

11. INSURED'S POLICY GROUP OR FECA NUMBER

a. OTHER INSURED'S POLICY OR GROUP NUMBER

a. EMPLOYMENT? (Current or Previous) ☐YES ☐NO

a. INSURED'S DATE OF BIRTH MM DD YY — SEX M☐ F☐

b. RESERVED FOR NUCC USE

b. AUTO ACCIDENT? PLACE (State) ☐YES ☐NO

b. OTHER CLAIM ID (Designated by NUCC)

c. RESERVED FOR NUCC USE

c. OTHER ACCIDENT? ☐YES ☐NO

c. INSURANCE PLAN NAME OR PROGRAM NAME

d. INSURANCE PLAN NAME OR PROGRAM NAME

10d. CLAIM CODES (Designated by NUCC)

d. IS THERE ANOTHER HEALTH BENEFIT PLAN? ☐YES ☐NO *If yes,* complete items 9, 9a, and 9d.

READ BACK OF FORM BEFORE COMPLETING & SIGNING THIS FORM.

12. PATIENT'S OR AUTHORIZED PERSON'S SIGNATURE I authorize the release of any medical or other information necessary to process this claim. I also request payment of government benefits either to myself or to the party who accepts assignment below.

SIGNED _____ DATE _____

13. INSURED'S OR AUTHORIZED PERSON'S SIGNATURE I authorize payment of medical benefits to the undersigned physician or supplier for services described below.

SIGNED _____

14. DATE OF CURRENT ILLNESS, INJURY, or PREGNANCY (LMP) MM DD YY QUAL.

15. OTHER DATE QUAL. MM DD YY

16. DATES PATIENT UNABLE TO WORK IN CURRENT OCCUPATION FROM MM DD YY TO MM DD YY

17. NAME OF REFERRING PROVIDER OR OTHER SOURCE 17a. 17b. NPI

18. HOSPITALIZATION DATES RELATED TO CURRENT SERVICES FROM MM DD YY TO MM DD YY

19. ADDITIONAL CLAIM INFORMATION (Designated by NUCC)

20. OUTSIDE LAB? ☐YES ☐NO $ CHARGES

21. DIAGNOSIS OR NATURE OF ILLNESS OR INJURY Relate A-L to service line below (24E) ICD Ind.

A. ____ B. ____ C. ____ D. ____
E. ____ F. ____ G. ____ H. ____
I. ____ J. ____ K. ____ L. ____

22. RESUBMISSION CODE ORIGINAL REF. NO.

23. PRIOR AUTHORIZATION NUMBER

24. A. DATE(S) OF SERVICE From / To MM DD YY MM DD YY	B. PLACE OF SERVICE	C. EMG	D. PROCEDURES, SERVICES, OR SUPPLIES (Explain Unusual Circumstances) CPT/HCPCS MODIFIER	E. DIAGNOSIS POINTER	F. $ CHARGES	G. DAYS OR UNITS	H. EPSDT Family Plan	I. ID. QUAL.	J. RENDERING PROVIDER ID. #
1									NPI
2									NPI
3									NPI
4									NPI
5									NPI
6									NPI

25. FEDERAL TAX I.D. NUMBER SSN EIN	26. PATIENT'S ACCOUNT NO.	27. ACCEPT ASSIGNMENT? (For govt. claims, see back) ☐YES ☐NO	28. TOTAL CHARGE $	29. AMOUNT PAID $	30. Rsvd for NUCC Use

31. SIGNATURE OF PHYSICIAN OR SUPPLIER INCLUDING DEGREES OR CREDENTIALS (I certify that the statements on the reverse apply to this bill and are made a part thereof.)

SIGNED _____ DATE _____

32. SERVICE FACILITY LOCATION INFORMATION

a. **NPI** b.

33. BILLING PROVIDER INFO & PH # ( )

a. **NPI** b.

NUCC Instruction Manual available at: www.nucc.org — *PLEASE PRINT OR TYPE*

© *Courtesy of the Centers for Medicare and Medicaid Services, www.cms.gov.*

Vertical right margin labels: CARRIER — PATIENT AND INSURED INFORMATION — PHYSICIAN OR SUPPLIER INFORMATION

HEALTH INSURANCE CLAIM FORM

APPROVED BY NATIONAL UNIFORM CLAIM COMMITTEE (NUCC) 02/12

| | PICA | | | | | | | PICA | | |

CARRIER

1. MEDICARE MEDICAID TRICARE CHAMPVA GROUP HEALTH PLAN FECA BLK LUNG OTHER
☐ (Medicare#) ☐ (Medicaid#) ☐ (ID#/DoD#) ☐ (Member ID#) ☐ (ID#) ☐ (ID#) ☐ (ID#)

1a. INSURED'S I.D. NUMBER   (For Program in Item 1)

2. PATIENT'S NAME (Last Name, First Name, Middle Initial)

3. PATIENT'S BIRTH DATE MM DD YY   SEX M ☐ F ☐

4. INSURED'S NAME (Last Name, First Name, Middle Initial)

5. PATIENT'S ADDRESS (No., Street)

6. PATIENT RELATIONSHIP TO INSURED
Self ☐ Spouse ☐ Child ☐ Other ☐

7. INSURED'S ADDRESS (No., Street)

CITY   STATE

8. RESERVED FOR NUCC USE

CITY   STATE

ZIP CODE   TELEPHONE (Include Area Code) ( )

ZIP CODE   TELEPHONE (Include Area Code) ( )

9. OTHER INSURED'S NAME (Last Name, First Name, Middle Initial)

10. IS PATIENT'S CONDITION RELATED TO:

11. INSURED'S POLICY GROUP OR FECA NUMBER

a. OTHER INSURED'S POLICY OR GROUP NUMBER

a. EMPLOYMENT? (Current or Previous)
☐ YES ☐ NO

a. INSURED'S DATE OF BIRTH MM DD YY   SEX M ☐ F ☐

b. RESERVED FOR NUCC USE

b. AUTO ACCIDENT?   PLACE (State)
☐ YES ☐ NO

b. OTHER CLAIM ID (Designated by NUCC)

c. RESERVED FOR NUCC USE

c. OTHER ACCIDENT?
☐ YES ☐ NO

c. INSURANCE PLAN NAME OR PROGRAM NAME

d. INSURANCE PLAN NAME OR PROGRAM NAME

10d. CLAIM CODES (Designated by NUCC)

d. IS THERE ANOTHER HEALTH BENEFIT PLAN?
☐ YES ☐ NO *If yes*, complete items 9, 9a, and 9d.

READ BACK OF FORM BEFORE COMPLETING & SIGNING THIS FORM.
12. PATIENT'S OR AUTHORIZED PERSON'S SIGNATURE I authorize the release of any medical or other information necessary to process this claim. I also request payment of government benefits either to myself or to the party who accepts assignment below.

SIGNED _____ DATE _____

13. INSURED'S OR AUTHORIZED PERSON'S SIGNATURE I authorize payment of medical benefits to the undersigned physician or supplier for services described below.

SIGNED _____

PATIENT AND INSURED INFORMATION

14. DATE OF CURRENT ILLNESS, INJURY, or PREGNANCY (LMP) MM DD YY QUAL.

15. OTHER DATE MM DD YY QUAL.

16. DATES PATIENT UNABLE TO WORK IN CURRENT OCCUPATION
FROM MM DD YY TO MM DD YY

17. NAME OF REFERRING PROVIDER OR OTHER SOURCE

17a.
17b. NPI

18. HOSPITALIZATION DATES RELATED TO CURRENT SERVICES
FROM MM DD YY TO MM DD YY

19. ADDITIONAL CLAIM INFORMATION (Designated by NUCC)

20. OUTSIDE LAB? ☐ YES ☐ NO $ CHARGES

21. DIAGNOSIS OR NATURE OF ILLNESS OR INJURY Relate A-L to service line below (24E)   ICD Ind.
A. _____ B. _____ C. _____ D. _____
E. _____ F. _____ G. _____ H. _____
I. _____ J. _____ K. _____ L. _____

22. RESUBMISSION CODE   ORIGINAL REF. NO.

23. PRIOR AUTHORIZATION NUMBER

24. A. DATE(S) OF SERVICE From To MM DD YY MM DD YY	B. PLACE OF SERVICE	C. EMG	D. PROCEDURES, SERVICES, OR SUPPLIES (Explain Unusual Circumstances) CPT/HCPCS MODIFIER	E. DIAGNOSIS POINTER	F. $ CHARGES	G. DAYS OR UNITS	H. EPSDT Family Plan	I. ID. QUAL.	J. RENDERING PROVIDER ID. #
1								NPI	
2								NPI	
3								NPI	
4								NPI	
5								NPI	
6								NPI	

25. FEDERAL TAX I.D. NUMBER SSN ☐ EIN ☐

26. PATIENT'S ACCOUNT NO.

27. ACCEPT ASSIGNMENT? (For govt. claims, see back) ☐ YES ☐ NO

28. TOTAL CHARGE $

29. AMOUNT PAID $

30. Rsvd for NUCC Use

31. SIGNATURE OF PHYSICIAN OR SUPPLIER INCLUDING DEGREES OR CREDENTIALS (I certify that the statements on the reverse apply to this bill and are made a part thereof.)

SIGNED _____ DATE _____

32. SERVICE FACILITY LOCATION INFORMATION

a. **NPI** b.

33. BILLING PROVIDER INFO & PH # ( )

a. **NPI** b.

PHYSICIAN OR SUPPLIER INFORMATION

NUCC Instruction Manual available at: www.nucc.org   *PLEASE PRINT OR TYPE*

HEALTH INSURANCE CLAIM FORM

APPROVED BY NATIONAL UNIFORM CLAIM COMMITTEE (NUCC) 02/12

▢▢ PICA ▢▢   PICA ▢▢▢

1.	MEDICARE	MEDICAID	TRICARE	CHAMPVA	GROUP HEALTH PLAN	FECA BLK LUNG	OTHER	1a. INSURED'S I.D. NUMBER	(For Program in Item 1)
	▢ (Medicare#)	▢ (Medicaid#)	▢ (ID#/DoD#)	▢ (Member ID#)	▢ (ID#)	▢ (ID#)	▢ (ID#)		

2. PATIENT'S NAME (Last Name, First Name, Middle Initial)

3. PATIENT'S BIRTH DATE MM | DD | YY SEX M ▢ F ▢

4. INSURED'S NAME (Last Name, First Name, Middle Initial)

5. PATIENT'S ADDRESS (No., Street)

6. PATIENT RELATIONSHIP TO INSURED Self ▢ Spouse ▢ Child ▢ Other ▢

7. INSURED'S ADDRESS (No., Street)

CITY   STATE

8. RESERVED FOR NUCC USE

CITY   STATE

ZIP CODE   TELEPHONE (Include Area Code) ( )

ZIP CODE   TELEPHONE (Include Area Code) ( )

9. OTHER INSURED'S NAME (Last Name, First Name, Middle Initial)

10. IS PATIENT'S CONDITION RELATED TO:

11. INSURED'S POLICY GROUP OR FECA NUMBER

a. OTHER INSURED'S POLICY OR GROUP NUMBER

a. EMPLOYMENT? (Current or Previous) ▢ YES ▢ NO

a. INSURED'S DATE OF BIRTH MM | DD | YY SEX M ▢ F ▢

b. RESERVED FOR NUCC USE

b. AUTO ACCIDENT? PLACE (State) ▢ YES ▢ NO

b. OTHER CLAIM ID (Designated by NUCC)

c. RESERVED FOR NUCC USE

c. OTHER ACCIDENT? ▢ YES ▢ NO

c. INSURANCE PLAN NAME OR PROGRAM NAME

d. INSURANCE PLAN NAME OR PROGRAM NAME

10d. CLAIM CODES (Designated by NUCC)

d. IS THERE ANOTHER HEALTH BENEFIT PLAN? ▢ YES ▢ NO *If yes*, complete items 9, 9a, and 9d.

READ BACK OF FORM BEFORE COMPLETING & SIGNING THIS FORM.
12. PATIENT'S OR AUTHORIZED PERSON'S SIGNATURE I authorize the release of any medical or other information necessary to process this claim. I also request payment of government benefits either to myself or to the party who accepts assignment below.

SIGNED _____ DATE _____

13. INSURED'S OR AUTHORIZED PERSON'S SIGNATURE I authorize payment of medical benefits to the undersigned physician or supplier for services described below.

SIGNED _____

14. DATE OF CURRENT ILLNESS, INJURY, or PREGNANCY (LMP) MM | DD | YY QUAL.

15. OTHER DATE QUAL. MM | DD | YY

16. DATES PATIENT UNABLE TO WORK IN CURRENT OCCUPATION FROM MM | DD | YY TO MM | DD | YY

17. NAME OF REFERRING PROVIDER OR OTHER SOURCE

17a.
17b. NPI

18. HOSPITALIZATION DATES RELATED TO CURRENT SERVICES FROM MM | DD | YY TO MM | DD | YY

19. ADDITIONAL CLAIM INFORMATION (Designated by NUCC)

20. OUTSIDE LAB? ▢ YES ▢ NO $ CHARGES

21. DIAGNOSIS OR NATURE OF ILLNESS OR INJURY Relate A-L to service line below (24E) ICD Ind. |

A. |_____ B. |_____ C. |_____ D. |_____
E. |_____ F. |_____ G. |_____ H. |_____
I. |_____ J. |_____ K. |_____ L. |_____

22. RESUBMISSION CODE ORIGINAL REF. NO.

23. PRIOR AUTHORIZATION NUMBER

24. A. DATE(S) OF SERVICE From MM DD YY To MM DD YY	B. PLACE OF SERVICE	C. EMG	D. PROCEDURES, SERVICES, OR SUPPLIES (Explain Unusual Circumstances) CPT/HCPCS	MODIFIER	E. DIAGNOSIS POINTER	F. $ CHARGES	G. DAYS OR UNITS	H. EPSDT Family Plan	I. ID. QUAL.	J. RENDERING PROVIDER ID. #
1										NPI
2										NPI
3										NPI
4										NPI
5										NPI
6										NPI

25. FEDERAL TAX I.D. NUMBER SSN ▢ EIN ▢

26. PATIENT'S ACCOUNT NO.

27. ACCEPT ASSIGNMENT? (For govt. claims, see back) ▢ YES ▢ NO

28. TOTAL CHARGE $

29. AMOUNT PAID $

30. Rsvd for NUCC Use

31. SIGNATURE OF PHYSICIAN OR SUPPLIER INCLUDING DEGREES OR CREDENTIALS (I certify that the statements on the reverse apply to this bill and are made a part thereof.)

SIGNED _____ DATE _____

32. SERVICE FACILITY LOCATION INFORMATION

a. **NPI**   b.

33. BILLING PROVIDER INFO & PH # ( )

a. **NPI**   b.

NUCC Instruction Manual available at: www.nucc.org   *PLEASE PRINT OR TYPE*

HEALTH INSURANCE CLAIM FORM

APPROVED BY NATIONAL UNIFORM CLAIM COMMITTEE (NUCC) 02/12

NUCC Instruction Manual available at: www.nucc.org   **PLEASE PRINT OR TYPE**

© *Courtesy of the Centers for Medicare and Medicaid Services, www.cms.gov.*

CARRIER

| | PICA | | | | | | | | PICA | |

1. MEDICARE ☐ *(Medicare#)* MEDICAID ☐ *(Medicaid#)* TRICARE ☐ *(ID#/DoD#)* CHAMPVA ☐ *(Member ID#)* GROUP HEALTH PLAN ☐ *(ID#)* FECA BLK LUNG ☐ *(ID#)* OTHER ☐ *(ID#)*

1a. INSURED'S I.D. NUMBER (For Program in Item 1)

2. PATIENT'S NAME (Last Name, First Name, Middle Initial)

3. PATIENT'S BIRTH DATE MM | DD | YY   SEX M ☐ F ☐

4. INSURED'S NAME (Last Name, First Name, Middle Initial)

5. PATIENT'S ADDRESS (No., Street)

6. PATIENT RELATIONSHIP TO INSURED Self ☐ Spouse ☐ Child ☐ Other ☐

7. INSURED'S ADDRESS (No., Street)

CITY STATE

8. RESERVED FOR NUCC USE

CITY STATE

ZIP CODE TELEPHONE (Include Area Code) ( )

ZIP CODE TELEPHONE (Include Area Code) ( )

9. OTHER INSURED'S NAME (Last Name, First Name, Middle Initial)

10. IS PATIENT'S CONDITION RELATED TO:

11. INSURED'S POLICY GROUP OR FECA NUMBER

a. OTHER INSURED'S POLICY OR GROUP NUMBER

a. EMPLOYMENT? (Current or Previous) YES ☐ NO ☐

a. INSURED'S DATE OF BIRTH MM | DD | YY   SEX M ☐ F ☐

b. RESERVED FOR NUCC USE

b. AUTO ACCIDENT? PLACE (State) YES ☐ NO ☐

b. OTHER CLAIM ID (Designated by NUCC)

c. RESERVED FOR NUCC USE

c. OTHER ACCIDENT? YES ☐ NO ☐

c. INSURANCE PLAN NAME OR PROGRAM NAME

d. INSURANCE PLAN NAME OR PROGRAM NAME

10d. CLAIM CODES (Designated by NUCC)

d. IS THERE ANOTHER HEALTH BENEFIT PLAN? YES ☐ NO ☐ *If yes,* complete items 9, 9a, and 9d.

READ BACK OF FORM BEFORE COMPLETING & SIGNING THIS FORM.
12. PATIENT'S OR AUTHORIZED PERSON'S SIGNATURE I authorize the release of any medical or other information necessary to process this claim. I also request payment of government benefits either to myself or to the party who accepts assignment below.

SIGNED _____ DATE _____

13. INSURED'S OR AUTHORIZED PERSON'S SIGNATURE I authorize payment of medical benefits to the undersigned physician or supplier for services described below.

SIGNED _____

PATIENT AND INSURED INFORMATION

---

14. DATE OF CURRENT ILLNESS, INJURY, or PREGNANCY (LMP) MM | DD | YY   QUAL.

15. OTHER DATE QUAL. MM | DD | YY

16. DATES PATIENT UNABLE TO WORK IN CURRENT OCCUPATION FROM MM | DD | YY TO MM | DD | YY

17. NAME OF REFERRING PROVIDER OR OTHER SOURCE 17a. 17b. NPI

18. HOSPITALIZATION DATES RELATED TO CURRENT SERVICES FROM MM | DD | YY TO MM | DD | YY

19. ADDITIONAL CLAIM INFORMATION (Designated by NUCC)

20. OUTSIDE LAB? YES ☐ NO ☐ $ CHARGES

21. DIAGNOSIS OR NATURE OF ILLNESS OR INJURY Relate A-L to service line below (24E) ICD Ind. |

A. |____ B. |____ C. |____ D. |____
E. |____ F. |____ G. |____ H. |____
I. |____ J. |____ K. |____ L. |____

22. RESUBMISSION CODE ORIGINAL REF. NO.

23. PRIOR AUTHORIZATION NUMBER

24. A. DATE(S) OF SERVICE						B. PLACE OF SERVICE	C. EMG	D. PROCEDURES, SERVICES, OR SUPPLIES (Explain Unusual Circumstances) CPT/HCPCS	MODIFIER	E. DIAGNOSIS POINTER	F. $ CHARGES	G. DAYS OR UNITS	H. EPSDT Family Plan	I. ID. QUAL.	J. RENDERING PROVIDER ID. #
From MM	DD	YY	To MM	DD	YY										
1														NPI	
2														NPI	
3														NPI	
4														NPI	
5														NPI	
6														NPI	

25. FEDERAL TAX I.D. NUMBER SSN ☐ EIN ☐

26. PATIENT'S ACCOUNT NO.

27. ACCEPT ASSIGNMENT? (For govt. claims, see back) YES ☐ NO ☐

28. TOTAL CHARGE $

29. AMOUNT PAID $

30. Rsvd for NUCC Use

31. SIGNATURE OF PHYSICIAN OR SUPPLIER INCLUDING DEGREES OR CREDENTIALS (I certify that the statements on the reverse apply to this bill and are made a part thereof.)

SIGNED _____ DATE _____

32. SERVICE FACILITY LOCATION INFORMATION

a. **NPI** b.

33. BILLING PROVIDER INFO & PH # ( )

a. **NPI** b.

PHYSICIAN OR SUPPLIER INFORMATION

Patient Billing, Posting Patient Payments, and Collecting Fees

Words to Know Challenge

Spelling: Each line contains three spellings of a word. Underline the correctly spelled word. Identify the following correctly spelled Words to Know.

1. bankrupcy   bankruptcy   bankurptcy

2. idol   idel   idle

3. outsourcing   outsourching   outsorcing

4. termination   ternimation   terminiation

5. vibility   viabality   viability

6. expanded   expender   expended

Matching: Match each term in column I to its meaning in column II.

COLUMN I	COLUMN II
____ 1. Bankruptcy	A. Seeking a name by entering in a system the first few letters of the name
____ 2. Viability	B. Accounts due from the provider's patients to the practice
____ 3. Account history	C. Date of service
____ 4. Termination	D. Practice management software
____ 5. Alpha search	E. Legal petition to the courts if one is unable to pay creditors
____ 6. Expended	F. Harmless, ineffectual, meaningless
____ 7. Third-party	G. Contracting work out
____ 8. Accounts receivable	H. Patient who has moved to avoid payments
____ 9. YTD	I. An act enforced by the FTC
____ 10. PM software	J. At the time of service
____ 11. Idle	K. Used up or spent

(continues)

223

____ 12. Aging of accounts   L. Capable of success or continuing effectiveness; practicable

____ 13. DOS   M. One other than the individuals involved in an account

____ 14. Skip   N. System used to analyze A/Rs on past due

____ 15. Outsourcing   O. A period starting January 1 of the current year and ending today (example)

____ 16. Truth in Lending   P. Computer term for a patient ledger

____ 17. ATOS   Q. End in time or existence

Chapter Review

Short Answer

1. What are the typical results of outsourcing physician office work?

   _____

   _____

   _____

2. Describe practice management software.

   _____

   _____

   _____

3. What types of services do PM software systems offer?

   _____

   _____

   _____

4. What is a third-party check?

   _____

   _____

   _____

5. Describe the use of an alpha search.

   _____

   _____

   _____

6. List the three forms of payment described in this chapter.

   _____

   _____

   _____

7. What should you do when a credit balance is discovered on a patient account?

   _____

   _____

   _____

8. List both the positive and negative terms that should or should not be used in a collection letter.

   _____

   _____

   _____

Matching: Match each item in column I to its meaning in column II.

COLUMN I	COLUMN II
___ 1. Cycle billing	A. Billing method more efficient in small practices
___ 2. Patient payments	B. Computer terminology for a patient ledger
___ 3. Antagonizing terms	C. NSF
___ 4. Truth in Lending Act	D. Neglect, ignored, failure
___ 5. Fair Debt Collection Practices Act	E. Specifies agreement between patient and physician regarding installments and finance charge disclosure
___ 6. Monthly billing	F. Establishes number of years during which legal collection procedures may be filed against a patient
___ 7. Statutes of limitation	G. Vital for the financial success of a medical facility
___ 8. Account history	H. Prohibits debt collectors from abusive, unfair, or deceptive collection practices
___ 9. Proper collection letter terms	I. Billing commonly used in large practices
___ 10. Nonsufficient funds	J. Missed, overlooked, forgotten

Chapter Application

Case Study with Critical Thinking Questions

Chris, the billing person at Bonita Medical Clinic, is responsible for all patient billing and bookkeeping. He has fallen behind on his daily posting and is having trouble catching up. His totals are not balancing for accounts receivable, and he is frustrated.

1. When should posting be done? _____
_____

2. In what order should the entries be placed? _____
_____

3. What could be the possible outcomes of sloppy bookkeeping practices? _____
_____

4. What should Chris do in this situation? _____
_____
_____
_____

Competency Practice

1. **Obtain accurate patient billing information, post Nonsufficient Funds (NSF) Checks and Collection Agency Payments Utilizing EMR and Practice Management Systems.** Use the detailed instructions and rationales outlined in Procedure 31–1 as a guideline and post NSF checks and collection agency payments. Students can download the patient ledger card from the Student Companion website to complete this activity and use as work product for this procedure. Use the following scenario information to complete the activity.

Scenario

Your office recently placed several accounts with an outside collection agency the practice uses for collection efforts when it has been unsuccessful in collecting the debt from the patient. One of the accounts was turned over to the agency because the patient had a habit of presenting checks that bounced due to lack of funds in the account to cover the amount the checks were issued for. Today, you received another NSF check written for payment on this patient's account. You also received the first collection agency payment on this same account.

- Use yourself as the patient and your provider's name as the physician.
- Use today's date.
- The NSF check amount is for the $20 co-pay check payment accepted on 2/1/20XX as listed on the patient ledger.
- Collection agency payment is for $15.

2. **Process a Credit Balance and Refund.** Use the detailed instructions and rationales outlined in Procedure 31–2 as a guideline and process a credit balance and refund. Students can download the patient ledger and blank check from the Student Companion website to complete this activity and use as work product for this procedure. Use the following scenario information to complete the activity.

- Use yourself as the patient and your provider's name as the physician.
- Use today's date.

Scenario

During a recent audit, your office discovered changes in insurance plans that resulted in different co-pay, out-of-pocket, and insurance amounts than were collected/recorded. Record the adjustment to the patient account and refund (or bill) the difference. The co-payment was discovered by the medical assistant to be $10 rather than the accepted check for $20. The overpayment amount is for $10 from the $20 co-pay check payment accepted on 2/1/20XX as listed on the patient ledger.

Banking and Accounting Procedures

Banking Procedures

Words to Know Challenge

Spelling: Each line contains three spellings of a word. Underline the correctly spelled word.

1.	reconcilling	reconciling	recountciling
2.	negotiable	negoshiable	necotible
3.	denomanation	demonination	denomination
4.	withdralle	withdrawl	withdrawal
5.	endorsement	endorcement	endorsment
6.	currensy	currency	currancy
7.	deposite	diposit	deposit
8.	registre	register	registir
9.	transaction	trensaction	transacion

Matching: Match the terms in column I to their meanings in column II.

	COLUMN I	COLUMN II
____	1. Agent	A. An amount of money (cash or checks) placed in a bank account
____	2. Endorser	B. A check generally made out to the patient by someone unknown to you
____	3. Deposit slip	C. An amount beyond what is currently in the account
____	4. Withdrawal	D. A fee charged by the bank for services rendered
____	5. Third-party check	E. Used when an error is made on a check
____	6. Outstanding	F. An itemized list of cash and checks deposited into an account
____	7. Deposit	G. A person authorized to act for another person

(continues)

____   8. VOID   H. Removal of funds from an account

____   9. Service charge   I. Payee

____   10. Overdraft   J. A check that has been written but that does not appear on the bank statement

Chapter Review

Short Answer

1. Explain the handling of currency in the office.

_____

_____

_____

2. List the seven components of a check you must examine to ensure that it is valid.

_____

_____

_____

3. List five pieces of information a bank needs to stop payment on a check. For what reasons may a payment be stopped?

_____

_____

_____

4. Name the two types of endorsements and explain what each means.

_____

_____

_____

_____

5. Briefly describe a bank statement.

_____

_____

_____

Labeling: Identify each component on the following check.

a. _____

b. _____

c. _____

d. _____

e. _____

Chapter Application

Case Study with Critical Thinking Question

Patient Jane Johansen called the office today after receiving a statement in the mail showing her balance due as $47.00 after the insurance company had paid its portion. Ms. Johansen tells you that she stopped by the office last Monday and paid the balance in cash and wants to know why she is still receiving a bill. During the discussion she tells you she cannot find the receipt and does not recall the name of the person she gave the money to.

1. What steps should you take to resolve the issue?

2. What can you do to prevent this happening in the future?

Competency Practice

1. **Prepare a Check.** Using Procedure 32–1 as a guideline, practice writing checks. Use the following information to write a check to Physician's Supply, Inc. for $125.50, using the sample check provided in Work Product 32–1. Use the current date and sign the checks with the physician's name provided, with your name below the line. Complete the stub end, subtracting each subsequent check with the initial total starting balance of $8,480.64. *Work product forms are provided at the end of the chapter.*

2. **Prepare a Deposit Slip.** Using Procedure 32–2 as a guideline, practice preparing a deposit slip. Use the following list of cash and check payments to prepare a bank deposit slip, provided in Work Product 32–2. Use today's date as the deposit date. *Work product forms are provided at the end of the chapter.*

Currency/coin	1 – $50.00 bill; 6 – $20.00 bills; 15 – $10.00 bills; 17 – $5.00 bills; 14 – $1.00 bills; 4 – quarters
Checks	Smith, check #1458: $40.00
	Manolo, check #501: $425.00
	Vronski, check #998: $220.00
	Leu, check #4010: $25.00
	Wallace, check #1155: $150.00
Money orders	Jones: $15.00

3. **Reconcile a Bank Statement**. Using Procedure 32–3 as a guideline, practice reconciling a bank statement. Use the information below to reconcile the bank account on Work Product 32–3. (You may assume the opening balance agrees with the previous statement.) *Work product forms are provided at the end of the chapter.*

Checkbook (Register)

Ending balance: $3173.71
Checks written during the month:

Check #	Amount	√	Check #	Amount	√
201	25.00		217	785.00	
202	600.00		218	28.37	
203	75.00		219	60.00	
204	37.54		220	36.30	
205	30.00		221	115.45	
206	95.94		222	35.00	
207	73.87		223	95.94	
208	44.00		224	19.00	
209	130.00		225	75.00	
210	95.94		226	400.00	
211	500.00		227	78.37	
212	18.22		228	95.94	
213	133.28		229	200.00	
214	57.50		230	33.60	
215	38.60		231	1200.00	
216	500.00		232	100.00	

Deposits made during the month:

Deposit Date	Amount	√
6-02	500.00	
6-03	750.00	
6-06	350.00	
6-07	700.00	
6-09	335.00	
6-12	500.00	
6-14	440.50	
6-15	180.00	
6-18	175.00	
6-19	520.00	
6-20	522.50	
6-22	720.00	
6-25	600.00	
6-27	662.00	
6-30	191.00	

Account Statement

THE NEVER FAIL BANK

NEVER FAIL ACCOUNT

ANYWHERE BRANCH
0000 THIS STREET
ANYTOWN, STATE 00000-0000

CUSTOMER SERVICE 24 HOURS A DAY, 800-000-0000

JANE D. CUSTOMER
1234 HOME STREET
ANYTOWN, STATE 00000-0000

ACCOUNT
12345-678910
STATEMENT PERIOD
6-1-20xx TO 7-1-20xx

ACCOUNTS SUMMARY

CHECKING		SAVINGS
BEGINNING BALANCE	1840.57	
DEPOSITS	6955.00	
CHECKS PAID	3715.32	
ATM & DEBIT CARD WITHDRAWALS	0.00	
SERVICE CHARGES/FEES	3.27	
ENDING BALANCE	5076.98	

CHECKING ACTIVITY

DEPOSITS POSTED	AMOUNT	DESCRIPTION
6-03	500.00	ATM DEPOSIT
6-04	750.00	ATM DEPOSIT

6-07	350.00	DEPOSIT
6-08	700.00	DEPOSIT
6-10	335.00	DEPOSIT
6-13	500.00	ATM DEPOSIT
6-15	440.50	ATM DEPOSIT
6-16	180.00	DEPOSIT
6-19	175.00	DEPOSIT
6-20	520.00	DEPOSIT
6-21	522.50	DEPOSIT
6-23	720.00	DEPOSIT
6-26	600.00	DEPOSIT
6-28	662.00	ATM DEPOSIT

CHECKS PAID CHECK #	AMOUNT
201	25.00
202	600.00
203	75.00
205	30.00
206	95.94
207	73.87
208	44.00
209	130.00
210	95.94
211	500.00
212	18.22
213	133.28
214	57.50
215	38.60
216	500.00
218	28.37
219	60.00
220	36.30
221	115.45
222	35.00
223	95.94
224	19.00
226	400.00
227	78.37
228	95.94
229	200.00
230	33.60
232	100.00

CHECKING SERVICES CHARGE AND FEE SUMMARY

AMOUNT	DESCRIPTION
3.27	MONTHLY SERVICE CHARGE

Work Product Forms

Work Product 32–1

1490	BAL. BRO'T FORD			
_____ 20___		DEPOSITS		
TO _____				
FOR _____				
	TOTAL			
	THIS CHECK			
	BALANCE			

ELIZABETH R. EVANS, M.D.
SUITE 205 100 E. MAIN ST.
YOURTOWN, US 98765-4321

1490
25-64/440

_____ 20 _____

PAY
TO THE
ORDER OF _____ $ _____

_____ DOLLARS

THE NEVER FAIL BANK
ANYWHERE, U.S.A 00000

7-68-25

FOR _____

|:00006 7894|: 12345678;' 01491 ;0000039158;

Work Product 32–2

I.M. Healthy, M.D.
101 Fitness Lane
Anywhere, U.S.A. 00000

DATE_____20____

_____

The Never Fail Bank
Anywhere, U.S.A.

:04400002 4|: 0 2894 11086 1|"

CHECKS AND OTHER ITEMS ARE RECEIVED FOR DEPOSIT SUBJECT TO THE PROVISIONS OF THE UNIFORM COMMERCIAL CODE OR ANY APPLICABLE COLLECTION AGREEMENT

CASH	CURRENCY		
	COIN		
LIST CHECKS SINGLY			
TOTAL FROM OTHER SIDE			
TOTAL			USE OTHER SIDE FOR ADDITIONAL LISTING
◆ LESS CASH RECEIVED			
NET DEPOSIT			BE SURE EACH ITEM IS PROPERLY ENDORSED

CHECKS LIST SINGLY	DOLLARS	CENTS
1		
2		
3		
4		
5		
6		
7		
8		
9		
10		
11		
12		
13		
14		
15		
16		
17		
18		
19		
TOTAL		
ENTER TOTAL ON THE FRONT OF THIS TICKET		

Work Product 32–3

RECONCILING THE BANK STATEMENT

Bank Statement Balance $ _____

(+) Plus Deposits not shown

_____

Total _____ $ _____

(−) Less Outstanding Checks

     # _____

     # _____

     # _____

     # _____

Total _____ $ _____

CORRECTED BANK STATEMENT BALANCE	$ _____

Checkbook Balance $ _____

(−) Less Bank Charges $ _____

CORRECTED CHECKBOOK BALANCE	$ _____

CHAPTER 33

Accounts Payable and Accounting Procedures

Words to Know Challenge

Spelling: Each line contains three spellings of a word. Underline the correctly spelled word.

1. ecquity   eqity   equity
2. voucher   vowcher   voutcher
3. writ-offs   rite-offs   write-offs
4. cost raetio   cost rashio   cost ratio
5. manegerial   managerial   manigerial
6. account payable   accounts payable account payabel
7. balence sheet   balanse sheet   balance sheet

Matching: Match the terms in column I to their meanings in column II.

COLUMN I	COLUMN II
____ 1. A/P	A. Debts or A/P owed by the business
____ 2. Expenditure	B. Adjusted collection ratio
____ 3. Petty cash	C. Current A/R balance ÷ average monthly gross production
____ 4. Net worth	D. Allows for program evaluation
____ 5. Assets	E. Document with itemized goods or services
____ 6. Net collection ratio	F. Assets – liability
____ 7. Invoice	G. Small amount of stored money, ranging from $25 to $75
____ 8. Liabilities	H. An acquired material in exchange for money
____ 9. A/R ratio	I. Total amounts owed by practice to supplier
____ 10. Income statement	J. The money and items of value in a business
____ 11. Cost-benefit analysis	K. Demonstrates the profit and expenses for a given time period

Chapter Review

Short Answer

1. Explain why comparing shipments to packing lists or invoices is important.

   _____

   _____

   _____

2. Describe what should be done when a shipment item does not match the invoice.

   _____

   _____

   _____

3. For what purpose is a petty cash fund used?

   _____

   _____

   _____

4. Explain why it is important to know the net worth of a business.

   _____

   _____

   _____

5. Explain why collection ratios might be important to a physician's office.

   _____

   _____

   _____

6. What are charges considered when deemed uncollectible? Provide two examples.

   _____

   _____

   _____

7. What are the three steps of cost-benefit analysis?

   _____

   _____

   _____

8. Explain what income statements and balance sheets demonstrate to a medical practice.

   _____

   _____

   _____

9. Name the two types of collection ratios most frequently used in a medical office.

   _____

   _____

   _____

Matching: Match the ratios in column I to their formulas in column II.

	COLUMN I	COLUMN II
____	1. A/R ratio	A. Assets – Liabilities = Net Worth
____	2. Cost ratio	B. Total Payments (A/R) ÷ Total Charges – Write-Offs
____	3. Basic accounting formula	C. Current A/R Balance ÷ Average Monthly Gross Production
____	4. Gross collection ratio	D. Total Expenses ÷ Total Number of Procedures for One Month
____	5. Net collection ratio	E. Total Payments (A/R) ÷ Total Charges

Chapter Application

Case Study with Critical Thinking Questions

Sabrina Holton is the office manager, and Dr. Imel asks her to report back on whether the use of the contracted diabetic educator is cost effective to house in the office. The educator has been teaching patients for one month in a small office space rented by Dr. Imel and, during that month, has taught 20 patients. The educator bills the physician $30.00 per patient. Additional details: The rental of the office space is $100 per month; electricity and Internet service for the space is $50; office supplies are $15.

1. What ratio formula will MA Sabrina use to calculate this loss or gain and why?

_____

_____

_____

2. Calculate the answer to the ratio formula you identified.

_____

_____

_____

Competency Practice

Establish and Maintain a Petty Cash Fund. Using Procedure 33–1 as a guide, use Work Product 33–1 and the following amounts to establish and maintain a petty cash fund, which was opened on 9/19 (current year) with an opening balance of $25.00. When the petty cash fund decreases below $5.00, a new check should be written to bring the fund back up to the $25.00 level.

a. Bill: postage $5.00, 9/20

b. Voucher 1: charity donation $10.00, 9/23

c. Bill: envelopes and pens $8.00, 9/24

d. Voucher 2: mileage $5.00, 9/27

e. Bill: postage $8.50, 9/30

Work Product 33–1

PETTY CASH FORM			
Date	Bill/Voucher Description	Amount	Balance

SECTION 4

The Back Office

11

Preparing for Clinical Procedures

CHAPTER 35

The Medical History and Patient Screening

Words to Know Challenge

Spelling: Each line contains three spellings of a word. Underline the correctly spelled word.

1.	emergant	emergent	emirgent
2.	familiel	femelial	familial
3.	genogram	geneogram	jeanogram
4.	treage	triage	treeage
5.	clinical diagnoses	clinical diagnosis	clinicle diagnosis
6.	alergies	allergys	allergies
7.	objective	abjective	objectiev
8.	sabjective	subjactive	subjective
9.	patronizing	patranizing	peitronizing
10.	remadies	remedies	remedys

Fill in the Blank

1. Our beliefs and values tend to provide _____ in how we view others.

2. An unexpected occurrence or situation demanding immediate action is considered _____ .

3. _____ can cause an abnormal reaction by the body to substances that are normally harmless.

4. Providers who treat _____ disorders and diseases may also use another type of history form called a _____ .

5. _____ can be described as anything that relieves or cures a disease.

6. Treating a patient condescendingly is known as _____ .

7. _____ symptoms are felt by the individual but are not perceptible to others.

8. A provider will arrive at a _____ from facts obtained through the medical history, physical exam, and lab testing.

9. You may need to use _____ skills to determine the order of importance of tasks at the medical office.

Chapter Review

Short Answer

1. Name five areas of knowledge that you should have to provide good patient screening. _____
_____
_____

2. If a patient complains of pain, what additional questions do you need to ask? _____
_____
_____
_____

3. Why might a health history form not be filled out entirely by the patient? _____
_____
_____

4. What is the goal of patient screening? _____
_____
_____

5. Why do some offices send out health history forms to the patient prior to the appointment? _____
_____
_____

6. Where should the medical assistant interview patients to obtain the health history information? _____
_____
_____

7. What is a genogram and why is it helpful to providers? _____
_____
_____

8. Why should you ask a patient whether he or she has any allergies, and how should you note it in the patient's medical record? _____
_____
_____

9. After obtaining a patient's chief complaint, the medical assistant should do what next? _____
_____
_____

10. Explain why health history forms vary in detail and length. _____
_____
_____

Matching: Match the term in column I to its definition in column II.

	COLUMN I	COLUMN II
____	1. Screening	A. Symptoms that can be observed
____	2. Triage	B. Referring to accessible, nonprescription drugs
____	3. Chief complaint (CC)	C. Beliefs that influence observations
____	4. Interview	D. Any perceptible change in the body that indicates disease
____	5. Over-the-counter	E. Process of obtaining information from patient
____	6. Prioritizing	F. Main reason for office visit
____	7. Symptoms	G. Talking to patients one on one and asking questions
____	8. Objective	H. Sort and assess injury
____	9. Biases	I. Arranging in order of importance

Chapter Application

Case Studies with Critical Thinking Questions

Scenario 1

When obtaining a patient's chief complaint of fatigue and dizziness, you also notice that he is short of breath and is having difficulty breathing. The patient doesn't mention these symptoms in his chief complaint and talks only about the fatigue and dizziness.

1. What should you do about the apparent symptoms of shortness of breath and dyspnea? _____

_____

_____

2. Should you chart your observed symptoms with the patient's chief complaint? _____

_____

_____

3. Should you discuss this information with the provider? _____

_____

_____

Scenario 2

A patient is scheduled to see the provider today for a sore throat and a low-grade fever, which he has had for about five days. While interviewing the patient, he tells you he has also been having chest pains and difficulty breathing and would like the provider to check him for these complaints as well.

1. Will the provider be able to address all the patient's complaints in the time allotted? _____

_____

_____

_____

2. What should you tell the patient regarding the additional complaints? _____

_____

_____

3. Should you document only the complaints for which the appointment time was scheduled? _____

_____

_____

Scenario 3

Amy, the medical assistant, is reviewing a completed medical history form with Mrs. Leonard. She reviews the list of medications Mrs. Leonard has listed and notices that no over-the-counter medications have been included. When Amy questions Mrs. Leonard, she says that she takes no OTC meds, even though she takes some herbal supplements and vitamins on a daily basis.

1. What should Amy have included in her questions about OTC medications? _____

_____

_____

2. Why should vitamins and herbal supplements be included in the history form? _____

_____

_____

3. What are possible implications of not including this information on the history form? _____

_____

_____

Scenario 4

Mr. Anthony is being seen by the provider for his annual physical. While screening the patient's history form, you notice that he has left the social history section blank. This is the section that includes information about alcohol and tobacco use. Mr. Anthony was told by the provider to stop smoking and drinking alcohol last year.

1. What should you do about the missing information? _____

_____

2. How should you approach the subject? _____

_____

_____

3. Why is it important to obtain information concerning the patient's habits? _____

_____

_____

Scenario 5

While assisting Mrs. Juarez with her health history forms you get to the section on family health history. This data in addition to the physical examination not only will assist the provider with the information necessary to arrive at a diagnosis and treatment for the current complaint but may also forewarn and possibly prevent future conditions that tend to develop within families.

1. What family members should be included in this history? _____

_____

2. What type of information should be provided regarding these members? _____

_____

_____

3. Providers who treat familial disorders and diseases may also use a special type of history form. What is the specific form and what it is used for? _____

_____

_____

Competency Practice

1. **Perform Patient Screening.** With a partner, choose an illness to portray and practice taking chief complaints. Develop the complaint, using the characteristics in the textbook to make them as complete as possible to provide the provider with the most information about what is troubling the patient. Using the mock chart below or EHR software, document the chief complaint. Refer to the textbook for charting examples. Use Procedure 35–1 as a guide.

PROGRESS NOTE		
Patient Name:		DOB
DATE/TIME	PROGRESS NOTES	ALLERGIES

2. **Obtain and Record a Patient Health History.**

   a. Select a disease condition and complete a health history form (download Procedure Form 35–2 from the Student Companion website). Have another student check the form for accuracy.

   b. With a partner, have one person be the patient and the other be the medical assistant. In a private setting, practice interviewing the patient and completing the health history forms. Be as thorough as possible, using all the techniques provided in the textbook. Use Procedure 35–2 as a guide. See whether you can anticipate what type of examination and testing the provider may need to do.

Body Measurements and Vital Signs

Words to Know Challenge

Spelling: Each line contains three spellings of a word. Underline the correctly spelled word.

1. afibrile   afebrile   effebrial

2. aral   oural   aural

3. bradypnea   bradipenia   braedypenia

4. fatil   fatal   fatel

5. ideopathic   idiopathic   edeopathic

6. menstration   menstruation   mensuration

7. orthostatic   orthastatic   orthostatec

8. pirogen   pyragen   pyrogen

9. sphygmomanometer   spygmonometer   spygmomanometer

10. sistole   systole   systoli

Fill in the Blank: Complete the following sentences with Words to Know from this chapter.
(*Hint*: You will use some correctly spelled words from the preceding Spelling section.)

1. Identify the four vital signs in the following sentences, indicating which body function is being measured:

   a. _____ measures the force of the heart.

   b. _____ measures the body's heat.

   c. _____ measures the action of the heart.

   d. _____ measures action of the lungs (breathing).

2. One respiration is the combination of one total inspiration and one total expiration. Two other terms that are frequently used and have the same meaning are _____ and _____ .

3. Patients with difficult or labored breathing are said to have _____ .

4. The absence of breathing is known as _____ .

5. Blood pressure is measured using a(n) _____ and a(n) _____ .

6. A sphygmomanometer has a(n) _____ dial.

7. An elevated pressure without apparent cause is said to be _____ or _____ hypertension.

8. Excessively rapid and deep respirations are known as _____ .

9. Taking a patient's temperature in the armpit is also known as the _____ method.

10. Another term for a patient running a fever is _____ .

Chapter Review

Short Answer: Using material from the chapter, provide a short answer in the space provided.

1. Name five types of mensurations. Why are mensurations particularly important with infants and children?

   _____

   _____

   _____

2. Explain why and when a patient's height and weight are measured.

   _____

   _____

   _____

3. If a patient measures 70 inches, how much is that in feet and inches?

   _____

   _____

   _____

4. List five types of thermometers.

   _____

   _____

   _____

5. Name at least three situations in which oral temperature measurement is contraindicated.

   _____

   _____

   _____

6. Identify when a patient may be asked to monitor his or her weight at home. What suggestions could you make to a patient about measuring his or her weight?

   _____

   _____

   _____

7. What is the normal adult rate pulse range? Discuss how pulse rate is determined and list five factors that affect the pulse rate.

   _____

   _____

   _____

8. Name two qualities of the heartbeat that must be observed, defining the terms and listing the words to describe the characteristics.

   a. _____
   _____
   _____

   b. _____
   _____
   _____

9. Why are respirations measured as the pulse is being measured?

   _____
   _____
   _____

10. What is the normal respiration rate for an adult?

    _____
    _____
    _____

11. Define *blood pressure* and then name the two phases of blood pressure, describing the corresponding action that occurs and the relative amount of pressure with each phase.

    _____
    _____
    _____

12. Define "auscultatory gap." _____

    _____
    _____

13. Explain indications for apical pulse measurements.

    _____
    _____
    _____
    _____

14. Identify normal and abnormal blood pressure, including factors affecting blood pressure.

    _____
    _____
    _____
    _____

Matching: Match the routes of measuring temperature listed in column I with the corresponding normal average temperature for that route in column II.
(*Hint*: Answers in column II may be used more than once.)

COLUMN I	COLUMN II
____ 1. Aural temperature	A. 97.6°F
____ 2. Axillary temperature	B. 98.6°F
____ 3. Oral temperature	C. 99.1°F
____ 4. Temporal artery temperature	D. 99.6°F
____ 5. Rectal temperature	

Labeling: Identify the labels in the following diagram, indicating the different sites where the pulse rate may be measured. Give an explanation for when or why the site is used.

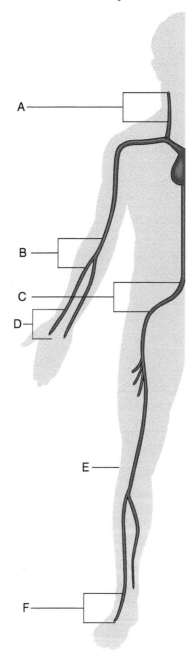

a. _____

b. _____

c. _____

d. _____

e. _____

f. _____

Chapter Application

Case Studies with Critical Thinking Questions

Scenario 1

The medical assistant is having difficulty taking Mrs. Anderson's pulse and respirations. She finally locates the radial pulse and then begins to count. There are some irregularities in the pulse, so the medical assistant counts it for one full minute. Mrs. Anderson is somewhat alarmed at how long this is taking and asks the medical assistant if something is wrong. The medical assistant then takes her finger off the pulse and tells Mrs. Anderson to breathe normally while she is counting the respirations.

1. Should the medical assistant tell the patient about her irregular pulse? _____
    _____
    _____

2. How could knowing this information affect the patient? _____
    _____
    _____

3. What mistake did the medical assistant make when counting the respirations? _____
    _____
    _____
    _____

Scenario 2

Carter always had trouble hearing blood pressures when he was in school, and the problem has carried over to his job. He cannot hear the blood pressure on a geriatric patient and is scared to admit this difficulty since this is only his second week on the job. Carter tries twice and gives up. He looks up the patient's last few readings and comes up with an average reading that he documents in the chart.

1. What should Carter do about his problem with hearing blood pressures? _____
    _____
    _____

2. Was it permissible for him to document the reading he averaged? _____
    _____
    _____

3. What possible implications might his actions have on the patient? _____
    _____
    _____
    _____

Conversion Exercises

1. Convert the following Celsius temperatures to Fahrenheit:

    a. 36.5°C = _____ °F   b. 35.7°C = _____ °F

    c. 39.5°C = _____ °F   d. 36.8°C = _____ °F

    e. 38.8°C = _____ °F   f. 37.4°C = _____ °F

2. Convert the following Fahrenheit temperatures to Celsius:

    a. 96.8°F = _____ °C   b. 99.2°F = _____ °C

    c. 97.4°F = _____ °C   d. 100.2°F = _____ °C

    e. 98.6°F = _____ °C   f. 102.4°F = _____ °C

3. The National Institutes of Health has published a BMI index chart that is easy to use, and many providers prefer to have this chart posted near the scale and in the exam rooms. You can access a copy of this chart on their website at www.nih.gov. Using the chart or calculation from the textbook and the following weights and heights, calculate the BMI for each:

a. 150 lbs/5'7 = _____   b. 212 lbs/5'4 = _____

c. 98 lbs/4'10 = _____   d. 260 lbs/6'1 = _____

e. 167 lbs/5'3 = _____   f. 137 lbs/5'1 = _____

Competency Practice

1. **Measure Height and Weight Using a Balance Beam Scale.** With a partner, practice setting the height bar and weights at different measurements and have the other partner read them. Then switch roles. When you get 10 in a row each correct, measure heights and weights on each other. In a mock patient chart or on HER software, document the height and weight. Refer to the textbook for charting examples. Use Procedure 36–1 as a guide.

2. **Measure and Record Oral, Axillary, Tympanic (core body), and Temporal Artery Temperatures.** Using all the types of thermometers available (disposable plastic, digital, electronic with oral probe, tympanic, and temporal artery), make a chart on a piece of paper, and obtain five of each temperature on different classmates. When finished, document two of the readings on a mock patient chart and two of the readings in an HER (if available). Use procedures that correspond as guides.

3. **Measure and Record Rectal Temperature with an Electronic Thermometer.** Using a mannequin, demonstrate the technique on obtaining a rectal temperature. Have a partner watch, critique, and provide feedback. Discuss when you should and should not use the rectal route to obtain the temperature. When finished, document on a mock patient chart or an HER. Use Procedure 36–3 as a guide.

4. **Measure the Apical Pulse.** With a partner, locate the apex of the heart and obtain an apical pulse on each other. Document your results on a mock patient chart or an HER. Use Procedure 36–7 as a guide.

5. **Measure Radial Pulse and Respirations.** With a partner, have one be the patient and the other be the medical assistant. Take turns performing the following exercises and then measure each other's pulse and respirations. Note the variations in the characteristics of your patient's pulse and respirations. Use Procedure 36–8 as a guide.

Sit in a chair quietly for three minutes.	
Walk around the classroom for a minute.	
Run in place for three minutes.	

6. **Measure Blood Pressure.** Obtain 10 blood pressures on different people and document on the following chart. Be sure to chart all the information requested. Use Procedure 36–9 as a guide.

Gender (male or female)	Age	Position (sitting, standing, or lying down)	Blood Pressure Result	Arm Used (right or left)

CHAPTER 37

Preparing for Examinations

Words to Know Challenge

Spelling: Each line contains three spellings of a word. Underline the correctly spelled word.

1. anatomical	annatomical	anatonical
2. dypsnea	dypnsea	dyspnea
3. fenastrated	fenetrated	fenestrated
4. lithotamy	lithotomy	litothomy
5. recumbent	recumbant	recunbant
6. supin	soopine	supine
7. Trendalenburg	Trendelenburg	Trendelenberg
8. aunterior	anteriour	anterior
9. incompatent	incompetent	incompetant
10. Fowler's	Fawler's	Foyler's

Fill in the Blank: Complete the following sentences with Words to Know from this chapter.

1. _______________ pertains to the back.
2. If someone is lying flat and even, level, and parallel to the plane of the horizon, he or she is said to be _______________.
3. The _______________ position is used for rectal or _______________ examinations and occasionally for a _______________ if a special table is not available.
4. The Trendelenburg position is most commonly used for a patient suffering from _______________.
5. _______________ pertains to the anterior or front side of the body.
6. If a patient is lying horizontal, with his or her face down, he or she is said to be in the _______________ position.
7. The _______________ position is an examination position in which the patient is lying on his or her left side.

Chapter Review

Short Answer

1. For what purpose is each of the following examination positions used?

   a. Horizontal recumbent or supine _____

   _____

   b. Dorsal recumbent _____

   _____

   c. Prone _____

   _____

   d. Anatomical _____

   _____

   e. Sims' or lateral _____

   _____

   f. Knee-chest _____

   _____

   g. Fowler's _____

   _____

   h. Lithotomy _____

   _____

   i. Trendelenburg _____

   _____

   j. Jackknife or Kraske _____

2. What safety precautions must be observed for protection of both the patient and you when moving patients?

   _____

   _____

3. Why is a drape used when positioning patients?

   _____

   _____

4. What support is used for the feet in the lithotomy position?

   _____

   _____

5. What is the name of the drape that has an opening for examination?

   _____

   _____

6. It is routine to check for supplies when preparing an examination room. List 13 supplies you must routinely check for.

   _____

   _____

7. Explain exam room cleanup and equipment that may need to be disinfected following patient examination.

   _____

   _____

   _____

   _____

   _____

   _____

   _____

   _____

Labeling: Label the following illustrations, indicating the various examination positions.

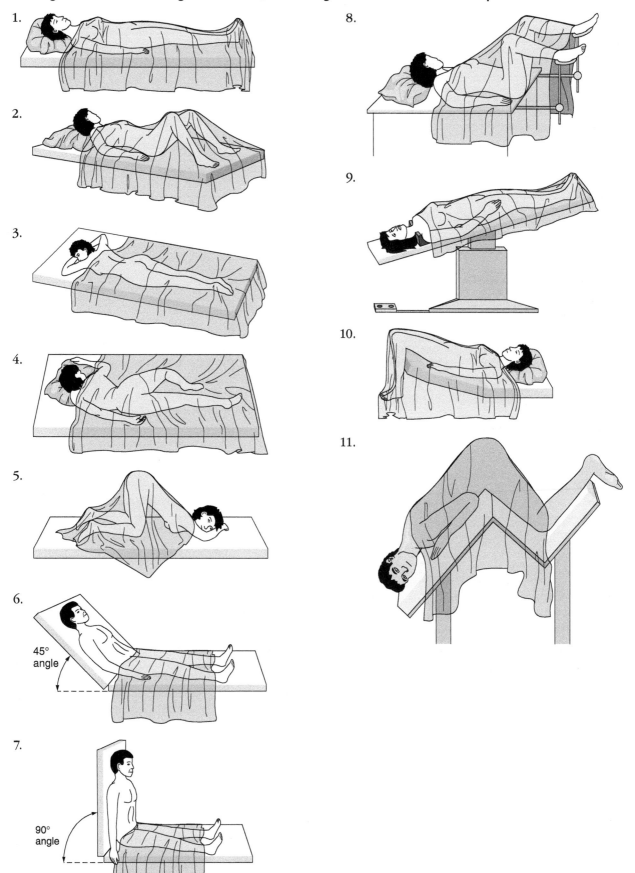

1.

2.

3.

4.

5.

6.

45°
angle

7.

90°
angle

8.

9.

10.

11.

1. _____
2. _____
3. _____
4. _____
5. _____
6. _____
7. _____
8. _____
9. _____
10. _____
11. _____

Chapter Application

Case Studies with Critical Thinking Questions

Scenario 1

Kelly escorts Mrs. Leonard into the exam room for her yearly Pap test and pelvic exam. Kelly didn't have time to clean the room before escorting Mrs. Leonard to the back office, so she asks her to have a seat on the stool while she tidies the room. She disposes of the used gown and table paper and sets up all the supplies. She then asks Mrs. Leonard to disrobe and prepares her for the exam.

1. What was Kelly's first *big* mistake? _____
   _____
   _____

2. What should Mrs. Leonard have been instructed to do before disrobing? _____
   _____
   _____

3. Should equipment and supplies be set up in the presence of the patient? _____
   _____
   _____

Scenario 2

Mr. Johnson is being seen in the office for a sigmoidoscopy. The medical assistant gives Mr. Johnson disrobing instructions and leaves the room for a few minutes. When she returns, she places Mr. Johnson in the knee-chest position, and he complains about how uncomfortable it is for him. The medical assistant assures the patient that it will be only a few more minutes before the provider is ready.

1. When should the patient have been placed into the position for the exam? _____
   _____
   _____
   _____

2. What should the medical assistant have done to make the patient more comfortable? _____
   _____
   _____

3. What is an alternative position that can be used for this procedure? _____
   _____
   _____

Competency Practice

1. **Prepare and Maintain Examination and Treatment Areas.** With a partner, practice setting up an examination room for a patient coming in for a complete physical examination. Be sure to include all the supplies and equipment needed. On a blank sheet of paper, design a checklist that can be used for cleaning, maintenance, and inventory for the room. Use critical thinking skills to determine what the list should include. Use Procedure 37–1 as a guide.

2. **Transfer a Patient from a Wheelchair to the Examination Table.** Using a classmate for a partner, demonstrate the proper technique for transferring a patient from a wheelchair to the examination table. Try practicing with two people assisting the transfer. This may be needed if you are working with a large patient or with a patient who is unable to bear weight at all. Use Procedure 37–2 as a guide.

3. **Transfer a Patient from the Examination Table to a Wheelchair.** Using a classmate for a partner, demonstrate the proper technique for transferring a patient from the examination table to a wheelchair. Try practicing with two people assisting the transfer. This may be needed if you are working with a large patient or with a patient who is unable to bear weight at all. Use Procedure 37–3 as a guide.

4. **Positioning the Patient for an Exam.** Using either a classmate or a mannequin, demonstrate placing the patient into a variety of positions that may be used for the provider examination. Be sure to use proper draping techniques as well. Use Procedure 37–4 as a guide.

Assisting with Examinations

The Physical Exam

Words to Know Challenge

Spelling: Each line contains three spellings of a word. Underline the correctly spelled word.

1.	auscultation	auscutatuion	asscultation
2.	menipulation	manipulation	maniputation
3.	bimanual	bymanual	bimanule
4.	bruet	bruit	brute
5.	gate	gait	gaite
6.	hurnia	hernea	hernia
7.	scribe	ascribe	scrabe
8.	psyical	fisicle	physical
9.	inspection	inspecktion	inspecscion
10.	pelpation	palpation	pallpation

Matching: Match the term in column I to its definition in column II.

COLUMN I

COLUMN II

____ 1. Physical

A. Pertains to a portion of the nervous system

____ 2. Bimanual

B. Measures the volume of inhaled and exhaled air

____ 3. Bruits

C. Two-handed; with both hands

____ 4. Spirometer

D. One part exactly corresponds to another in size, shape, and position

____ 5. Symmetry

E. Pertaining to the body; used for the examination of the body

____ 6. Peripheral

F. Projection of a part from its normal location

____ 7. Hernias

G. Obscure; hidden

____ 8. Occult

H. An adventitious sound of venous or arterial origin heard on auscultation

Fill in the Blank: Complete the following sentences with Words to Know from this chapter.

1. _____ , quality, _____ , and _____ are terms that refer to _____ .

2. _____ is a visual exam of the body's various parts.

3. The heel-to-shin test and the heel-to-toe test are used to check the patient's _____ .

4. Using one finger of a gloved hand, the provider will perform a _____ to palpate the rectum to check for abnormalities.

5. When performing percussion, the provider listens to the sounds to determine the size, density, and location of underlying _____ organs.

6. _____ of the skin is measured by pinching the back of the hand and observing the length of time for it to return to normal.

7. The _____ documents the provider's dictation during an exam.

8. _____ is used to screen for occult blood in the stool.

Chapter Review

Short Answer

1. Describe the role of the medical assistant in the patient examination process. _____
   _____
   _____

2. During the physical exam, what might your role entail regarding patient education?
   _____
   _____
   _____

3. Name the six examination techniques and provide an example of each.
   a. _____
   b. _____
   c. _____
   d. _____
   e. _____
   f. _____

4. Name four areas of the body that will be examined during the review of systems, and describe the patient's position and equipment and supplies needed for each.
   _____
   _____
   _____

5. Describe the six steps included when performing patient education for the breast self-examination (BSE).

   a. _____

   b. _____

   c. _____

   d. _____

   e. _____

   f. _____

6. Describe the five steps included when performing patient education for the testicular self-examination (TSE).

   a. _____

   b. _____

   c. _____

   d. _____

   e. _____

On the following table, enter the organs in the abdominal area in which they are primarily located.

ascending colon	appendix	cecum
descending colon	gallbladder	left ovary
left spermatic cord	liver	pancreas
pregnant uterus	right ovary	right spermatic cord
sigmoid colon	spleen	stomach
transverse colon	urinary bladder	

Abdominal Area	Organs
Right hypochondriac	
Epigastric	
Left hypochondriac	
Right lumbar	
Umbilical	
Left lumbar	
Right inguinal	
Hypogastric	
Left inguinal	

Chapter Application

Case Studies with Critical Thinking Questions

Scenario 1

The medical assistant escorts Mr. Carter into the examination room to prepare him for a complete physical exam. He tells the assistant that he hasn't been seen by a physician for 10 years. After weighing the patient and taking his vital signs, she instructs Mr. Carter to use the restroom and collect a clean catch sample. Mr. Carter is confused and can't possibly remember all those instructions, so he just collects a specimen in a cup. She then tells Mr. Carter to disrobe and wait for the provider. Mr. Carter says he is anxious and doesn't understand why he has to do all these things. The medical assistant tells him to just relax and that the provider will be in soon.

1. List some reasons the patient might be anxious. _____

_____

_____

2. Will the specimen Mr. Carter collected be accurate for testing? _____

_____

_____

3. What should the medical assistant have done to calm Mr. Carter's fears? _____

_____

_____

Scenario 2

Mrs. Karnes is being seen today because she found a lump in her breast. When the provider enters the room, he finds Mrs. Karnes in tears. She is still in her street clothes, and the provider is quite upset that his normally efficient medical assistant did not properly prepare this patient for an exam.

1. How should the patient have been prepared for the exam? _____

_____

_____

2. What can this do to the provider's schedule? _____

_____

_____

3. How might the medical assistant have served the needs of the patient better? _____

_____

_____

_____

Competency Practice

1. **Prepare a Patient for and Assist with a Routine Physical Examination.** Create a table listing all the parts of a complete physical exam, along with the medical assisting duties for each part. Include a review of systems and be sure to list the medical assisting duties for each system. Use Procedure 38–1 as a guide.

Specialty Examinations and Procedures

Words to Know Challenge

Spelling: Each line contains three spellings of a word. Underline the correctly spelled word.

1. <u>acuity</u>   acuety   acuitie
2. tonameter   <u>tonometer</u>   tonnameter
3. <u>Jaeger chart</u>   Jagger chart   jayger chart
4. Escihara   <u>Ishihara</u>   Ischihara
5. pulse oxemetry   <u>pulse oximetry</u>   pulse auximetry
6. ennima   enima   <u>enema</u>
7. <u>laxative</u>   laxetive   laxitive
8. luman   luemen   <u>lumen</u>
9. <u>mucosa</u>   mucousa   mycousa
10. obtruator   <u>obturator</u>   abturator
11. evakuant   evacuent   <u>evacuant</u>
12. <u>occluder</u>   ocluder   aucluder

Matching: Match the term in column I to its definition in column II.

COLUMN I	COLUMN II
____ 1. Audiometer	A. Means "to wash out"
____ 2. Acuity	B. Unit for measuring volume of sound
____ 3. Cerumen	C. Medical term for earwax
____ 4. Decibel	D. Another word for lavage
____ 5. Irrigate	E. Clarity/sharpness of perception
____ 6. Lavage	F. Instrument that measures hearing

(continues)

275

© 2017 Cengage Learning. All Rights Reserved. May not be scanned, copied or duplicated, or posted to a publicly accessible website, in whole or in part.

____	7. Snellen Chart	G.	A screening tool for near vision acuity
____	8. Jaeger Chart	H.	A screening tool for distant visual acuity
____	9. Guaiac test paper	I.	Test for occult blood in stool
____	10. Enema	J.	Part of preparation for sigmoidoscopy

Fill in the Blank: Complete the following sentences with Words to Know from this chapter.

1. Screening patients for color vision acuity is done with _____ color plates.

2. In the Weber test, the vibrating tuning fork is held against the _____ or against the skull or forehead in the midline.

3. Rectal examinations may be performed by using a _____ or a _____ to get a better view of the colon.

4. An evacuant is used to expel _____ matter from the colon.

5. Side vision while looking straight forward is known as _____ vision.

6. Lung capacity can be measured by a _____ or a _____ meter.

7. As part of an eye examination, _____ and _____ are recommended every four years for patients past 40 years old.

8. The patient covers one eye with an _____ so each eye may be tested individually when performing the Snellen exam.

9. _____ is defined as the greatest volume of air that can be expelled during a complete, slow, unforced expiration following a maximum inspiration.

10. A simple, noninvasive test that measures the patient's pulse rate and oxygen saturation level in the blood is known as a _____ test.

Chapter Review

Short Answer

1. What must the medical assistant remember to do with the ophthalmoscope and otoscope in preparing for eye and ear examinations? _____

_____

_____

2. What types of patients will require testing for visual acuity with the letter E chart? _____

_____

_____

3. What is the Ishihara screening method, and why is it administered to patients? _____

_____

_____

4. What is the purpose of eye irrigation? _____

_____

_____

5. What is cerumen? Why must impacted cerumen be softened and irrigated from the ear?

_____

_____

_____

6. Describe the Rinne test for hearing. _____

_____

_____

7. Describe the Weber test for hearing. _____

_____

_____

8. List common behaviors that can indicate hearing loss. _____

_____

_____

9. List common complaints that can indicate visual disturbances. _____

_____

_____

10. What is the purpose of the audiometer? _____

_____

_____

Chapter Application

Case Studies with Critical Thinking Questions

The provider asks the medical assistant to irrigate a patient's ear for removal of impacted cerumen. She prepares the irrigating solution but can't find the thermometer to check the temperature of the solution. She inserts the syringe straight into the ear and begins irrigation. While the medical assistant is irrigating the patient's ear, the patient complains of pain and a burning sensation in the ear. The medical assistant continues the irrigation anyway, despite the patient's complaints, because the provider is in a hurry and is running behind.

1. Should the medical assistant have continued with the irrigation after the patient complained about pain and a burning sensation? _____

_____

_____

2. What could be the outcome of continuing with the irrigation? _____

_____

_____

3. Did the medical assistant have the syringe properly positioned? _____

_____

_____

Competency Practice

1. **Irrigate the Ear.** Using a mannequin, demonstrate the technique for irrigating the ear. Have a partner watch, critique, and provide feedback. Discuss the equipment available for use to perform the procedure and what the pros and cons are for each. When finished, document in a mock patient chart or an EHR. Use Procedure 39–1 as a guide.

2. **Perform Audiometry Screening.** In pairs, have one student be the patient and the other be the medical assistant. Take turns screening hearing with an audiometer. When finished document in a mock patient chart or EHR. Use Procedure 39–2 as a guide.

3. **Irrigate the Eye.** In pairs, have one student be the patient and the other be the medical assistant. The medical assistant should set up all the necessary equipment and supplies for eye irrigation and mimic the procedure without actually using any solution. Discuss the importance of irrigating from the inner canthus to the outer canthus and reasons the eye(s) might need irrigation. When finished, document in a mock patient chart or an EHR. Use Procedure 39–3 as a guide.

4. **Screen Visual Acuity with a Snellen Chart.** In pairs, have one student be the patient and the other be the medical assistant. Take turns screening visual acuity with a Snellen chart. When finished, document in a mock patient chart or an EHR. Use Procedure 39–4 as a guide.

5. **Screen Visual Acuity with the Jaeger System.** In pairs, have one student be the patient and the other be the medical assistant. Take turns screening visual acuity with a Jaeger chart. When finished, document in a mock patient chart or an EHR. Use Procedure 39–5 as a guide.

6. **Determine Color Vision Acuity by the Ishihara Method.** In pairs, have one student be the patient and the other be the medical assistant. Take turns screening color vision with the Ishihara method. Discuss the importance of color vision testing and make a list of the occupations in which color vision is critical. When finished, document in a mock patient chart or an EHR. Use Procedure 39–6 as a guide.

7. **Perform Spirometry Testing.** In pairs, have one student be the patient and the other be the medical assistant. Take turns performing spirometry testing on each other. Be sure when you are the MA to coach the patient to assist in obtaining the best results possible. When finished, document in a mock patient chart or an EHR. Use Procedure 39–7 as a guide.

8. **Perform Peak Flow Testing.** In pairs, have one student be the patient and the other be the medical assistant. Take turns educating each other on how to perform a peak flow measurement and how to obtain the patient's personal best. Discuss what the three zones are and what a patient would be advised, depending on which zone his or her result was in. When finished, document in a mock patient chart or an EHR. Use Procedure 39–8 as a guide.

9. **Measure and Record Pulse Oximetry Testing.** In pairs, have one student be the patient and the other be the medical assistant. Take turns performing a pulse oximetry measurement on each other. Discuss what you would need to do if the patient was an infant, had dark nail polish on, or had calloused fingers. When finished, document in a mock patient chart or an EHR. Use Procedure 39–9 as a guide.

10. **Assist with a Flexible Sigmoidoscopy.** Using a mannequin and a classmate, role-play one being the provider and the other the MA. Demonstrate assisting the provider with a flexible sigmoidoscope. Use your critical thinking skills to determine what would be the next steps and what your role is. Discuss the equipment used to perform the procedure and what the cleanup process is after the procedure is complete, including chemically sterilizing the scope. Use Procedure 39–10 as a guide.

CHAPTER 40

OB/GYN Examinations

Words to Know Challenge

Spelling: Each line contains three spellings of a word. Underline the correctly spelled word.

1. cervical   servical   cervacal

2. fundas   fundes   fundus

3. gestation   jestation   guestation

4. Lamazae   Lamaze   Lemaze

5. trymester   triemister   trimester

Matching: Match the term in column I to its definition in column II.

	COLUMN I	COLUMN II
____	1. Atypical	A. Fetus in the uterus
____	2. Cytology	B. Not the usual
____	3. Douche	C. Before birth
____	4. Endocervical	D. Cells shedding
____	5. Exfoliated	E. Method to estimate expected date of delivery
____	6. Naegele's rule	F. Physician who developed cervical cancer test
____	7. Papanicolaou	G. Within the cervix
____	8. Pregnancy	H. Cleansing the vagina
____	9. Prenatal	I. Inflammation of the vagina
____	10. Vaginitis	J. Study of cells

Fill in the Blank: Complete the following sentences with Words to Know from this chapter.

1. In place of the conventional Pap test, many providers are now using a liquid-based method known as _____ .

2. Another name for a birth class is _____ .

3. Pap smears are sent to the _____ department to be analyzed.

4. During the prenatal examination, you assist the provider as appropriate for the _____ of the patient's _____ .

5. A flexible centimeter tape is used to measure the height of the _____ from the symphysis pubis bone to evaluate the growth of the fetus.

6. Women should be especially conscientious in scheduling Pap tests if they have a family history of uterine or _____ cancer.

7. Patients should be advised not to _____ for 48 hours prior to their Pap test because it could wash away _____ cells.

Chapter Review

Short Answer

1. List five reasons the liquid-based Pap test is preferred.

   a. _____

   b. _____

   c. _____

   d. _____

   e. _____

2. When is the FocalPoint (AutoPap) used? _____
   _____
   _____
   _____

3. Identify the four main guidelines regarding patient preparation for a Pap test.

   a. _____

   b. _____

   c. _____

   d. _____

4. Why should you have a female patient empty her bladder before a pelvic exam?
   _____
   _____
   _____

5. Why is BSE necessary when a patient has an annual provider examination?
   _____

6. What are the three main categories for reporting Pap results?

   a. _____

   b. _____

   c. _____

7. List the responsibilities of the medical assistant during a prenatal office visit.

_____
_____
_____
_____

8. How can pregnancy be confirmed?

_____
_____

Fill in the Blank: Using material from the chapter, fill in the answers in the space provided.

1. Initial Pap screening should begin after a female patient turns _____ years old.

2. At 30 years old, if the woman has had _____ normal tests in a row, she may get screened every _____ to _____ years unless she has _____ factors.

3. Women over 30 may elect to have screenings every _____ years if they also have the _____ test.

4. If 65 or older, women who have had _____ Pap test findings in _____ years in a row and no _____ findings in _____ years, and do not have any _____ factors, may stop Pap screenings.

5. Women with total _____ may stop screenings unless the surgery was done to treat _____ .

6. Gynecological instruments, in addition to the speculum, are used for examinations and procedures. The _____ measures uterine depth. The _____ scrapes the lining for a specimen. A small piece of tissue may be removed with the _____ .

Chapter Application

Case Studies with Critical Thinking Questions

Scenario 1

Lyn is being seen today for her Pap test and pelvic exam. She was given preparation instructions prior to her appointment. After the medical assistant prepares Lyn for her exam, Lyn says she is on the last day of her period and figured it would be fine to have the Pap test anyway, since her flow was light. Lyn also tells the medical assistant that she and her husband are trying to get pregnant and have been having intercourse every night for the past month.

1. Will the physician be able to collect a specimen for the Pap test? _____

_____
_____

2. What should the medical assistant have done before prepping the patient for the exam? _____

_____
_____

3. When is the best time for the patient to have her Pap test? _____

_____
_____

Scenario 2

Amanda calls the office to report that she is cramping and spotting. She is at 28 weeks' gestation. The first available appointment the provider has is two days from now. Amanda is very anxious and asks if she is having a miscarriage.

1. What should the office scheduling person have done about an appointment time for Amanda? _____

_____

_____

2. What should the medical assistant tell Amanda about her condition? _____

_____

_____

3. Who should the medical assistant consult about Amanda's problems? _____

_____

_____

Competency Practice

1. Prepare the Patient for and Assist with a Gynecological Exam and Pap Test.

In groups of four, role-play preparing the patient and assisting the provider with a gynecological exam and Pap test. Assign each person in the group to one of the following roles: narrator, provider, MA, and patient. Using Procedure 40–1 and the evaluation form below, evaluate the group's performance of the procedure (including completeness and preparedness) and communication skills (verbal and nonverbal). The final calculated grade or evaluation will be determined by your evaluation, the instructor's evaluation, and the group's evaluation. The instructor will use this same evaluation form, and a combined evaluation will be used for feedback to the group.

Group Project Evaluation

Prepare the Patient for and Assist with a Gynecological Exam and Pap Test

Based on the performance, give feedback and rate your group according to the following scale:

1 = poor	2 = fair	3 = good	4 = exceptional

Verbal Communication	1	2	3	4

- Communication was complete and concise with only necessary information given to the patient.
- The information given to the patient was clear (using good diction and enunciating each word distinctly). The message was audible. The MA did not use technical terms with patient.
- Patient was allowed time to process the message and verify its meaning.
- MA established rapport with the patient, acknowledging the patient by name.

Feedback: _____

_____

_____

_____

Nonverbal Communication	1	2	3	4

- MA smiled when greeting patient, used appropriate facial expression according to the situation, and maintained appropriate eye contact.
- Maintained a close but comfortable position facing the patient without standing over her; respected patient's personal space.
- Used appropriate gestures to enhance communication, used appropriate touch, and displayed empathy with the patient.
- Respected patient privacy by keeping patient covered during exam.

Feedback: _____

_____

_____

_____

_____

Performance	1	2	3	4

- Group performed the procedure within 25 minutes.
- MA performed or role-played each step within Procedure 41–1. (Refer to competency assessment.)
- MA carried out each step correctly, including positioning the patient.
- Group members acted professionally.

Feedback: _____

_____

_____

_____

_____

Preparedness	1	2	3	4

- Equipment and supplies were gathered prior to procedure.
- Group members seemed well-prepared.
- Procedure and scenario flowed naturally.
- Each member was aware of his or her role and responsibilities.

Feedback: _____

_____

_____

_____

_____

Final Score _____ / **16 pts**

Pediatric Examinations

Words to Know Challenge

Spelling: Each line contains three spellings of a word. Underline the correctly spelled word.

1. circumfrence   circumference   circumphrence

2. attachment   attachtment   atachtment

3. listlessness   listlesness   lislessness

4. prevantive   preventive   preventiv

5. intercede   interceed   intersceed

6. suscpicion   suspiscion   suspicion

7. malnutrition   mallnutrition   malnutrision

8. letharjic   lethargic   lethargick

Matching: Match the key term in column I to its definition in column II.

COLUMN I	COLUMN II
____ 1. Pediatrics	A. Attachment of two persons
____ 2. Apgar	B. Inflicting emotional, physical, or sexual injury
____ 3. Child neglect	C. Lack of or withholding of care
____ 4. Child abuse	D. Advancement of abilities and knowledge
____ 5. Development	E. Scoring system used on infants after birth
____ 6. Bonding	F. Specialty medical practice that cares for infants and children
____ 7. Caregiver	G. Arrangement of events or dates in order of occurrence
____ 8. Chronologic	H. Person responsible for another's care and well-being
____ 9. Percentile	I. Lack of vigorous growth
____ 10. Failure to thrive	J. Used on a growth chart to compare a child to his or her peers

Chapter Review

Fill in the Blank: Use information from the chapter to fill in the blank space in the sentence.

1. The American Academy of Pediatrics (AAP) has established _____ _____, a chart that outlines the types and frequency of examinations to provide preventive care for normally developing, healthy children.

2. Pediatric care is usually continued until age _____ or upon high school graduation.

3. An infant's growth refers to changes in _____ and _____.

4. An infant should be examined at _____ month intervals for the first 18 months of life.

5. Poor hygiene, inadequate clothing size, and apparent malnutrition are signs of _____.

6. Infants usually crawl at _____ months of age.

7. Most infants will walk between _____ months of age.

8. The _____ program, Medicaid's comprehensive and preventive child health program, is for individuals under the age of _____.

9. An infant's weight should be taken with his or her _____ removed.

10. Children older than _____ months can have their height measured on an upright scale.

Short Answer

1. Explain the difference between child abuse and neglect. _____
   _____
   _____

2. List five signs of abuse.
   _____
   _____
   _____

3. List five signs of neglect.
   _____
   _____
   _____

4. Explain the difference between a well-child and a sick-child visit. _____
   _____
   _____
   _____
   _____
   _____

5. List five responsibilities of the medical assistant when assisting with pediatric exams. _____
   _____
   _____

6. Identify immunizations given to infants and children at various ages according to the Childhood and Adolescent Immunization Schedule. _____
   _____
   _____

7. Identify two charts that assess pediatric vision acuity and explain how each is used.
   _____
   _____
   _____

Chapter Application

Case Studies with Critical Thinking Questions

Scenario 1

Jane, the medical assistant, escorts a 19-year-old single mother and her 6-month-old infant to the exam room. Jane observes that both the mother and child are wearing soiled clothing. The mother's hygiene is poor, and the infant has dried mucus around his nose and food stuck to his cheeks. While weighing and measuring the infant, Jane notices red marks on his bottom and his thigh.

1. What could Jane's observations indicate? _____

   _____

   _____

2. What should Jane do about what she has observed? _____

   _____

   _____

Scenario 2

Mrs. Leonard brings her son, Carter, into the office for his well-child checkup. He is very agitated today, and Amy, the medical assistant, is having a great deal of difficulty measuring and weighing him. Amy tries to measure his recumbent length with a tape measure but is not sure whether she can obtain an accurate measurement because she is unable to straighten the child's legs. Carter is squirming on the scale, and it is difficult to balance it. When Amy attempts to record the measurement on Carter's growth chart, she finds that the measurements are lower than at his last visit.

1. What should Amy do about the discrepancy in the measurements? _____

   _____

   _____

2. Were Amy's methods of measurement accurate? _____

   _____

   _____

3. What could Amy have done to help remedy the situation? _____

   _____

   _____

Competency Practice

1. **Measure Length, Weight, and Head and Chest Circumference of an Infant or Child.** Use infant and child mannequins and practice obtaining the length, weight, head circumference, and chest circumference. Use Procedure 41–1 as a guide. Document a mock patient chart entry in the following space, or enter into an EMR and on a growth chart. You can download appropriate growth charts from the CDC's website at www.cdc.gov.

2. **Plot Data on a Growth Chart.** Use the following scenario information and a growth chart to practice plotting measurements on growth charts for both female and male patients and age groups. Be sure also to fill in the data on the bottom of the growth chart with the measurements provided. Use Procedure 41–2 as a guide. You can download appropriate growth charts from the CDC's website at www.cdc.gov.

A. Use a growth chart for **GIRLS** to plot the following measurements.

Age	Weight	Length
1 month	8 lb. 10 oz.	21"
2 months	11 lb. 6 oz.	22 ½"
3 months	14 lb. 8 oz.	24"
6 months	18 lb.	26 ½"
9 months	23 lb. 4 oz.	28 ¼"
12 months	24 lb. 7 oz.	31 ½"
15 months	26 lb. 10 oz.	32"

B. Use a growth chart for **BOYS** to plot the following measurements.

Age	Head Circumference Measurement
1 month	14 ¾"
6 months	17 ½"
12 months	18 ½'
20 months	19 ¼"
24 months	20"

C. Calculate the percentile of WEIGHT FOR LENGTH and plot, using the example growth chart for **BOYS**. Use rounded numbers to the nearest 5% (e.g., 10%, 15%, 20%; not 13%).

Weight	Length	Percentile
8#	20 ½"	_____
12#	24"	_____
25#	30 ¾"	_____
28#	32"	_____
36#	38"	_____

3. **Screen Pediatric Visual Acuity with a Modified Snellen Chart.** With a partner, have one person role-play a child patient and the other person the medical assistant. Take turns screening visual acuity with one of the modified Snellen charts listed in the chapter. When finished, document a mock patient chart entry in the following space or enter into an EMR. Use Procedure 41–3 as a guide.

Laboratory Procedures

CHAPTER 42

The Physician's Office Laboratory

Words to Know Challenge

Spelling: Each line contains three spellings of a word. Underline the correctly spelled word.

1. binnoculir	binocular	binoculare
2. compensate	conpemsate	compensait
3. prophicent	proficient	proficiant
4. microscopie	microscopee	microscopy
5. monocular	moncular	nomocular
6. waved	waived	wiaved
7. assurance	asurance	asurrance

Matching: Match each part of the microscope in column I with its description in column II.

COLUMN I	COLUMN II
_____ 1. Condenser	A. The result of combining the ocular and the lens for observation of a specimen
_____ 2. Objectives	B. An adjective describing the size of articles examined microscopically
_____ 3. Hpf	C. Part of the substage that regulates the amount of light directed on a specimen
_____ 4. Ocular	D. The part of the microscope on which slides are placed for viewing
_____ 5. Magnification	E. Part of the microscope that helps bring the specimen on the slide into sharper view
_____ 6. Minute	F. Three or four small lenses that have different magnifying powers
_____ 7. Stage	G. Magnifies an object about 10 times
_____ 8. Lpf	H. Magnifies an object about 40 times

Chapter Review

Short Answer

1. Explain why quality assurance (QA) and quality control (QC) are of the utmost importance in any laboratory setting.

   _____

   _____

   _____

   _____

2. Identify three categories of testing within the laboratory setting.

   a. _____

   b. _____

   c. _____

3. List four forms of basic recommended personal protective equipment (PPE) that can be used when collecting specimens from patients.

   a. _____

   b. _____

   c. _____

   d. _____

4. Why is proper hand washing an important consideration when working in the laboratory and with patients?

   _____

   _____

   _____

5. List and define two of the regulatory bodies the POL falls under.

   a. _____

   b. _____

6. Describe the process in compliance reporting of unsafe activities, errors in patient care, and incident reports.

   _____

   _____

   _____

   _____

7. Describe the importance of safety data sheets (SDS) in a health care setting.

   _____

   _____

8. Discuss protocols for disposal of biological chemical materials.

   _____

   _____

   _____

9. Describe three examples of evaluating the medical office environment for safety compliance.

   _____

   _____

   _____

   _____

Chapter Application

Case Studies with Critical Thinking Questions

Scenario 1

As Mary Ramirez, the medical assistant, escorts the first patient into the exam room, she notices that the room is disorganized and that there is evidence of the last patient from the day before. Mary needs to take the patient's vitals and notices that the blood pressure cuff is missing, so she leaves the room to find it.

1. What might the patient's impression of the office be? _____
_____
_____

2. What should the medical assistant have done before bringing the patient to the exam room? _____
_____
_____

3. How can this situation be prevented in the future? _____
_____
_____

Scenario 2

While carrying a rack full of tubes containing blood to be discarded in the biohazard container, Jennifer slips and falls. The tubes scatter everywhere, but, fortunately, only three of them break. This accident occurred in the main hallway, so Jennifer needs to think fast and get this mess cleaned up.

1. What PPE should Jennifer apply? _____
_____
_____

2. Describe the steps Jennifer should use to clean up the spilled blood. _____
_____
_____
_____
_____

3. Where should the tubes be discarded? _____
_____
_____

Competency Practice

1. **Complete an Incident Report Related to an Error in Patient Care**. Using the following scenario, fill out an Unusual Occurrence Report (UOR) form. Use Procedure 42–1 as a guide. You can download the UOR form from the Student Companion website.

   Today's Date: Wednesday, October 3, 20XX

   Dominic Delgado is a certified medical assistant working for Dr. Roy Johnson in a busy pediatric family practice clinic. He begins his shift at 9 a.m. At 10:15 a.m., Dr. Johnson (the patient PCP) orders a pneumococcal vaccination for his patient, Tabitha Briggs, an alert, 65-year-old woman who is being seen for an annual physical examination. Dominic prepared the injection and administered it to the patient. After completion, while he was charting the injections in the patients' medical record, he realized that he administered an incorrect vaccine. He administered a flu vaccination instead of the pneumococcal vaccination that was ordered. Dominic alerted the provider immediately and reported the incident to the clinic manager, Alicia Smith, who requested the UOR form to be filled out. The provider disclosed the error to the patient, who was very understanding and did not appear to be too concerned as she was planning to get the flu shot at her next visit.

Employee Information:

Name: Dominic Delgado CMA

Patient Information:

Name: Tabitha Briggs

Address: 232 Cooper Lane

                   Wichita KS, 55119

Phone: (563) 555-1234

Employer Information:

Name: Wichita Family Practice

DOB: 05/05/XX

Health Plan: BXBS ID#26354 (HMO)

2. **Comply with Safety Signs, Symbols, and Labels.** Obtain a set of Hazardous Communications pictograms from www.osha.gov and cut them out. Paste them to a plain piece of paper, and list all of the areas that would be appropriate for the sign to be placed. Use Procedure 42–2 as a guide.

3. **Clean a Spill.** Gather all of the supplies and equipment needed to clean a spill, and practice cleaning up mock materials properly. Use Procedure 42–3 as a guide.

4. **Demonstrate Proper Use of Eyewash Equipment.** Use Procedure 42–4 as a guide and complete the steps included in using the eyewash equipment. Have a classmate or partner check off the steps and critique your process as you complete the task.

5. **Demonstrate Fire Preparedness.** Using Procedure 42–5 as a guide, complete the scenarios and steps included. Have a classmate or partner check off the steps and critique your process as you complete the task.

6. **Use a Microscope.** Practice the steps on how to use a microscope. Use Procedure 42–6 as a guide. Use slides that have already been prepared with specimens, or cut out letters from a magazine and tape to the slide for focusing purposes.

CHAPTER 43

Specimen Collection and Processing

Words to Know Challenge

Spelling: Each line contains three spellings of a word. Underline the correctly spelled word.

1. guiac   gauiac   <u>guaiac</u>

2. <u>bilirubin</u>   billirubin   biliribun

3. urineanalysis   urinalisys   <u>urinalysis</u>

4. hemoturia   <u>hematuria</u>   hemituria

5. uribilinogen   uribilinogin   <u>urobilinogen</u>

Fill in the Blank: Complete the following sentences with Words to Know from this chapter.

1. Substance used to encourage bacterial growth: _____

2. The final step in the culture, during which various antibiotics are tested for bacterial inhibition: _____

3. Bacterial staining characteristic that yields a pinkish-red color: _____

4. Bacterial staining characteristic that yields a bluish-purple color: _____

5. Drainage from a wound or affected area: _____

6. The first step in the process to isolate and identify bacterial infections: _____

7. The destruction of red blood cells present in culture media: _____

Chapter Review

Short Answer

1. What is a culturette?

_____

_____

_____

2. When obtaining a throat swab for group A strep screening, what is the proper procedure for performing the swab?

_____

_____

_____

3. Identify three elements of a complete urinalysis. _____

_____

_____

4. Discuss the differences among random, first morning, clean-catch midstream, and 24-hour urine specimens.

    a. Random: _____

    _____

    b. First morning specimen: _____

    _____

    _____

    c. Clean-catch midstream: _____

    _____

    d. 24-hour specimen: _____

    _____

    _____

5. Name the three morphologic shapes and provide a description of each.

_____

_____

_____

6. Identify types of pathogens that can be checked for in fecal specimens.

_____

_____

_____

7. Which conditions might be diagnosed in a sputum specimen?

_____

_____

_____

Matching: Match the item in column I with its description in column II.

COLUMN I	COLUMN II
____ 1. Normal fecal occult blood	A. Confirmatory test for urinary ketones
____ 2. Specific gravity	B. Blood in the urine
____ 3. pH	C. Normal urine, slightly acidic
____ 4. Bilirubin	D. Positive in starvation
____ 5. Ketones	E. Confirmatory test for urinary protein
____ 6. SSA	F. Confirmatory test for urinary bilirubin
____ 7. Acetest	G. Pregnancy
____ 8. Ictotest	H. Negative
____ 9. Hematuria	I. Might indicate liver disease when detected
____ 10. Human chorionic gonadotropin	J. Concentration or dilution of urine specimen

Chapter Application

Case Studies with Critical Thinking Questions

Scenario 1

You are working in a multipractice clinic that has an in-house laboratory, including a microbiology lab. Part of your duties in the laboratory includes checking and recording temperatures for all refrigerators, freezers, and incubators used in the facility. You are checking the microbiology incubators and discover that one of them is registering a temperature of 10° Celsius.

1. Should you report this to anyone and, if so, who?

_____

_____

_____

2. What is a possible result of this temperature decrease?

_____

_____

_____

Scenario 2

You are working in the laboratory in the late afternoon and perform a pregnancy test on a patient of Janna Aron, the nurse practitioner at your clinic. The patient's test comes back negative, but the patient is adamant that she has already missed two menstrual periods and knows that she is pregnant.

1. What should you do next, and what might be the problem?

_____

_____

_____

2. What other options does the patient have?

_____

_____

_____

Competency Practice

1. **Instruct a Patient on the Collection of a Clean-Catch, Midstream Urine Specimen.** With a partner, gather the supplies needed to instruct a patient on the steps of collecting a midstream urine specimen, and role-play with one being the MA and one being the patient. Use Procedure 43–1 as a guide.

2. **Perform Screening for Pregnancy.** Using random urine specimens provided by classmates, urine QC (Quality Controls), and a waived pregnancy test kit, practice the process for completing controls and screening for pregnancy. Use Procedure 43–2 as a guide.

3. **Test Urine with Reagent Strips.** Using random urine specimens provided by classmates, urine QC, and a bottle of Multistix 10 SG reagent strips, practice testing urine controls and samples. Use Procedure 43–3 as a guide.

4. **Obtain Urine Sediment for Microscopic Examination.** Using Procedure 43–4 as a guide, practice preparing slides for microscopic examination using random urine samples from classmates.

5. **Screen and Follow Up Test Results.** Download a variety of test result documents from www.labtestsonline.org or obtain them from your instructor, and practice identifying any abnormalities by highlighting them or underlining them with a red pen. With a partner, simulate receiving orders from the provider and calling the patient with results and orders. Use Procedure 43–5 as a guide.

6. **Instruct a Patient to Collect a Stool Specimen.** Using the Procedure 43–6 as a guide, gather the supplies needed and with a partner simulate the instructions for collecting a sputum specimen.

7. **Perform an Occult Blood Test.** Obtain a fecal occult kit and with a partner simulate going over the patient education required for this test and instructions for collecting the specimens for this test. Using Procedure 43–7 as a guide, perform the steps required to test for fecal occult blood.

8. **Instruct a Patient to Collect a Sputum Specimen.** With a classmate, simulate the process of instructing a patient on how to obtain a sputum specimen. Use Procedure 43–8 as a guide.

9. **Perform a Wound Collection for Microbiologic Testing.** With a classmate or using an anatomical body part, simulate the collection process for obtaining a wound culture. Use Procedure 43–9 as a guide.

10. **Obtain a Throat Culture.** With a partner, practice obtaining throat cultures on each other and process to send out to a reference lab. Use Procedure 43–10 as a guide.

11. **Perform a Rapid Strep Screening Test for Group A Strep.** Using a waived rapid strep kit, practice performing rapid strep controls and tests on a partner. Use Procedure 43–11 as a guide.

Role-Play Activities

1. Research the health risks of untreated streptococcal infections. Write a short narrative of your findings and why these types of infections should be treated.

2. With a partner, role-play as a medical assistant and patient and take turns explaining the various types of urine collection.

CHAPTER 44

Blood Specimen Collection

Words to Know Challenge

Spelling: Each line contains three spellings of a word. Underline the correctly spelled word.

1. hemotoma   hematoma   hemitoma

2. tourniquet   tournequet   tournequette

3. flebotomy   phelbotomy   phlebotomy

4. elasticity   elastizity   ilasticity

5. plazma   palasma   plasma

Matching: Match the term in column I to its description in column II.

COLUMN I	COLUMN II
____ 1. Venipuncture	A. Without any organisms
____ 2. Sterile	B. To scatter or spread
____ 3. Lancet	C. Pertaining to a vein
____ 4. Diffuse	D. Used for a skin puncture
____ 5. Puncture	E. The size of a needle bore
____ 6. Venous	F. A hole made by something pointed
____ 7. Gauge	G. The surgical puncture of a vein

Chapter Review

Short Answer

1. Why is it important for the lancet to be positioned to cut across the fingerprints rather than parallel to them?

_____

_____

_____

2. Why should the lateral sides of the infant's heel be used for capillary puncture?

_____

_____

_____

3. Why is the first drop of blood wiped away from the capillary puncture site?

_____

_____

_____

4. Identify the acceptable sites to perform a capillary puncture on a patient's hand.

_____

5. During the venipuncture procedure, the tourniquet should not remain on the patient's arm for more than how long?

_____

6. What is the medical term for abnormal collection of blood immediately below the surface of the skin?

_____

7. The destruction of red blood cells is known as what?

_____

Matching: Match the item in column I with its description in column II.

COLUMN I	COLUMN II
____ 1. EDTA	A. Sodium heparin
____ 2. Gray stopper	B. Hematology testing, purple stopper
____ 3. Syringe	C. Blood cultures
____ 4. Butterfly	D. Serum separator tube (SST)
____ 5. Yellow stopper	E. Evacuated tube holder
____ 6. Red stopper	F. Prevents clotting
____ 7. Mustard or speckled stopper	G. Multisample needle for small veins
____ 8. Green stopper	H. Sodium fluoride, blood glucose
____ 9. Multisample capability	I. No additive
____ 10. Anticoagulant	J. Single-use venous collection device
____ 11. Blue stopper	K. Anticoagulant tubes
____ 12. Plasma	L. Sodium citrate, coagulation studies

Chapter Application

Case Studies with Critical Thinking Questions

Scenario 1

Ben has arrived for a venous blood test to check his liver function levels and glucose. In the process of collecting the specimen, you notice a hematoma is beginning to form and you have not completed filling all the necessary tubes for the tests.

1. Why would a hematoma develop as a result of phlebotomy?

   _____
   _____
   _____

2. What should you do?

   _____
   _____
   _____

Scenario 2

Mrs. Johnson has a laboratory order for you to collect a capillary specimen for a random blood glucose level. You assemble your supplies in preparation for collecting and testing the specimen; when you grasp her hand, you notice it is exceptionally cold.

1. What do Mrs. Johnson's cold hands indicate?

   _____
   _____
   _____

2. What instructions should you give Mrs. Johnson?

   _____
   _____
   _____

Competency Practice

1. **Puncture Skin with a Sterile Lancet.** Place the following steps of the capillary puncture procedure in their proper order from 1 to 10. Use Procedure 44–1 as a guide.

   _____ 1. Collect the specimen.

   _____ 2. Introduce yourself and identify the patient.

   _____ 3. Assemble the necessary supplies.

   _____ 4. Wipe away the first drop of blood.

   _____ 5. Provide the patient with a clean gauze to apply pressure to the site.

   _____ 6. Perform the puncture with the lancet, penetrating across the fingerprints.

   _____ 7. Allow the selected site to dry.

   _____ 8. Disinfect the site with alcohol.

   _____ 9. Don gloves.

   _____ 10. Dispose of lancet and contaminated materials in the appropriate biohazard containers.

2. **Obtain Venous Blood with a Sterile Needle and Syringe.** Working with a partner, practice how you would explain the venipuncture procedure using a sterile needle and syringe. Use Procedure 44–2 as a guide.

3. **Obtain Venous Blood with a Vacuum Tube.** Using an anatomical blood drawing arm or a classmate, practice performing venipuncture with a vacuum tube system. Use Procedure 44–3 as a guide.

4. **Obtain Venous Blood with the Butterfly Needle Method.** Using an anatomical blood drawing arm or a classmate, practice performing venipuncture with a butterfly system using both syringes and vacuum tubes. Use Procedure 44–4 as a guide.

CHAPTER 45

Diagnostic Testing

Words to Know Challenge

Spelling: Each line contains three spellings of a word. Underline the correctly spelled word.

1. poloysithemia | policythemia | polycythemia
2. wheel | wheal | weal
3. allergie | alergy | allergy
4. glycohemoglobin | glycohemaglobin | glycohemeglobin
5. esinofil | esinophil | eosinophil
6. imunology | immoonology | immunology
7. mononuclosis | mononucleosis | mononucleusis

Matching: Match the term in column I with its description in column II.

COLUMN I	COLUMN II
____ 1. Antibody	A. Released in allergic and inflammatory reactions
____ 2. Immune	B. Of or pertaining to the whole body
____ 3. Venom	C. Immunizing agent that produces antibodies
____ 4. Histamine	D. Protected or exempt from disease
____ 5. Systemic	E. A protein substance carried by cells to counteract effects of an antigen
____ 6. Antigen	F. A substance distilled or drawn out of another substance
____ 7. Extract	G. A poisonous toxin produced by several groups of animal species

Chapter Review

Short Answer

1. What two tests are commonly used in screening for anemia?

2. What test is used for diagnosis of diabetes mellitus?

3. Name two diseases associated with hypercholesterolemia.

4. Name two tests that may be performed in the POL for immunology testing.

5. What are the proper units of measurement for reporting hemoglobin and hematocrit results?

6. Describe patient education regarding allergy injections.

7. What are signs and symptoms of anaphylactic shock? What can be injected to prevent anaphylactic shock?

8. When performing intradermal tests, the antigen is introduced into the dermal layer of skin in what dosages?

9. From the following test results, place an X next to the values that would be considered a panic value.
   a. Hemoglobin (male), test result 10 g/dL: _____
   b. Hematocrit (female), test result 40%: _____
   c. Total cholesterol, test result 150 mg/dL: _____
   d. Sodium (Na), test result 160 mEq/L: _____
   e. BUN, test result 15 mg/dL: _____
   f. Potassium (K), test result 6.0 mEq/L: _____

Matching I: Match the items in column I to their descriptions in column II.

COLUMN I	COLUMN II
____ 1. Normal male hemoglobin	A. 4.0 to 5.5 million/cubic mm
____ 2. Normal WBC	B. Type of allergy test
____ 3. Normal female ESR	C. Virus that causes infectious mononucleosis
____ 4. PKU	D. 13–17 g/dL
____ 5. Normal glucose	E. ESR
____ 6. Normal cholesterol	F. 4.5 to 6.0 million/cubic mm
____ 7. Normal female hemoglobin	G. 12–16 g/dL
____ 8. Normal male ESR	H. Measures glycosylated hemoglobin
____ 9. Normal female Hct	I. Required in all states and Canada
____ 10. Normal male RBC	J. 0–10 mm/hr
____ 11. Normal male Hct	K. Below 200 mg/dL fasting
____ 12. Normal female RBC	L. Requires immediate attention by the health care provider
____ 13. Polycythemia	M. 42–52%
____ 14. Test for nonspecific tissue damage	N. Glucose
____ 15. Screen for diabetes	O. Abnormal increase in all blood cells
____ 16. Equals Hgb x 3 + 3	P. Below 126 mg/dL fasting
____ 17. Epstein-Barr virus	Q. Hematocrit
____ 18. RAST	R. 36–48%
____ 19. Hemoglobin A1C	S. 4500–11,000
____ 20. Panic value	T. 0–20 mm/hr

Chapter Application

Case Studies with Critical Thinking Questions

Scenario 1

Amy has come to the laboratory requesting that you check her hemoglobin level because she is feeling tired, is short of breath, and is sleeping more than usual. After checking with the health care provider in your office, you perform a hemoglobin test on Amy and find that her hemoglobin result is 6.0 mg/dL.

1. What does this result indicate? _____

_____

_____

2. What action should you take? _____

_____

_____

_____

Scenario 2

Mrs. Morris brings her seven-year-old son to your office to be tested for allergies. He seems to be having a lot of difficulty with congestion, sneezing, and coughing. You administer the scratch test and have been told to watch the patient closely for any severe reactions. Almost immediately, wheals begin to develop, and several swell to a +4 in a very short period of time. Mrs. Morris' son complains that his tongue feels big, and he can't breathe very well.

1. Based on the skin reactions, what could be happening to the patient? _____

_____

_____

2. What will the provider most likely do to help the patient? _____

_____

_____

Competency Practice

1. **Determine Hemoglobin Using a Hemoglobinometer.** With a partner, demonstrate the proper steps for performing a capillary puncture and performing a CLIA-waived hemoglobin. Use Procedure 45–1 as a guide.

2. **Determine Hematocrit (Hct) Using a Microhematocrit Centrifuge**. With a partner, demonstrate the proper steps for performing a capillary puncture and performing a CLIA-waived hematocrit. Use Procedure 45–2 as a guide.

3. **Perform an Erythrocyte Sedimentation Rate (ESR).** Gather all of the supplies and equipment needed to perform a sed rate. You will also need a filled lavender-top blood tube. Demonstrate the proper steps for performing a CLIA-waived sed rate. Use Procedure 45–3 as a guide.

4. **Screen Blood Sugar (Glucose) Level.** With a partner, demonstrate the proper steps for performing a capillary puncture and performing a CLIA-waived glucose screening using a glucometer. Use Procedure 45–4 as a guide.

5. **Perform Hemoglobin A1C (Glycosylated Hemoglobin) Screening.** With a partner, demonstrate the proper steps for performing a capillary puncture and performing a CLIA-waived hemoglobin A1C screening. Use Procedure 45–5 as a guide.

6. **Perform a Cholesterol Screening.** With a partner, demonstrate the proper steps for performing a capillary puncture and performing a CLIA-waived cholesterol screening. Use Procedure 45–6 as a guide.

7. **Perform a Screening for Infectious Mononucleosis.** With a partner, demonstrate the proper steps for performing a capillary puncture and performing a CLIA-waived mononucleosis test. Use Procedure 45–7 as a guide.

Cardiology and Radiology Procedures

CHAPTER 47

Radiology Procedures

Words to Know Challenge

Spelling: Each line contains three spellings of a word. Underline the correctly spelled word.

1. distenze   <u>distends</u>   destends
2. <u>flatus</u>   flates   flatis
3. <u>iodine</u>   eyeodine   iodyne
4. rentgen   <u>roentgen</u>   reantgen
5. macherity   <u>maturity</u>   michrity
6. systoscopy   cystascopy   <u>cystoscopy</u>
7. <u>electron</u>   electran   elecktron
8. ennema   enama   <u>enema</u>
9. <u>conjunction</u>   congunction   cunjunction
10. flexable   <u>flexible</u>   flecksable
11. fluroscope   floroscope   <u>fluoroscope</u>
12. thareputic   theraputic   <u>therapeutic</u>
13. radiopaqe   radiopaiqe   <u>radiopaque</u>

Matching: Match the key term in column I to its definition in column II.

COLUMN I

_____ 1. Maturity

_____ 2. Claustrophobia

_____ 3. Sonogram

_____ 4. Therapeutic radiation

_____ 5. Mammography

_____ 6. Evacuants

_____ 7. IVP

_____ 8. KUB

_____ 9. Contrast media

_____ 10. Retrograde pyelogram

COLUMN II

A. Fear of being enclosed

B. Used to treat cancer

C. Laxatives and enemas

D. Flat plate of abdomen

E. Perform with sterile catheter in conjunction with cystoscopy

F. Barium and water mixture

G. Defines structures of the urinary system

H. X-ray of different angles of breast tissue

I. High-frequency sound waves conducted through a transducer

J. Full development

Chapter Review

Fill in the Blank: Use information from the chapter to fill in the blank space in the sentence.

1. Diagnostic X-rays are _____ in pregnant women, especially during the first trimester.

2. Carbonated and alcoholic beverages should be avoided prior to X-rays of the visceral organs because they produce _____.

3. A voiding cystogram may be ordered along with a(n) _____.

4. Nuclear medicine uses _____ in the diagnosis and treatment of patients.

5. A _____ X-ray is helpful in determining the position of an intrauterine device (IUD).

6. Breast self-examination is recommended _____ for women of all ages.

7. An upper GI series is also referred to as a barium _____.

8. To reduce the possible effects of swelling and soreness often caused by compression of the breasts during mammography, instruct the patient to omit _____ from her diet 7 to 10 days prior to examination. Compression of the breasts during mammography allows a much clearer picture of breast tissue and requires less _____.

Short Answer

1. What are roentgen rays? _____
   _____
   _____

2. What are therapeutic X-rays used for? _____
   _____
   _____

3. What types of symptoms do patients experience if the gallbladder malfunctions? _____
   _____
   _____

4. What food should patients avoid if they have gallbladder trouble? _____
   _____
   _____

5. Why must the digestive tract be free of foods during an upper GI series? _____
_____
_____

6. Why is air contrast sometimes ordered with a barium enema examination? _____
_____
_____

7. What is an IVP? _____
_____
_____

8. Describe the method of radiology called a CT (computerized tomography) scan. _____
_____
_____

9. Explain why pregnant women should not have X-rays. _____
_____
_____

10. List X-ray procedures that do not require patient preparation. _____
_____
_____

Chapter Application

Case Studies with Critical Thinking Questions

Scenario 1

Cynthia needs to be scheduled for an MRI of her head and neck. You are responsible for scheduling the test and explaining the procedure to the patient. After you have explained the procedure to Cynthia, she tells you she is extremely claustrophobic and doesn't think she can have the MRI.

1. What special preparation instructions should be given to the patient? _____
_____
_____

2. To whom should you relay the information regarding the patient's claustrophobia? _____
_____
_____

3. What could be done to help combat the claustrophobia? _____
_____
_____

Scenario 2

A 55-year-old male calls the office to say that he had a barium enema this morning. He says that he is nauseated, bloated, and constipated and wants to know what he should do.

1. Who will determine how to treat the patient's complaint? _____
_____
_____

2. Why can't you tell the patient what he should do about his situation? _____
_____
_____

Scenario 3

A 35-year-old female with upper-right quadrant pain is scheduled for an ultrasound this morning. When she arrives at the facility, she is questioned about her preparation for the procedure, and it is determined that she cannot have the ultrasound because she ate a liquid, fat-free breakfast. The patient calls your office and is quite upset because she had to reschedule her appointment. She claims that the medical assistant never told her that she couldn't have anything to eat or drink after midnight. However, the medical assistant did explain all preparation instructions and gave her printed instructions to take with her.

1. How might this situation be handled in a professional manner? _____
_____
_____

2. How might this error have been prevented? _____
_____
_____

Role-Play Activity

Working in pairs, have one partner portray the medical assistant while the other partner portrays the patient. Choose any of the radiographic examinations in the chapter and provide patient education to the patient with the instructions for the preparation and explaining to the patient what to expect with the examination and procedure. After completion, change roles and choose another topic to repeat the activity.

Minor Surgical Procedures

CHAPTER 48

Preparing for Surgery

Words to Know Challenge

Spelling: Each line contains three spellings of a word. Underline the correctly spelled word.

1. anticeptic   antiseptic   anticeptik

2. micorganism   mickroorganism   microorganism

3. ratchet   rachet   rachette

4. contamination   contaminition   cantamination

5. serattions   serrations   cearations

6. asceptic   aseptic   aseptick

7. forseps   forsepts   forceps

8. microbial   microrbial   microrbital

9. skrub   sgrub   scrub

Fill in the Blank: Complete the following sentences with correctly spelled words from the Spelling section.

1. Because body hair encourages _____ accumulation, it is sometimes shaved.

2. The process of maintaining sterility throughout the surgical procedure is known as _____ technique.

3. The _____ is the locking mechanism of an instrument.

4. _____ are etchings located on the blade of an instrument to keep it from slipping.

5. A _____ is performed prior to surgery to remove all microorganisms and aid in keeping the microbial count low.

6. _____ occurs when fluid penetrates a sterile package or sterile tray and field.

7. Prepping the skin with an _____ solution should begin at the center of the incision site and proceed outward in one continuous circular motion as shown.

8. In compliance with standard precautions, proper barriers, such as gloves, gown, and face mask or shield, must be worn to protect the health care staff from possible _____ while performing these procedures.

Chapter Review

Short Answer

1. When scheduling the patient for surgery, identify at least four items the medical assistant should advise the patient of.

   _____

   _____

   _____

   _____

2. Explain how to care for surgical instruments before and following use.

   _____

   _____

   _____

3. The three instrument classifications are: _____

   _____

   _____

4. Discuss the four sterilization techniques and identify the method most widely used.

   _____

   _____

   _____

   _____

5. List three examples of when the sterile tray or field would become contaminated.

   _____

   _____

   _____

6. List the items included in the basic setup for most minor surgical procedures.

   _____

   _____

   _____

7. List five guidelines to follow when draping a patient.

   _____

   _____

   _____

8. Describe what needs to be done when the patient arrives for the appointment.

   _____

   _____

   _____

9. Select the order of procedures to prepare the skin for surgery from the following list:
   a. _____
   b. Apply antiseptic solution, cleanse, rinse, shave, drape
   c. Shave, cleanse, rinse, drape, apply antiseptic solution

10. What is the purpose of the skin preparation before a surgical procedure?

    _____

    _____

    _____

11. Why must the medical assistant be extremely careful to avoid nicking the patient's skin when performing a skin preparation?

    _____

    _____

    _____

Matching: Match the classification to each instrument in the list. (*Hint:* Classifications may be used more than once.)

INSTRUMENT	CLASSIFICATION
____ 1. Forceps	A. Cutting and dissecting
____ 2. Retractors	B. Clamping or grasping
____ 3. Hemostats	C. Dilating, probing, and visualizing
____ 4. Scissors	
____ 5. Specula	
____ 6. Scalpels	
____ 7. Needle holders	
____ 8. Sounds	

Chapter Application

Case Study with Critical Thinking Questions

Madison has not had time to sterilize the surgical instruments on the counter from an earlier procedure because she has been so busy with patient care. A coworker says that his provider needs the instruments for a procedure right away. Madison explains that the instruments have been cleaned and disinfected but not sterilized.

1. What should Madison tell her coworker? _____

_____

_____

2. Should these instruments be used anyway? _____

_____

_____

3. What would the repercussions be if the instruments were used prior to being sterilized? _____

_____

_____

Competency Practice

1. **Prepare Sterile Field.** Assemble all of the supplies needed and demonstrate how to set up for a minor surgery procedure. Discuss what steps would be needed to take if a contamination breach occurs. Use Procedure 48–1 as a guide.

2. **Hand Washing for Surgical Asepsis.** Using an appropriate surgical scrub agent, demonstrate the procedure of surgical hand washing and discuss when it is appropriate for this type of hand washing. Use Procedure 48–2 as a guide.

3. **Sterile Gloving.** Selecting the appropriate sterile glove size for your hands, demonstrate the technique for applying and removing sterile gloves. Discuss when it is appropriate to wear sterile gloves. Use Procedure 48–3 as a guide.

4. **Prepare Skin for Minor Surgery.** With a partner or an anatomical body part, practice preparing the skin for minor surgery. Use Procedure 48–4 as a guide.

Assisting with Minor Surgery

Words to Know Challenge

Spelling: Each line contains three spellings of a word. Underline the correctly spelled word.

1. biopsy	biopsie	biopcie
2. cyrosrurgery	kryosrusery	cryosurgery
3. electocautery	electrocautery	elecktrocautery
4. coagalate	coagulate	cogulate
5. hemophilia	hemophillia	hemopilia
6. anathesia	anesthesia	anathesia
7. exudate	exadate	exadite
8. sewture	suwture	suture
9. hypoalerrgenic	hypoallergenik	hypoallergenic
10. exision	excision	excison

Fill in the Blank: Complete the following sentences with correctly spelled words from the Spelling section.

1. Destruction of tissue and skin lesions using extremely cold temperatures is the procedure known as _____.

2. In a needle _____, fluid or tissue cells are aspirated through a needle into a syringe for microscopic examination.

3. A biopsy is an _____ of a small amount of tissue for microscopic examination.

4. _____ means to clot.

5. When performing a wound collection, the swab should not touch any part of the wound except the _____.

6. A _____ is a type of thread that joins skin of a wound.

7. When something is _____, it is unlikely to cause an allergic reaction.

8. _____ is a hereditary condition causing inability to clot blood.

Chapter Review

Short Answer

1. Discuss some of the reasons behind the upsurge in outpatient and ambulatory surgery.

   _____
   _____
   _____

2. Identify the two most common local anesthetic agents.

   _____
   _____
   _____

3. What is the purpose of an electrocautery device in minor surgical procedures performed in the office?

   _____
   _____
   _____

4. Discuss general postop instructions that should be given to a patient following a minor surgery performed in the office.

   _____
   _____
   _____

5. List unusual patient symptoms that should be reported to the provider following a surgical procedure.

   _____
   _____
   _____

6. List the important information that must be recorded on the patient's chart regarding a surgical procedure.

   _____
   _____
   _____

7. Why are follow-up visits necessary in patient care? Other than the scheduled postop visit, what can the medical assistant do to follow up with patients?

   _____
   _____
   _____

8. Explain how to remove sutures properly and why they should be removed.

   _____
   _____
   _____
   _____

9. Describe how to remove skin staples.

   _____
   _____
   _____

10. Describe skin closures and how they are applied.

   _____
   _____
   _____

Matching: Match the procedure in column I to its description in column II.

	COLUMN I	COLUMN II
____	1. Sebaceous cyst removal	A. Closing a wound or laceration by placing sutures or stitches or staples in the skin to hold the edges of the wound together
____	2. Laceration repair	B. Fluid or tissue cells aspirated through a needle into a syringe for microscopic examination
____	3. Chemical destruction	C. Incision in a localized infection, such as an abscess, to drain the exudates from the area
____	4. Laser surgery	D. Excision of a small, painless sac containing a buildup of sebum, the secretion from a sebaceous gland
____	5. I&D	E. Tissue destroyed by applying silver nitrate to the area
____	6. Needle biopsy	F. A concentrated, intense light beam destroys a target area without harming the surrounding tissue

Chapter Application

Case Studies with Critical Thinking Questions

Scenario 1

A surgical procedure was performed at the outpatient surgery center, and the patient was instructed to return to the office for removal of the staples. When you take the bandage off, you notice that the site is infected.

1. What should you do first? _____

_____

_____

2. Describe the procedure the provider might ask you to perform. _____

_____

_____

_____

Scenario 2

Joshua Leonard is having a sebaceous cyst removed from his scalp today. While you are performing the skin prep, he tells you that he is a little nervous about having the procedure because he has hemophilia.

1. What should you do with this information? _____

_____

_____

2. What are the risks while having this procedure? _____

_____

_____

Competency Practice

1. **Perform Wound Collection.** Using an anatomical body part, mannequin, or partner, practice the process of wound collection. Use Procedure 49–1 as a guide.

2. **Assist with Minor Surgery.** Gathering all of the supplies and equipment needed for various surgical procedures as discussed in the textbook, role-play with a partner the process of assisting the provider. Use Procedure 49–2 as a guide.

3. **Assist with Suturing a Laceration.** Using an anatomical body part, mannequin, or partner, practice the process of assisting the provider with suturing a laceration. Role-play various types of lacerations and tetanus vaccine history to determine whether the patient will need an updated vaccine. Use Procedure 49–3 as a guide.

4. **Remove Sutures or Staples.** Practice removing sutures from an artificial arm or a suture pillow. Document the number of sutures placed and the number of sutures removed. Use Procedure 49–4 as a guide.

16

Medication Administration Procedures

CHAPTER 50

Pharmacology Fundamentals

Words to Know Challenge

Spelling: Each line contains three spellings of a word. Underline the correctly spelled word.

1. aganest   aganist   <u>agonist</u>
2. <u>generic</u>   generic   jenerik
3. prescibption   <u>prescription</u>   priscription
4. <u>vial</u>   vile   vyle
5. <u>narcotic</u>   norcatic   narcotek
6. pharmocology   pharmecolagy   <u>pharmacology</u>
7. sinergistic   <u>synergistic</u>   synergistic
8. antigonist   antaganist   <u>antagonist</u>
9. allergie   <u>allergy</u>   allurgy

Fill in the Blank: Complete the following sentences with Words to Know from this chapter.

1. A _____ drug enhances the effects of another drug, whereas a drug that prevents the action of another drug or chemical is referred to as a(n) _____ .

2. A controlled class of drugs used to relieve pain is called a _____ .

3. The study of medications and uses is also referred to as _____ .

4. A reaction to a medication that causes an immune response is called a(n) _____ , whereas a(n) _____ to a medication can be only a symptom, such as an upset stomach, that can be controlled by taking the medication at a different time.

5. The _____ name of a medication is also its official name.

6. The _____ name of a medication is a label assigned by the manufacturer.

7. Drugs that have the potential for abuse or addiction are known as _____ .

8. Instructions written by a provider to the pharmacist for preparing, labeling, and dispensing medications that will be self-administered by a patient are called a _____ .

Chapter Review

Short Answer

1. Circle one: There are (1, 2, 3, 4, 5) basic categories of insulins.

2. What is meant by *generic* drug name? What is the difference between a generic name and a trade name?

   _____

   _____

   _____

3. Explain why the correct spelling is so important when dealing with drugs.

   _____

   _____

   _____

4. The _____ is responsible for regulation and oversight of controlled substances; the _____ monitors drug safety and clinical trials and verifies that medications are safe for consumption based on available data.

5. What is a controlled substance? Describe the proper storage requirements of controlled substances in the medical office.

   _____

   _____

   _____

   _____

6. Name at least five print or online drug reference sources that are used in the medical office.

   _____

   _____

   _____

7. Describe how refrigerated medications should be stored and handled.

   _____

   _____

   _____

   _____

Matching: Drug Classifications

Match the drug classifications in column I with their description in column II.

COLUMN I	COLUMN II
_____ 1. Anesthetic	A. Thins mucous
_____ 2. Chemotherapeutics	B. Controls cardiac rhythm
_____ 3. Antiemetic	C. Relieves muscle spasms
_____ 4. Anticonvulsant	D. Produces a calming effect
_____ 5. Antiarrhythmic	E. Increases production of urine
_____ 6. Antianxiety	F. Interferes with body's ability to experience pain
_____ 7. Diuretic	G. Cures infections
_____ 8. Expectorant	H. Prevents or relieves seizures
_____ 9. Antibiotics	I. Cures cancer
_____ 10. Muscle relaxant	J. Stops or prevents nausea and vomiting

Matching: Controlled Substances

Match the description items in column I with the corresponding schedule in column II.
(*Hint:* There might be multiple answers for items in Column I.)

COLUMN I

_____ 1. Not able to be refilled

_____ 2. Limited risk for physical dependence; Phenobarbital

_____ 3. Illegal drugs

_____ 4. Low risk of addiction, small amounts of codeine in cough syrups

_____ 5. Can be refilled up to five times in six months

_____ 6. Requires a signed prescription to be presented with 72 hours of a phoned prescription

_____ 7. Legal drug but carries severe risk for psychic and physical addiction

_____ 8. Marijuana, heroin

_____ 9. Prescriptions may be written or phoned in

COLUMN II

A. Schedule I

B. Schedule II

C. Schedule III

D. Schedule IV

E. Schedule V

Matching

Recognize and describe medical, legal, and ethical concerns regarding medications and appropriate actions to be taken for each.
Hint: Each can have more than one answer. Be prepared to discuss your answers and rationales in class.

COLUMN I

_____ 1. Medical assistant notices that a medication prescribed is on the list of patient's allergies.

_____ 2. Birth control pills prescribed for mentally challenged patient 14 years old.

_____ 3. Immunizations given to a child with permission of the babysitter.

_____ 4. Narcotics stored alongside blood pressure medications in common office cabinet.

_____ 5. Alzheimer's patient who does not have a reported injury or pain problem is prescribed a narcotic pain patch to help calm her down.

_____ 6. Prescriptions for two patients are mixed up at the time of discharge. One is for antibiotic and one is for heart rhythm control.

_____ 7. Prescribing antibiotics for an ear infection in a child because the parent insists rather than because it is clinically necessary.

_____ 8. Medical personnel's objection to participating in administration or dispensing of morning-after pill.

COLUMN II

A. Ethical concern is on the list of patient's allergies.

B. Legal concern patient 14 years old.

C. Medical issue babysitter.

Chapter Application

Case Study with Critical Thinking Questions

An elderly patient presents for a new patient appointment and has brought with her a paper bag with assorted bottles: prescription, over-the-counter, and herbal remedies. Some pills are loose and unlabeled.

1. How might you help determine which medications the patient is using, and how might you identify them to arrive at an accurate medication list?

   _____
   _____
   _____
   _____

2. What safety precautions might you discuss with the patient?

   _____
   _____
   _____
   _____

Competency Practice

1. **Use the PDR or Other Drug Reference to Find Medication Information.**

   a) Using the PDR or other drug reference, fill in the missing information. Use Procedure 50–1 as a guide.

	Trade name	Generic Name	Recommended Dose and Route	Common side effects
a.	Captopril			_____
b.		alendronate sodium		_____ _____ _____
c.	Lexapro			_____ _____

   b) Using Procedure 50–1 as a guide, use the most current PDR or other drug reference available to find the following information and be prepared to discuss your findings in class:
   - Determine the manufacturer for Aricept and determine if it is the generic or trade name.
   - Note the appearance of the drug.
   - Determine pregnancy category ratings.

CHAPTER 51

Measurement Systems, Basic Mathematics, and Dosage Calculations

Words to Know Challenge

Spelling: Each line contains three spellings of a word. Underline the correctly spelled word.

1. decimal   decemul   decimol
2. dividend   dividened   dividind
3. devisor   diviser   divisor
4. product   produouct   prodact
5. extreems   extremes   extrimes
6. fraktion   fracshun   fraction
7. means   miens   meens
8. metric system   mitric system   metrik system
9. nomerator   numerater   numerator
10. purcentage   percentage   percentige
11. denuminater   denominator   dinominater
12. rashio   rachio   ratio
13. purportion   perportion   proportion

Fill in the Blank: Complete the following sentences with correctly spelled words from the Spelling section.

1. A _____ is the result of multiplying two numbers together.

2. The number *to be* divided is the _____, and the _____ is the number *used to divide* another number.

3. A _____ indicates part of a whole number and is written with a _____ as the top number and a _____ as the bottom number.

4. A number expressed as part of 100 is called a _____.

5. A _____ expresses the relationship between two components.

6. The relationship between two ratios is a _____.

7. The _____ is based on multiples of ten; it is the most commonly used system of measurement in health care.

Chapter Review

Short Answer

1. Write out the formula for the basic method of calculating dosages and explain what each component of the formula means.

   _____
   _____
   _____

2. What are the three steps required for calculating dosages in the ratio and proportion method? What is the formula for this method?

   _____
   _____
   _____

3. What are the three basic units used in the metric system?

   _____
   _____
   _____

4. Why is it necessary for all health care personnel to use the same system of measurement when prescribing or administering medications?

   _____
   _____
   _____

5. Fill in the blanks: An _____ fraction has a numerator larger than the denominator, and a _____ fraction includes a whole number along with a fraction.

6. Explain why household measurement devices, such as teaspoons and tablespoons, should be avoided.

   _____
   _____
   _____

7. What is the purpose of learning to convert medication dosages from different units?

   _____
   _____
   _____

Abbreviations Review: Write out the following abbreviations and then tell which system of measurement it belongs to.

1. gtt _____

2. g _____

3. gr _____

4. fl oz _____

5. lb _____

6. mL _____

7. kg _____

8. pt _____

Matching: Match the *measurement* with the appropriate *system* of measurement.
(*Hint:* The systems will be used more than once, and there may be more than one answer for some.)

____	1. Cup	A. Metric
____	2. Dram	B. Household
____	3. Liter	C. Apothecary
____	4. Grain	
____	5. Gram	
____	6. Drop	
____	7. Pint	
____	8. Quart	
____	9. Meter	
____	10. Teaspoon	

Chapter Application

Case Study with Critical Thinking Questions

A patient in the clinic just received her regular allergy shot injections and immediately shows symptoms of an anaphylaxis reaction including difficulty breathing, a weak and rapid pulse, and dizziness. You are asked to prepare epinephrine 0.3 mg for subcutaneous injection by the provider. The epinephrine is supplied as a 1:1000 solution in a 30 mL vial containing 1 mg/mL.

1. Describe the proper way to label the syringe. _____
   _____
   _____
   _____

2. Calculate the dose. What is the correct volume? _____

Competency Practice

1. **Calculate Proper Dosages of Medication for Administration.** Using the steps outlined in Procedure 51–1, complete the following math review exercises:

   1. How many tsp make 180 gtt? _____
      _____

   2. Convert 3 tsp into mL. _____
      _____

   3. Convert 150 pounds into kg. _____
      _____

   4. How many cups are in 2 quarts? _____
      _____

   5. Based on the information found in the chapter, what conversions need to be performed to find the number of gtts in 20 mL?
      _____
      _____
      _____

6. Add the following. Show your work.
   a. 1¼ + 68% + 0.7 = _____
   b. 3/8 + 0.42 + 13.5% = _____

7. Identify the means and extremes of the following proportions.
   a. 4:5 = 12:15 _____
   b. 1:3 = 3:9 _____

Solving Proportions and Equations: Solve the following proportions and equations. Show your work.

1. $1{:}4 = 3{:}x$ _____

2. $3{:}9 = x{:}12$ _____

3. $25 + x = 175$ _____

4. $1.35 - 0.67 = x$ _____

5. $4.3 \times 2.1 = x$ _____

6. $4 \times \frac{1}{2} = x$ _____

7. $150 \div 3 = x$ _____

8. $75 \times \frac{1}{2} = x$ _____

Dosage Calculation Exercises: Determine the correct dosages. Use either method presented in the chapter but show your work.

1. Order: Novolin R 10 units SubQ now
   Supplied as 100 units per 1 mL
   What is the correct volume to be administered? _____

2. Order: Aspirin 162 mg po chew and swallow now for chest pain
   Supplied as 81 mg tablets
   What is the correct amount? _____

3. Order: Benadryl 100 mg IM now for acute allergic reaction
   Supplied as 50 mg per mL
   What is the correct amount? _____

4. Order: Amoxicillin 500 mg po
   Supplied in dry powder form; when reconstituted, solution contains 200 mg per 5 mL
   What is the correct volume to be administered? _____

5. Order: Terbutaline 0.25 mg IM
   Supplied as 1 mg/mL vial.
   What is the correct volume? _____

6. Order: Digitek 250 mcg po as a loading dose.
   Supplied as 0.125 mg tablets
   What is the correct amount? _____

7. Order: Dexamethasone 5 mg po now
   Supplied to your office in 0.5 mg and 2 mg tablets
   What is the correct amount? _____

CHAPTER 52

Administering Oral and Noninjectable Medications

Words to Know Challenge

Spelling: Each line contains three spellings of a word. Underline the correctly spelled word.

1. <u>narcotic</u>   narcotec   nercotic

2. seppository   <u>suppository</u>   sopository

3. sublingal   subblingual   <u>sublingual</u>

4. rectul   <u>rectal</u>   rictal

5. <u>prescription</u>   proscription   priscription

6. <u>topical</u>   typical   topicul

7. parental   perinteral   <u>parenteral</u>

8. transdirmel   <u>transdermal</u>   trensindermal

9. <u>buccal</u>   buckal   buckle

10. mediation order   <u>medication order</u>   medicaton order

11. dispanse   dispence   <u>dispense</u>

Fill in the Blank: Complete the following sentences with Words to Know from this chapter.

1. A _____ is a written or transmitted instruction to the pharmacist for preparing and dispensing a medication to a patient for self-administration.

2. A written instruction composed by a physician or licensed practitioner for administering medications directly to a patient is a _____.

3. DAW stands for _____.

4. Oral medications are intended for absorption through the digestive system; other methods are said to be _____, or intended for absorption from outside the digestive system.

5. _____ medications are placed under the tongue; _____ medications are placed between the cheek and gum.

6. A medication supplied as a dissolvable solid for rectal administration is called a _____ .

7. A(n) _____ could be used to introduce contrast material rectally for imaging of the lower intestinal tract.

8. _____ medications are those that are given by a route outside of the digestive system.

9. Patches give medications by the _____ route.

10. The _____ are the rules that ensure safe medication administration.

Chapter Review

Short Answer

1. Why are different medications used to treat the same symptoms?

   _____
   _____
   _____

2. A prescription is defined as _____

   _____
   _____

3. When preparing a prescription for signature, the medical assistant should always _____

   _____
   _____

4. What does DAW on a prescription stand for and what does it mean? _____

   _____
   _____

5. What action should be taken to avoid errors when calling in prescriptions to a pharmacy? _____

   _____
   _____

6. What information is required for a complete and accurate medication order?

   a. _____
   b. _____
   c. _____
   d. _____
   e. _____
   f. _____
   g. _____
   h. _____

7. What is the purpose of a medication order? _____

   _____
   _____

8. What must be performed before giving medications by ANY route?

   _____
   _____

9. When signing off a medication or other chart entry, how should you signify the end of the entry to prevent anyone else making an unauthorized addition to your note?

   _____
   _____
   _____

10. In the following chart, list the Seven Rights of medication administration and explain what each right means.

	Right	Description
1.	_____	_____ _____ _____
2.	_____	_____ _____ _____
3.	_____	_____ _____ _____
4.	_____	_____ _____ _____
5.	_____	_____ _____ _____
6.	_____	_____ _____ _____
7.	_____	_____ _____ _____

11. To avoid medication errors, when should the medical assistant check the order and the medication?
_____
_____

12. What steps should the medical assistant take in the event of a medication error? _____
_____
_____

13. List the elements required for a complete and accurate medication entry.

   a. _____
   b. _____
   c. _____
   _____
   d. _____
   e. _____
   _____

14. When should a medication entry be completed? _____
_____
_____

15. Why is oral administration the most commonly used route for medications?
_____
_____
_____

16. What information is required, in addition to the standard information, when documenting immunizations?

_____

_____

_____

17. What legislation requires health care providers to report adverse events following a vaccination? What is its purpose?

_____

_____

_____

18. Identify the routes by which a medical assistant is permitted to administer medications (unless otherwise designated by state laws).

_____

_____

_____

Matching: Routes of Administration

Match the routes of administration in column I with their descriptions in column II.

	COLUMN I	COLUMN II
____	1. Sublingual	A. Medication given in the ear canal
____	2. Buccal	B. Applied directly to the skin
____	3. Ointment	C. Placed between the cheek and gum for absorption through the mucous membranes in the mouth
____	4. Inhalation	D. Medication applied into the eyelid or opening in the corner of the eye
____	5. Otic	E. Emulsion of medication applied topically
____	6. Topical	F. Under the tongue
____	7. Ophthalmic	G. An adhesive patch containing medication worn on the skin
____	8. Intraosseous	H. Into the spinal column
____	9. Transdermal	I. Breathed in
____	10. Intrathecal	J. Medication given directly into the bone marrow

Matching: Acceptable Abbreviations

For each abbreviation listed, identify whether it is acceptable to use or is a Do Not Use abbreviation. Next to only the acceptable abbreviations, write what each stands for.

	Abbreviation	Abbreviation Written Out	Use or Do Not Use?
____	1. kg	_____	A. Use
____	2. QD	_____	B. Do Not Use
____	3. tsp	_____	
____	4. tinc	_____	
____	5. IU	_____	
____	6. STAT	_____	
____	7. U (unit)	_____	
____	8. IV	_____	
____	9. IM	_____	
____	10. MS	_____	

Chapter Application

Case Study with Critical Thinking Questions

Scenario 1

Kelly Anderson, 15 years old, is being seen for back pain. She strained muscles while playing volleyball at school. Her chart notes that she has an allergy to ibuprofen. The provider has seen her and left a prescription and an order for medication. You, the MA, prepare and administer Advil 600 mg, per the order. Within a few minutes, Kelly begins to complain of itching all over. When you go back to check the chart, you notice that both the chart and the prescription are for *Kevin* Anderson, another patient being seen across the hall.

1. What has occurred? _____

   _____

   _____

2. Describe how you will handle this situation. _____

   _____

   _____

   _____

   _____

3. Make a charting entry that outlines the incident and the steps taken.

   _____

   _____

   _____

   _____

   _____

   _____

   _____

   _____

   _____

   _____

   _____

   _____

   _____

   _____

   _____

   _____

Competency Practice

1. **Prepare a Prescription According to the Provider's Direction.** Using blank prescriptions in paper form (can be accessed on the Student Companion website) or using the prescription application in an EHR, complete a variety of prescriptions using medications provided from your instructor. Use a PDR or other resource for proper dosing information. Use Procedure 52–1 as a guide.

2. **Record a Medication Entry in the Patient's Chart.** Using the examples provided in the textbook or a list of medication orders from your instructor, document the medication entries in the patient's chart. Use Procedure 52–2 as a guide.

3. **Prepare and Administer Oral Medication.** With a partner, gather the supplies needed and role-play administering oral medications to a patient. Use Procedure 52–3 as a guide.

4. **Administer Eyedrops.** Using an anatomical model of the head, or a mannequin, practice administering eyedrops. Use Procedure 52–4 as a guide.

5. **Instill Drops in the Ears.** Using an anatomical model of the head, or a mannequin, practice instilling drops into the ear. Use Procedure 52–5 as a guide.

6. **Administer Rectal Medication.** Using an anatomical model of the buttocks, or a mannequin, practice administering a rectal medication. Use Procedure 52–6 as a guide.

CHAPTER 53

Administering Injections and Immunizations

Words to Know Challenge

Spelling: Each line contains three spellings of a word. Underline the correctly spelled word.

1.	neumonia	pnumonia	pneumonia
2.	meningytis	meningitis	miningitis
3.	wheel	weal	wheal
4.	intradermal	interdermal	intradurmol
5.	subceutaneous	subcutaneous	subcutanious
6.	incubation period	incubasion period	encubation period
7.	anaphylactic	anyphalactic	aniphylactic
8.	influensa	inflouinza	influenza
9.	hipatytis	hepatitis	hepititis
10.	immunization	emunization	immunozation

Matching: Match the words in column I with the definitions in column II.

	COLUMN I	COLUMN II
____	1. Hepatitis A	A. Vaccine
____	2. Incubation period	B. Whooping cough
____	3. Photosensitivity	C. Period when symptoms peak
____	4. Catarrhal stage	D. Chickenpox
____	5. Subcutaneous	E. Transmission occurs when fecal matter is ingested
____	6. Intramuscular	F. Sensitivity to light
____	7. Rubella	G. Time required for a disease to develop before symptoms present

(continues)

____ 8. Immunization   H. Period when disease is highly communicable

____ 9. Varicella   I. Flu

____ 10. Diphtheria   J. Beneath the skin

____ 11. Paroxysmal stage   K. Usually spread from blood, semen, or other body fluids

____ 12. Hepatitis B   L. Into the muscle

____ 13. Pertussis   M. German measles

____ 14. Influenza   N. Preventable disease that might require a tracheostomy and ventilatory support; highly contagious

____ 15. Anaphylactic   O. Also known as rubeola

____ 16. Incubation period   P. A complication of Haemophilus influenza type B or HIB

____ 17. Measles   Q. Time in which a virus or bacterium reproduces in the host before signs and symptoms of an illness appear.

____ 18. Meningitis   R. A serious allergic response that requires immediate treatment

Chapter Review

Short Answer

1. List three advantages of parenteral medications.

   _____

   _____

   _____

   _____

   _____

2. What is the difference between a tuberculin syringe and an insulin syringe? Can they be used interchangeably?

   _____

   _____

   _____

3. Fill in the blanks: Medical assistants _____ permitted to provide direct intravenous (IV) injections or to initiate an IV access. However, it is important to be able to _____ a problem and _____ it to the provider immediately.

4. Name at least one use for the intradermal route of medication administration.

   _____

   _____

   _____

5. Fill in the following table with the correct angles of injection for each type of injection listed.

Type of Injection	Angle of Injection
Subcutaneous	_____
Intradermal	_____
Intramuscular	_____
Z-Track IM	_____

6. Why are intramuscular injections given at the angle you listed?

_____
_____
_____

7. Describe the correct technique for giving a Z-track injection.

_____
_____
_____
_____

8. Name three actions that can be taken to avoid needlesticks.

_____
_____
_____
_____

9. What steps should be taken in the event of an accidental needlestick?

_____
_____
_____
_____

Labeling

1. Identify the parts of the needle pictured.

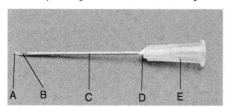

   a. _____
   b. _____
   c. _____
   d. _____
   e. _____

2. Identify the parts of a syringe.

   a. _____
   b. _____
   c. _____
   d. _____
   e. _____

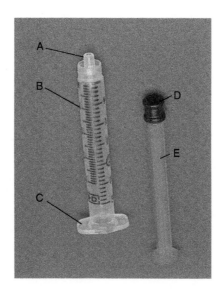

3. Next to each intramuscular injection site, identify the site name.

Injection Site	Site Name

Chapter Application

Case Studies with Critical Thinking Questions

Scenario 1

A mother brings her six-month-old in for a well-baby check. The child is playful, there is no sign of illness, and the baby's temperature is normal. Flu season is in full swing. When you ask the mother whether she is here for the baby's six-month vaccinations, she replies that she has no intention of vaccinating her baby.

1. How might you handle this conversation? (Select the best option.)
   a. Tell her that it is her legal obligation to vaccinate the baby.
   b. Give her a vaccination schedule and printed information and leave the room to hide your disapproval.
   c. Make a note in the chart and continue on with the visit.
   d. Ask her what her objections are to having vaccinations and offer to answer any questions.

2. Why did you choose this option?

   _____
   _____
   _____
   _____

3. After discussion, the mother decides she would like to proceed with an immunization schedule. Where might you find information on catching up the baby's immunizations?

   _____
   _____
   _____

Scenario 2

After preparing a vaccination for little Joey Jones, age 2, you discover that he feels warm and is just lying quietly on his mother's lap. The mother has signed the vaccination information and consent forms. The provider was about to see the baby but was called away on an emergency before seeing the child. The mother is looking at her watch and has indicated that she has another pressing appointment. Several other patients are waiting, and the provider's absence is going to put the appointment list behind schedule.

1. How will you address the situation?

   _____
   _____
   _____
   _____
   _____

Competency Practice

1. **Withdraw Medication from an Ampule.** Assemble the supplies and equipment needed. Practice opening an ampule properly and withdrawing the medication into a syringe for administration. Use Procedure 53–1 as a guide.

2. **Prepare Medication from a Multi- or Single-Dose Vial.** Assemble supplies and equipment needed. Practice using multi- or single dose vials to prepare a variety of medications for administration. Use Procedure 53–2 as a guide.

3. **Reconstitute a Powder Medication.** Using a vial of practi-powdered medication, and diluent, use a safety needle and syringe to reconstitute medication to prepare for administration. Use Procedure 53–3 as a guide.

4. **Administer an Intradermal Injection.** Gather the supplies and equipment needed for administering ID injections. Using an anatomical model, prepare and administer medication intradermally. Use Procedure 53–4 as a guide.

5. **Administer a Subcutaneous Injection.** Gather the supplies and equipment needed for administering Sub Q injections. Using an anatomical model, prepare and administer medication subcutaneously. Use Procedure 53–5 as a guide.

6. **Administer an Intramuscular Injection.** Gather the supplies and equipment needed for administering IM injections. Using an anatomical model, prepare and administer medication intramuscularly. Use Procedure 53–6 as a guide.

7. **Administer an Intramuscular Injection by Z-track Method.** Gather the supplies and equipment needed for administering Z-track injections. Using an anatomical model, prepare and administer medication intramuscularly using the Z-track Method. Use Procedure 53–7 as a guide.

First Aid and Responding to Emergencies

Emergencies in the Medical Office and the Community

Words to Know Challenge

Spelling: Each line contains three spellings of a word. Underline the correctly spelled word.

1. asperation   aspirashun   <u>aspiration</u>

2. <u>diaphoresis</u>   diephoresis   diaforesis

3. profalatic   frofalytic   <u>prophylactic</u>

4. <u>exhaustion</u>   eghaustion   egaustion

5. ammonea   <u>ammonia</u>   amoania

6. seezure   seazure   <u>seizure</u>

7. <u>cessation</u>   sessation   cesation

8. coraner   coriner   <u>coroner</u>

9. <u>intubation</u>   entubation   intobacion

10. poision   <u>poison</u>   poisen

11. sincope   syncape   <u>syncope</u>

12. <u>resuscitation</u>   resesutation   recessatation

Fill in the Blank: Complete the following sentences with Words to Know from this chapter.

1. A _____ is when someone is in an abnormally deep stupor from which he or she cannot be aroused by external stimuli.

2. If you should encounter any emergency situation or if you happen to come upon an unknown person who has become ill or lost _____, check for a universal emergency medical identification symbol.

3. _____, also known as _____, is caused by an increased amount of sugar in the blood.

4. Diabetic ketoacidosis (hyperglycemia) is caused by an increased amount of sugar in the blood. The patient might complain of confusion, dizziness, weakness, or nausea. Vomiting can occur. Respiration can be rapid and deep. The skin might be dry and _____.

5. The patient who is exposed to high temperatures for a long period in industry or at home might suffer from _____.

6. In _____, the skin is pale, cool, and moist and the body temperature is normal. The patient becomes overheated with profuse perspiration, usually after some form of vigorous exercise.

7. _____ is the most severe of the heat-related problems.

8. _____ occurs when the body loses heat faster than it can produce it, resulting in a dangerously low body temperature.

9. Exposure to freezing temperatures will often result in _____.

10. _____, also known as _____, can occur from an excess amount of insulin in the body.

11. One of the most common medical emergencies is an _____ airway. The most usual cause in adults is food that is aspirated while eating.

12. Poison can be _____, absorbed, inhaled, injected, or acquired from bites and stings.

Chapter Review

Short Answer

1. Identify five medical conditions for which a patient should wear an identification symbol.

_____

2. Name the three types of visible bleeding and the characteristics of each.

_____
_____

3. List the eight symptoms or stages that might occur with a seizure.

_____
_____

4. List at least seven symptoms of a heart attack.

_____
_____
_____

5. What are the symptoms of internal bleeding, and how is it initially and eventually treated?

_____
_____
_____

6. Describe the purpose of an AED and its capabilities.

_____
_____
_____
_____
_____

7. Explain instances when obstructive airway can occur in adults and children.

_____
_____
_____
_____

8. List at least 10 supplies that can be found on a crash cart.

_____
_____
_____
_____
_____
_____
_____

9. Compare and contrast the symptoms of hyperglycemia and hypoglycemia.

_____
_____
_____
_____
_____
_____
_____

Matching: Match the term in column I to its definition in column II.

COLUMN I	COLUMN II
____ 1. Chronic	A. Extensive, advanced
____ 2. Subtle	B. Requires intervention as soon as possible
____ 3. Urgent	C. Can cause death
____ 4. Sudden	D. Long, drawn out, not acute
____ 5. Acute	E. Provides vital health information
____ 6. Severe	F. Injury
____ 7. Life threatening	G. The act of reviving
____ 8. Universal emergency medical ID	H. Rapid onset, severe symptoms, short course
____ 9. Trauma	I. Unexpected occurrence needing immediate action
____ 10. Resuscitation	J. Another term for heart attack
____ 11. Bandage	K. Hidden, not apparent
____ 12. Myocardial infarction	L. Period after death
____ 13. Medical emergency	M. Occurring quickly, without warning
____ 14. Postmortem	N. A dressing

Chapter Application

Case Studies with Critical Thinking Questions

Scenario 1

Mr. Karnes, a diabetic patient, tells the receptionist that he is not feeling very well and wants to know if he can be taken to an exam room right away. He took his insulin this morning, but didn't have time to eat before his appointment. While waiting for the medical assistant to escort him to the room, Mr. Karnes becomes unconscious and falls to the floor in the waiting room. The medical assistant summons the provider and gets the crash cart, only to find that there is no glucose in the cart.

1. What must be done immediately after the emergency has been dealt with? _____

_____
_____

2. How can an inadequately stocked crash cart be prevented in the future? _____

_____

_____

Scenario 2

A frantic mother has just called your office and reports that her three-year-old son has just ingested household cleaner. She is hysterical and is asking questions so quickly that you can hardly understand what she is saying.

1. What information should be obtained from the caller? _____

_____

2. Who should the mother be instructed to call? _____

_____

Scenario 3

A patient in the waiting room is suffering with a hacking cough and is hurriedly trying to take a cough drop. A few seconds later, you look up and notice that the patient's face is red and she is giving the universal sign for choking.

1. What is the first thing you need to do? _____

_____

2. If the patient is indeed choking, how can you help? _____

_____

3. Should you try to dislodge the object in the patient's mouth? _____

_____

_____

Competency Practice

1. **Perform First Aid Procedures for Syncope (Fainting Episode).** With a partner, practice role-playing being the patient and the MA, and assist the patient as he or she has a syncope (fainting episode). Use Procedure 54–2 as a guide.

2. **Perform First Aid Procedures for Bleeding.** With a partner, practice role-playing being the patient and the MA, and assist the patient to control bleeding as he or she role-plays having a wound that is bleeding profusely. Use Procedure 54–3 as a guide.

3. **Perform First Aid Procedures for Seizures.** With a partner, practice role-playing being the patient and the MA, and assist the patient as he or she role-plays having a seizure. Use Procedure 54–4 as a guide.

4. **Perform an Abdominal Thrust on an Adult Victim with an Obstructed Airway.** With a partner, demonstrate how to perform abdominal thrusts. Explain what your next step would be if the patient loses consciousness. Use Procedure 54–5 as a guide.

5. **Perform First Aid Procedures for Shock.** With a partner, practice role-playing being the patient and the MA, and assist the patient as he or she role-plays being in shock. Use Procedure 54–6 as a guide.

6. **Develop Safety Plans for Emergency Preparedness.** Utilizing a website that specializes in emergency preparedness such as http://emergency.cdc.gov or www.fema.gov, develop safety plans for an environmental event (such as a tornado or flood), for personal safety on the job, and for personal safety at home. Use Procedure 54–7 as a guide.

First Aid for Accidents and Injuries

Words to Know Challenge

Spelling: Each line contains three spellings of a word. Underline the correctly spelled word.

1. anafalactic   anaphylactic   aniphylactic
2. avulsion   evulsion   avulzion
3. cravat   cravet   cravette
4. moltan   molten   moltin
5. superficiel   superficial   superfisual
6. thermel   theremal   thermal

Matching: Match the term in column I to its definition in column II.

	COLUMN I	COLUMN II
____	1. Abrasion	A. Smooth cut
____	2. Chemical	B. A brisk rubbing
____	3. Electrical	C. A hole
____	4. Friction	D. A tear
____	5. Immobilize	E. An injury
____	6. Incision	F. To prevent from moving
____	7. Laceration	G. Having a current
____	8. Puncture	H. Acid or alkaline substance
____	9. Foreign body	I. A scrape or scratch
____	10. Rabies	J. State of very low blood pressure, rapid pulse, pallor
____	11. Shock	K. Not normally found in the location; splinter, dirt
____	12. Splinter	L. Transmitted by an animal bite
____	13. Wound	M. Thin, sharp piece of wood

Chapter Review

Short Answer

1. How is a bee stinger removed? _____

2. When is antirabies serum required following an animal bite? _____
   _____
   _____

3. Name the three types of burns and give examples of each.
   a. _____
   _____
   b. _____
   c. _____

4. What is the first priority in the treatment of burns? _____

5. Compare the types of first aid treatment for the three degrees of burns.
   a. _____
   b. _____
   _____
   c. _____
   _____

6. What is the benefit of adding moisture to a heat treatment? _____
   _____

7. What action does the application of cold treatments have on the body? _____
   _____
   _____

8. What action does the application of heat treatments have on the body? _____
   _____
   _____

9. Name five types of wounds.
   _____

10. What four pieces of information are needed to determine the severity of an illness or injury?
    a. _____
    b. _____
    c. _____
    d. _____

Fill in the Blank: Use information from the chapter to complete the sentence.

1. The Rule of _____ is used to estimate the extent of a burn.

2. A _____ degree burn involves all three layers of the skin.

3. A break in the bone is also known as a _____.

4. Injury to a muscle or muscle group is known as a _____.

5. A _____ causes a ligament injury at the joint.

6. You would place a _____ over the wound before you cover it with a _____.

7. A scrape in the epidermis is also known as an _____.

8. A _____ degree burn causes white, leathery tissue.

9. You should flood a _____ burn with water for 15 minutes.

10. A _____ bandage should be used for an injury to the palm of the hand.

Chapter Application

Case Studies with Critical Thinking Questions

Scenario 1

Mrs. Leonard calls the office because her three-year-old child has been stung. She thinks it was a wasp, but she isn't sure. She says he is having trouble breathing, is very restless, his head hurts very badly, and his skin is becoming mottled and blue.

1. What is happening to the child? _____

2. If he is going into anaphylactic shock, what medication needs to be given immediately? _____

3. What instructions should be given to Mrs. Leonard? _____

Scenario 2

A patient rushes into the office with a severe burn to his left hand. He says that he was deep-frying some fish and spilled the hot grease on his hand. His skin is red and blistered.

1. Which class of burn is the patient suffering from? _____

2. What is another name for this degree burn? _____

3. What is the proper first aid? _____

_____

_____

Competency Practice

1. **Perform First Aid Procedures for Fractures.** With a partner, gather the needed equipment and supplies and role-play demonstrating the proper procedure for providing first aid for a fracture. One partner is the MA and the other the patient. Be sure to provide the patient with any education regarding the fracture. Use Procedure 55–1 as a guide.

2. **Perform wound care.** With a partner, gather the needed equipment and supplies and role-play demonstrating the proper procedure for cleaning a wound. One partner is the MA and the other the patient. Be sure to provide the patient with any education regarding the wound. Use Procedure 55–2 as a guide.

3. **Demonstrate Application of a Tube Gauze, Spiral, Figure-Eight, and Cravat Bandage.** With a partner, practice these bandaging techniques. Be sure to ask the instructor to check your work for correctness. Discuss any patient education that would be needed about the bandages. Use Procedures 55–3 through 55–6 as guides.

Rehabilitation and Healthy Living

Rehabilitation

Words to Know Challenge

Spelling: Each line contains three spellings of a word. Underline the correctly spelled word.

1. angel   angle   angul
2. crutches   crutzes   crutious
3. sling   sleng   slinge
4. suport   support   sapport
5. walcher   walker   wocker
6. weelchair   whealchair   wheelchair

Matching: Match the term in column I to its definition in column II.

	COLUMN I	COLUMN II
____	1. Ambulate	A. Proper positioning to reduce injury
____	2. Axilla	B. Manner of walking
____	3. Balance	C. A type of cane
____	4. Flexibility	D. To walk
____	5. Gait	E. Extent of movement
____	6. Mobility	F. Area under the arm
____	7. Quad-base	G. The ability to twist and bend
____	8. Range of motion	H. Equilibrium
____	9. Stabilize	I. Move about freely
____	10. Body mechanics	J. To hold secure

Chapter Review

Short Answer

1. Identify seven situations during which the use of some form of device might be indicated to assist patients with mobility.

   _____

   _____

   _____

2. Explain the importance of good body mechanics.

   _____

   _____

   _____

3. What are range-of-motion exercises?

   _____

   _____

   _____

4. When are range-of-motion exercises indicated?

   _____

   _____

5. Identify two guidelines concerning fitting a cane.

   (1) _____

   (2) _____

6. Explain the proper height for crutches.

   _____

7. List four factors that will increase safety for the patient at home.

   _____

   _____

   _____

Matching: Match the term in column I to its definition in column II.

COLUMN I	COLUMN II
____ 1. Abduction	A. A motion that turns a part on its axis
____ 2. Adduction	B. Bending movement that decreases the angle between two parts
____ 3. Dorsiflexion	C. The movement of the sole toward the median plane
____ 4. Extension	D. A motion that pulls a structure or part away from the midline of the body
____ 5. Flexion	E. Flexion of the entire foot inferiorly
____ 6. Hyperextension	F. A motion that pulls a structure or part toward the midline of the body or toward the midline of a limb
____ 7. Inversion	G. The opposite of flexion
____ 8. Plantar Flexion	H. Extension of the entire foot superiorly
____ 9. Pronation	I. A position of maximum extension
____ 10. Rotation	J. A rotation of the forearm that moves the palm from an anterior-facing position to a posterior-facing position
____ 11. Supination	K. The opposite of pronation

Chapter Application

Case Studies with Critical Thinking Questions

Scenario 1

Mr. Durst has twisted his knee and cannot walk very well. He says he has no balance and is afraid of falling again.

1. Which mobility device could be helpful to the patient? _____

2. If the provider instructs you to provide patient education regarding this mobility device, what information should be given to the patient? _____

_____

_____

Scenario 2

Sue Larson, an active 16-year-old, presented to the office with an ankle fracture. The provider has ordered you to help fit her for crutches. She states she has never had an injury like this before and that she doesn't think she needs assistance—it will be fun and easy to use the crutches.

1. What do you need to tell the patient about why you need to help with the crutch fitting? _____

_____

_____

2. What does the patient need to know about walking with the crutches? _____

_____

_____

3. What can you do to ensure patient compliance? _____

_____

_____

_____

Competency Practice

1. **Demonstrate Using Proper Body Mechanics.** With a partner or alone, practice lifting and moving various large objects, using the guidelines for proper body mechanics. For a variation, have students role-play, one being the patient and the other being the MA, and apply body mechanic principles in moving the patient. Use Procedure 56–1 as a guide.

2. **Demonstrate Application of an Arm Sling.** With a partner, demonstrate the proper application of a commercial arm sling on your partner. Be sure to choose the correctly fitting sling and go over patient education on proper use and how to watch for circulation impairment. Use Procedure 56–2 as a guide.

3. **Demonstrate Fitting and Instruction in Use of a Cane.** With a partner, demonstrate adjusting a cane to the proper height. Conduct patient education sessions on the proper use of a cane. Use Procedure 56–3 as a guide.

4. **Demonstrate Fitting and Instruction in Use of Crutches.** With a partner, practice adjusting crutches for one another. Then divide into three groups and have each group choose a crutch gait. Practice the gaits and demonstrate them to the class. Then rotate groups until each group has gotten to apply each one. Use Procedure 56–4 as a guide.

5. **Demonstrate Instruction in Use of a Walker.** With a partner, using both walkers with wheels and those without, adjust the height of the walker and practice ambulating with it. Role-play with each other instructing the patient on the proper way to walk, keeping safety in mind at all times. Discuss when a walker might be indicated for a patient. Use Procedure 56–5 as a guide.

Nutrition, Exercise, and Healthy Living

Words to Know Challenge

Spelling: Each line contains three spellings of a word. Underline the correctly spelled word.

1. anorexec   <u>anorexic</u>   annorhexic
2. <u>beriberi</u>   berryberry   baribari
3. <u>scurvy</u>   scurvey   skurvey
4. tactille   <u>tactile</u>   tacktile
5. sleep apnia   <u>sleep apnea</u>   sleep apniea
6. protine   proteen   <u>protein</u>
7. <u>obesity</u>   obeasety   obeesity
8. rickettes   ricettes   <u>rickets</u>
9. <u>dietitian</u>   diatician   diatichian
10. carbohidrate   <u>carbohydrate</u>   carbohydrat

Matching: Match the term in column I to its definition in column II.

	COLUMN I		COLUMN II
D	1. Amenorrhea	A.	Illness, disease
K	2. Anorexia nervosa	B.	Overeating and then initiating vomiting
B	3. Bulimia nervosa	C.	To rid body of food after eating
J	4. Deprivation	D.	Absence of menstruation
H	5. Emaciation	E.	To overindulge in food or drink
A	6. Infirmity	F.	Period of no breathing
C	7. Purge	G.	Non-rapid eye movement
F	8. Apnea	H.	Abnormal thinness

(continues)

E   9. Binge   I. Rapid eye movement

G   10. NREM   J. Having to do without or being unable to use

I   11. REM   K. No appetite, refusal to eat

Chapter Review

Short Answer

1. Identify three dos and three don'ts from the Guidelines for Good Health. _____
_____
_____
_____

2. Name the five sections in MyPlate, and list examples of foods in each section. _____

   Grains: Bread, Noodle, Whole Grain

   Vegetables: Beans, Peas, Lettuce

   Fruits: Bananas, Apple, Orange

   Dairy: Milk, Yogurt, Cheese

   Protein Foods: Meat, Poultry, Seafood, Nuts

3. Name the fat-soluble vitamins. _____

4. Name the water-soluble vitamins. _____

5. Name two essential minerals that are most often missing from the average diet. _____

6. List 10 diseases or conditions that can develop from poor diet and a sedentary lifestyle.

   a. _____
   b. _____
   c. _____
   d. _____
   e. _____
   f. _____
   g. _____
   h. _____
   i. _____
   j. _____

7. What are eight pieces of information included on food labels?

   a. Calorie
   b. Serving Size
   c. Fiber
   d. Carbs
   e. Sugar

f. Protein

g. Vitamins

h. Fat

8. What two eating disorders affect primarily teenagers, and what are the underlying causes of these conditions? _____

_____

9. Why is sleep necessary? _____

_____

_____

10. What happens after prolonged sleep deprivation? _____

_____

_____

Fill in the Blank: Use information from the chapter to complete the sentence.

1. A deficiency of vitamin D can cause rickets .

2. A deficiency of vitamin C can cause scurvy .

3. People who weigh 20 percent MORE than their ideal body weight are considered obese.

4. Generally, a(n) BRAT diet is recommended to patients at least every 2 hours the first 24 hours for patients with diarrhea.

5. The BRAT acronym stands for bananas , rice , applesauce , and toast .

6. The clear liquid diet is recommended for 24 hours as tolerated by patients after diarrhea stops, or as directed by the provider.

7. Those who have been sick and are just getting over an intestinal virus might find the soft diet to be tolerable.

8. Patients who wish to reduce their weight should exercise at least three times a week and follow a(n) low calorie diet.

9. Patients who have special dietary needs should consult with a(n) registered dietician .

10. insomnia describes the inability to sleep.

11. Lack of sleep is termed deprivation .

12. Research shows that a person needs both REM and NREM stages of sleep.

13. People who sleep at least six hours at a time generally feel good because they benefit from the effects of the proper sequence of sleep.

Chapter Application

Case Studies with Critical Thinking Questions

Scenario 1

Mrs. Anderson is being seen in the office to evaluate her general state of health. She is found to be malnourished and is suffering from lethargy and malaise. The provider suggests she should incorporate more protein in her diet, including some red meat, which has valuable amino acids and iron. The provider asks the medical assistant to provide Mrs. Anderson with a diet sheet listing certain meats and other foods high in protein. Mrs. Anderson tells the medical assistant she is a Seventh-Day Adventist and does not eat meat.

1. What should the medical assistant tell Mrs. Anderson about her dietary restrictions? _____

_____

_____

2. How can the dietary restrictions be dealt with? Should the medical assistant tell Mrs. Anderson about a dietary supplement that is very high in protein? _____

_____

_____

Scenario 2

Andrea, a 32-year-old in good health, calls the office to talk with the medical assistant about the diarrhea she has had for the past three days. She says she is eating only small portions of chicken noodle soup and drinking milk, but she can't seem to get over the diarrhea. She wants to know when she can expect to get better and when she can return to a normal diet.

1. With the provider's approval, what should Andrea's diet be until the diarrhea has stopped? _____

2. Which diet should Andrea follow for 24 hours after the diarrhea has stopped? _____

3. Before resuming a normal diet, which eating plan should be followed next? _____

Competency Practice

1. **Develop a Nutritional Meal Plan to Instruct Patients According to Dietary Needs.** With a partner, role-play being the MA and the patient, and instruct the patient on a meal plan you develop using the ChooseMyPlate.gov website. You can create a variety of plans. Use Procedure 57–1 as a guide.

Preparing for Employment

Workplace Readiness

Practicum and the Job Search

Words to Know Challenge

Spelling: Each line contains three spellings of a word. Underline the correctly spelled word.

1. resame   résumé   reesume
2. transscript   transcript   transcrip
3. practicum   practical   practicam
4. chronilogical   chonological   chronological
5. targeted   targited   tarrgated
6. extirnship   externshop   externship

Fill in the Blank: Complete the following sentences with correctly spelled words from the Spelling section.

1. The _____ is a period of time when a student is placed in an actual health care setting to practice skills that have been learned in the classroom. Another name for this experience is _____.

2. A _____ style résumé highlights your previous work experience related to the position you are seeking.

3. The goal of a _____ is to make a favorable impression so you will obtain an interview for a position.

4. This type of résumé lists education achievements followed by work experience, starting with the present or most recent job and progressing back in time. It is called a _____ style résumé.

5. The _____ style résumé will usually include a position statement.

6. An official copy of a student's educational record is known as a _____.

Chapter Review

Short Answer

1. Name three reasons participation in a practicum is beneficial to a student.

   _____
   _____
   _____

2. List at least six possible areas that might be included on an externship evaluation form.

_____

_____

_____

3. What is the goal of a résumé?

_____

_____

_____

4. What is the purpose of a cover letter?

_____

_____

_____

5. List the styles of résumés and the purpose of each.

_____

_____

_____

_____

6. List at least six places a medical assistant can find information about job opportunities.

_____

_____

_____

7. Why is it important to dress professionally for an interview?

_____

_____

_____

8. Name six things you need to remember to be prepared for your interview.

A. _____

B. _____

C. _____

D. _____

E. _____

F. _____

9. Why should you send a follow-up letter after an interview?

_____

_____

_____

10. What are six things you can do to advance in employment?

A. _____

B. _____

C. _____

D. _____

E. _____

F. _____

Matching: Identify the items in the following list as desirable skills or qualities that employers seek in employees.

____	1. Teamwork	A.	Desirable skill
____	2. Flexibility	B.	Desirable quality
____	3. Honesty		
____	4. Critical thinking/Problem solving		
____	5. Computer proficiency		
____	6. Responsible		
____	7. Time management		
____	8. Positive attitude		
____	9. Communication		
____	10. Punctuality		

Chapter Application

Case Studies with Critical Thinking Questions

Scenario 1

Avery is beginning her second week at her practicum. She has been given one of the best sites, where she will gain a lot of valuable experience. She is not happy about putting in hours and not getting paid for them. Avery feels that this is just another part of her school experience and, therefore, she can skip whenever she feels like it. She has already been 10 minutes late on three occasions and has missed one whole day.

1. What does her practicum performance say about her as a medical assistant? _____
   _____
   _____

2. What does her performance say about her school? _____
   _____
   _____
   _____

3. What impact could her performance have on her career? _____
   _____
   _____

Scenario 2

You are on your way to a job interview for a position you really want. You thought you allowed plenty of time for traffic and for any other problems that could arise. Traffic on the freeway is at a standstill because of an accident, and you realize you are going to be late for your interview.

1. What should you do? _____
   _____

2. What impact can this situation have if you arrive late without notifying the facility? _____
   _____
   _____

3. What impression could your late arrival give to your interviewer? _____
   _____
   _____

Scenario 3

You found an ad in the newspaper for a medical assisting position that you are really interested in. The ad instructed applicants to visit the clinic in person to fill out an application and drop off a résumé. You hurriedly print off a copy of your résumé and drive to the clinic, wearing clothes appropriate for the gym, since you'll be going there after. Upon arriving at the clinic, you find that there are five other people filling out applications. You hurry through your application to be the first one done, give the receptionist your résumé, and are told that they will be contacting qualified applicants for an interview next week. Three weeks later, you have not been contacted for an interview, and you are very disappointed.

1. If you could start this day over again, what would be the first thing you would do over? _____

_____

2. What are some other things that might have prevented you from receiving an interview? _____

_____

_____

3. What could you have done to get an interview? _____

_____

Competency Practice

Scenario: You read about an open position for a clinical medical assistant at Napa Valley Family Health Associates (Address: 101 Vine Street, Napa, CA 94558) and want to apply for the job. The practice manager is Takari Miata. Referring to the job description provided in Figure 58–7, prepare a résumé, cover letter, complete the job application, and prepare a follow-up letter.

1. **Prepare a Résumé**. Using Procedure 58–1 as a guideline, prepare a résumé for a position as a clinical medical assistant in a family practice clinic.

2. **Prepare a Cover Letter**. Using Procedure 58–2 as a guideline, prepare a cover letter for a position as a clinical medical assistant in a family practice clinic.

3. **Complete a Job Application**. Using Procedure 58–3 as a guideline, complete a job application for a position as a clinical medical assistant in a family practice clinic. Use Procedure Form 58–3 provided on the Student Companion website to complete this competency.

4. **Write an Interview Follow-Up Letter**. Using Procedure 58–4 as a guideline, prepare a follow-up letter for a position as a clinical medical assistant in a family practice clinic.

Managing the Office

Words to Know Challenge

Spelling: Each line contains three spellings of a word. Underline the correctly spelled word.

1. acounttant   accountant   accowntant
2. benefits   benifits   bennefits
3. complimentary   complamentary   complimentry
4. dissability   disability   disabbility
5. fring benafits   fringe bennefits   fringe benefits
6. Internal Revenue Service   Internal Revinue Service   Internal Revanue Service
7. profit shareing   profit sharing   profut sharing
8. berevement   bearevement   bereavement
9. collaborating   colaborating   colobarting
10. compitance   competence   compatance
11. conflect   conficlt   conflict
12. stratagy   strategie   strategy
13. stile   style   styel
14. salery   salary   sallary
15. owerly wage   hourly waje   hourly wage

Matching: Match the term in column I to its definition in column II.

	Column I	Column II
____	1. Site review	A. Freed from or not liable for something to which others are subject
____	2. Deductions	B. A long duration of life; lasting a long time
____	3. Exemption	C. The amount of work accomplished in a period of time
____	4. Gross	D. Settled; complete; absolute; continuous
____	5. Longevity	E. Exclusive of deductions; total, entire
____	6. Net	F. To pay back or compensate for money spent or losses or damages incurred
____	7. Productivity	G. To deduct or subtract; remove, take away
____	8. Reimbursement	H. Remaining after all deductions have been made; to clear as profit
____	9. Vested	I. An inspection to ensure compliance with regulations and policies

Chapter Review

Short Answer

1. Describe leadership and management styles. _____

_____

_____

_____

2. List legal and illegal applicant interview questions. _____

_____

_____

3. Describe types and reasoning behind training, motivation, and the nonpunitive work environment. ____

_____

_____

_____

_____

_____

_____

_____

_____

_____

_____

_____

_____

4. Explain the probationary period and employee counseling. _____

_____

_____

_____

_____

_____

_____

_____

5. Discuss conflict management. _____

_____

_____

_____
_____
_____

6. Describe six responsibilities a manager has to employees.

_____
_____
_____
_____

7. Describe how HIPAA has affected office policy.

_____
_____
_____

8. Define sexual harassment and the hostile work environment.

_____
_____
_____
_____
_____

9. Explain the purpose of W-4, W-2, and I-9 forms.

   a) W-4: _____
   _____

   b) W-2: _____
   _____

   c) I-9: _____
   _____
   _____

10. Differentiate between gross and net salary.

_____
_____
_____

11. Describe the office manager's role in staff meetings.

_____
_____
_____

12. Describe the office manager's role in employee evaluation and review.

_____
_____
_____

13. Describe the office manager's role in termination of employment.

_____
_____
_____

14. What are salary benefits? In your answer, identify six examples of benefits an employee might receive.

_____
_____
_____

15. Describe and list at least six responsibilities a manager has to the providers.

_____
_____
_____
_____
_____

16. In the following chart, place an X in the column next to items that would be included on a practice information brochure.

Lengthy physician biography	
After-hours policy	
Missed appointment policy	
Physician specialties	
Smoking policy	
Hospital affiliation	
Office hours	
Prescription refill policy	

17. List at least four organizations that inspect medical offices during site visits.

_____
_____
_____

Matching: For each item listed in column I, identify whether it is considered an office POLICY (A) or PROCEDURE (B). (*Note:* Answers in column II may be used more than once.)

COLUMN I

____ 1. Absenteeism

____ 2. Paid time off

____ 3. Opening and closing the office

____ 4. Harassment

____ 5. OSHA and CLIA requirements

____ 6. Confidentiality

____ 7. Laboratory tests

____ 8. Emergency procedures

____ 9. Employment evaluations

____ 10. Information technology

COLUMN II

A. Policy

B. Procedure

Matching: For each item listed in column I, identify whether it is considered the manager's responsibility to EMPLOYEE (A), PROVIDER (B), or FACILITY (C). (*Note:* Answers in column II may be used more than once.)

COLUMN I

____ 1. Subscriptions to magazines

____ 2. Conduct staff meetings to inform, discuss, and exchange information

____ 3. Assist in creating/updating business policies to increase efficiency

____ 4. Monitor and pay utilities

____ 5. Security (locks, alarms), privacy (HIPAA)

____ 6. Order CPT and ICD books annually to review for deleted or added codes

____ 7. Create, implement, and enforce work schedules

____ 8. Manage staff in most efficient and effective manner for provider productivity

____ 9. Information technology support

____ 10. Conduct performance evaluations

COLUMN II

A. Responsibility to employee

B. Responsibility to provider

C. Responsibility for facility

Chapter Application

Case Studies with Critical Thinking Questions

Scenario 1

A job applicant for the position of clinical medical assistant has passed the first interview and is handed a stack of paperwork to be filled out to ensure that she is eligible to work in this capacity and in this country. She is hired for the job, but at the end of the first two-week pay period, the person responsible for payroll in the office sends the clinical supervisor a note stating that the applicant cannot be paid.

1. Can you think of a reason the employee cannot be able to be paid? _____

_____

_____

2. Which form must be filled out before anyone can begin working in the United States? _____

_____

_____

Scenario 2

Maryn Leonard, a single mother of three, has just been hired to work as a medical assistant at the Downtown Clinic. She has completed all required documents for employment and has started working. Her first paycheck seems to be lower than what she expected, and she wants to know why.

1. How many dependent deductions can she claim? _____

_____

2. On which form would you check to ensure that the correct number of dependent deductions are claimed to raise her pay? _____

_____

Scenario 3

You have just been hired at Downtown Clinic as a clinical medical assistant. The office manager tells you that although the office carries liability insurance, you personally are not covered under the policy. You ask another medical assistant about whether she has insurance, and she tells you she does not. She says she hasn't looked into it, but she thinks it might be expensive. She says she's been working there for five years, and it's not a big deal whether you get the insurance. What should you do?

_____

_____

_____

Scenario 4

While a patient was leaving the exam room at the Downtown Clinic, she slipped and fell on a wet surface. You helped her up and discovered a large gash on her forehead. You contact the treating physician to attend to the patient and then immediately notify the practice manager of the incident and prepare an incident report. Why is office liability insurance important?

_____

_____

_____

Research Activity

1. Go to the IRS website (www.irs.gov) and locate an I-9 form. Locate "Section 2. Employer Review and Verification" on the form and the "List of Acceptable Documents." In the following chart, identify which types of documents are included in lists A, B, and C and then identify three documents within each category.
   Documents in List A are documents that establish _____
   Documents in List B are documents that establish _____
   Documents in List C are documents that establish _____

	List A	List B	List C
1.			
2.			
3.			

2. Go online and search for free employee evaluation form templates. Compare several forms and print out the form you think is the best. With a partner, complete the evaluation form based on your partner's performance in the classroom.

Competency Practice

1. **Conduct a Staff Meeting.** Using Procedure 59–1 as a guideline, create an agenda, conduct a staff meeting, and record minutes of meeting for the following scenario.

   SCENARIO: The office has been transitioning from paper to electronic health records. A meeting has been scheduled with the EHR vendor to make a presentation to the providers and staff, outlining new upgrades, workflows, practice management and electronic medical record features, and a time frame to complete the process.

   _____

Part 2

COMPETENCY CHECKLIST

Name: _____ Date: _____ Score: _____

Competency Checklist Tracking Sheet

Procedure Number and Title	School Date/Initials	Score	Practicum Date/Initials
Procedure 1–1: Demonstrate Professional Behavior			
Procedure 3–1: Perform Compliance Reporting Based on Public Health Statutes			
Procedure 3–2: Report an Illegal Activity in the Health Care Setting Following Proper Protocol			
Procedure 3–3: Apply HIPAA Rules to Release of Patient Information			
Procedure 3–4: Locate a State's Legal Scope of Practice for Medical Assistants			
Procedure 4–1: Develop a Plan for Separation of Personal and Professional Ethics			
Procedure 4–2: Demonstrate Appropriate Responses to Ethical Issues			
Procedure 5–1: Recognize and Respond to Nonverbal Communication			
Procedure 6–1: Coach Patients Regarding Health Maintenance, Disease Prevention, and Treatment Plans while Considering Cultural Diversity, Developmental Life Stages, and Communication Barriers.			
Procedure 22–1: Demonstrate Professional Telephone Techniques			
Procedure 22–2: Document Telephone Messages Accurately			
Procedure 22–3: Telephone a Patient with Test Results			
Procedure 22–4: Develop a Current List of Community Resources Related to Patients' Health Care Needs			
Procedure 22–5: Facilitate Referrals to Community Resources in the Role of a Patient Navigator			
Procedure 23–1: Compose Professional Correspondence Utilizing Electronic Technology			
Procedure 24–1: Open the Office and Evaluate the Work Environment to Identify Unsafe Working Conditions			
Procedure 24–2: Perform an Inventory of Equipment and Supplies with Documentation			
Procedure 24–3: Close the Office and Evaluate the Work Environment to Identify Unsafe Working Conditions			
Procedure 24–4: Use Proper Ergonomics			
Procedure 24–5: Perform Routine Maintenance of Administrative or Clinical Equipment			
Procedure 25–1: Manage the Appointment Schedule Using Established Priorities			
Procedure 25–2: Schedule a Patient Procedure			
Procedure 25–3: Apply HIPAA Rules in Regard to Patient Privacy and Release of Information When Scheduling a Patient Procedure			
Procedure 25–4: Explain General Office Policies to the Patient			
Procedure 26–1: Create and Organize a Patient's Medical Record			
Procedure 26–2: Use an Alphabetic Filing System			
Procedure 26–3: Use a Numeric Filing System			
Procedure 27–1: Verify Insurance Coverage and Eligibility for Services			
Procedure 27–2: Obtain Precertification or Preauthorization (Predetermination) and Inform a Patient of Financial Obligations for Services Rendered			
Procedure 28–1: Perform Procedural Coding			
Procedure 28–2: Utilize Medical Necessity Guidelines			
Procedure 28–3: Perform Diagnostic Coding			
Procedure 29–1: Perform Accounts Receivable Procedures to Patient Accounts, Including Posting Charges, Payments, and Adjustments			
Procedure 29–2: Inform a Patient of Financial Obligations for Services Rendered			
Procedure 30–1: Complete an Insurance Claim Form			

Name: _____   Date: _____   Score: _____

Procedure Number and Title	School Date/Initials	Score	Practicum Date/Initials
Procedure 30–2: Process Insurance Claims			
Procedure 31–1: Post Nonsufficient Funds (NSF) Checks and Collection Agency Payments Utilizing EMR and Practice Management Systems			
Procedure 31–2: Process a Credit Balance and Refund			
Procedure 32–1: Prepare a Check			
Procedure 32–2: Prepare a Deposit Slip			
Procedure 32–3: Reconcile a Bank Statement			
Procedure 33–1: Establish and Maintain a Petty Cash Fund			
Procedure 34–1: Participate in a Mock Exposure Event with Documentation of Specific Steps			
Procedure 34–2: Hand Washing for Medical Asepsis			
Procedure 34–3: Remove Nonsterile Gloves			
Procedure 34–4: Choose, Apply, and Remove Appropriate Personal Protective Equipment (PPE)			
Procedure 34–5: Sanitize Instruments			
Procedure 34–6: Disinfect (Chemical "Cold" Sterilization) Endoscopes			
Procedure 34–7: Wrap Items for Autoclaving			
Procedure 34–8: Perform Autoclave Sterilization			
Procedure 35–1: Perform Patient Screening			
Procedure 35–2: Obtain and Record a Patient Health History			
Procedure 36–1: Measure Height and Weight Using a Balance Beam Scale			
Procedure 36–2: Measure and Record Oral Temperature with an Electronic Thermometer			
Procedure 36–3: Measure and Record Rectal Temperature with an Electronic Thermometer			
Procedure 36–4: Measure Axillary Temperature			
Procedure 36–5: Measure Core Body Temperature with a Tympanic (Aural) Thermometer			
Procedure 36–6: Measure Temperature with a Temporal Artery Thermometer			
Procedure 36–7: Measure the Apical Pulse			
Procedure 36–8: Measure the Radial Pulse and Respirations			
Procedure 36–9: Measure Blood Pressure			
Procedure 37–1: Prepare and Maintain Examination and Treatment Areas			
Procedure 37–2: Transfer a Patient from a Wheelchair to the Examination Table			
Procedure 37–3: Transfer a Patient from an Examination Table to a Wheelchair			
Procedure 37–4: Positioning the Patient for an Exam			
Procedure 38–1: Prepare a Patient for and Assist with a Routine Physical Examination			
Procedure 39-1 Irrigate the Ear			
Procedure 39-2 Perform Audiometry Screening			
Procedure 39–3: Irrigate the Eye			
Procedure 39–4: Screen Visual Acuity with a Snellen Chart			
Procedure 39–5: Screen Visual Acuity with the Jaeger System			
Procedure 39–6: Determine Color Vision Acuity by the Ishihara Method			
Procedure 39–7: Perform Spirometry Testing			
Procedure 39–8: Perform Peak Flow Testing			
Procedure 39–9: Measure and Record Pulse Oximetry Testing			
Procedure 39–10 Assist with a Flexible Sigmoidoscopy			

391

Name: _____ Date: _____ Score: _____

Procedure Number and Title	School Date/Initials	Score	Practicum Date/Initials
Procedure 40–1: Prepare the Patient for and Assist with a Gynecological Exam and Pap Test			
Procedure 41–1: Measure Length, Weight, and Head and Chest Circumference of an Infant or Child			
Procedure 41–2: Plot Data on a Growth Chart			
Procedure 41–3: Screen Pediatric Visual Acuity with a Modified Snellen Chart			
Procedure 42–1: Complete an Incident Exposure Report Related to an Error in Patient Care			
Procedure 42–2: Comply with Safety Signs, Symbols, and Labels			
Procedure 42–3: Clean a Spill			
Procedure 42–4: Demonstrate Proper Use of Eyewash Equipment			
Procedure 42–5: Demonstrate Fire Preparedness			
Procedure 42–6: Use a Microscope			
Procedure 43–1: Instruct a Patient on the Collection of a Clean-Catch, Midstream Urine Specimen			
Procedure 43–2: Perform Screening for Pregnancy			
Procedure 43–3: Test Urine with Reagent Strips			
Procedure 43–4: Obtain Urine Sediment for Microscopic Examination			
Procedure 43–5: Screen and Follow Up Test Results			
Procedure 43–6: Instruct a Patient to Collect a Stool Specimen			
Procedure 43–7: Perform an Occult Blood Test			
Procedure 43–8: Instruct a Patient to Collect a Sputum Specimen			
Procedure 43–9: Perform a Wound Collection for Microbiologic Testing			
Procedure 43–10 Obtain a Throat Culture			
Procedure 43–11 Perform a Rapid Strep Screening Test for Group A Strep			
Procedure 44–1: Puncture Skin with a Sterile Lancet			
Procedure 44–2: Obtain Venous Blood with a Sterile Needle and Syringe			
Procedure 44–3: Obtain Venous Blood with a Vacuum Tube			
Procedure 44–4: Obtain Venous Blood with the Butterfly Needle Method			
Procedure 45–1: Determine Hemoglobin Using a Hemoglobinometer			
Procedure 45–2: Determine Hematocrit (Hct) Using a Microhematocrit Centrifuge			
Procedure 45–3: Perform an Erythrocyte Sedimentation Rate (ESR)			
Procedure 45–4: Screen Blood Sugar (Glucose) Level			
Procedure 45–5: Perform Hemoglobin A1C (Glycosylated Hemoglobin) Screening			
Procedure 45–6: Perform a Cholesterol Screening			
Procedure 45–7: Perform a Screening for Infectious Mononucleosis			
Procedure 46–1: Perform Electrocardiography			
Procedure 46–2: Holter Monitoring			
Procedure 48–1: Prepare a Sterile Field			
Procedure 48–2: Hand Washing for Surgical Asepsis			
Procedure 48–3: Sterile Gloving			
Procedure 48–4: Prepare Skin for Minor Surgery			
Procedure 49–1: Perform Wound Collection			
Procedure 49–2: Assist with Minor Surgery			
Procedure 49–3: Assist with Suturing a Laceration			
Procedure 49–4: Remove Sutures or Staples			

Name: _____ Date: _____ Score: _____

Procedure Number and Title	School Date/Initials	Score	Practicum Date/Initials
Procedure 50–1: Use the PDR or Other Drug Reference to Find Medication Information			
Procedure 51–1: Calculate Proper Dosages of Medication for Administration			
Procedure 52–1: Prepare a Prescription			
Procedure 52–2: Record a Medication Entry in the Patient's Chart			
Procedure 52–3: Prepare and Administer Oral Medication			
Procedure 52–4: Administer Eyedrops			
Procedure 52–5: Instill Drops in the Ears			
Procedure 52–6: Administer Rectal Medication			
Procedure 53–1: Withdraw Medication from an Ampule			
Procedure 53–2: Prepare Medication from a Multi- or Single-Dose Vial			
Procedure 53–3: Reconstitute a Powder Medication			
Procedure 53–4: Administer an Intradermal Injection			
Procedure 53–5: Administer a Subcutaneous Injection			
Procedure 53–6: Administer an Intramuscular Injection			
Procedure 53–7: Administer an Intramuscular Injection by Z-Track Method			
Procedure 54–1: Produce Up-To-Date Documentation of Provider/Professional Level CPR			
Procedure 54–2: Perform First Aid Procedures for Syncope (Fainting Episode)			
Procedure 54–3: Perform First Aid Procedures for Bleeding			
Procedure 54–4: Perform First Aid Procedures for Seizures			
Procedure 54–5: Perform an Abdominal Thrust on an Adult Victim with an Obstructed Airway			
Procedure 54–6: Perform First Aid Procedures for Shock			
Procedure 54–7: Develop Safety Plans for Emergency Preparedness			
Procedure 55–1: Perform First Aid Procedures for Fractures			
Procedure 55–2: Perform wound care			
Procedure 55–3: Apply a Tube Gauze Bandage			
Procedure 55–4: Apply a Spiral Bandage			
Procedure 55–5: Apply a Figure-Eight Bandage			
Procedure 55–6: Apply a Cravat Bandage to Forehead, Ear, or Eyes			
Procedure 56–1: Use Proper Body Mechanics			
Procedure 56–2: Apply an Arm Sling			
Procedure 56–3: Use a Cane			
Procedure 56–4: Use Crutches			
Procedure 56–5: Use a Walker			
Procedure 57–1: Instruct a Patient According to Special Dietary Needs			
Procedure 58–1: Prepare a Résumé			
Procedure 58–2: Prepare a Cover Letter			
Procedure 58–3: Complete a Job Application			
Procedure 58–4: Write an Interview Follow-Up Letter			
Procedure 59–1: Conduct a Staff Meeting			

Competency Checklist
Procedure 1–1 Demonstrate Professional Behavior

ABHES Curriculum

MA.A.1.11.b Demonstrate professional behavior

CAAHEP Core Curriculum

V.A.1.a Demonstrate empathy
V.A.1.b Demonstrate active listening
V.A.2 Demonstrate the principles of self-boundaries

Task:	To display professional qualities in all aspects of your position and thus be respected as a reputable medical assistant.
Supplies & Conditions:	Because this is more of a mindset than a procedure, the scenarios selected by your instructor will dictate conditions and supplies with which to practice this procedure. In general, you must exhibit a professional appearance and professional characteristics as you play out the scenarios selected by your instructor to measure each step. Some steps can be in the fashion of questions and answers rather than as an actual scenario.
Standards:	A maximum of three attempts may be used to complete the task. The time limit for each attempt is 20 minutes, with a minimum score of 100 percent. **Scoring:** Determine student's score by dividing points awarded by total points possible and multiplying results by 100.
Forms:	Optional: Procedure Scenario 1–1; procedure scenarios are found in the Instructor's Manual.

EVALUATION

Evaluator Signature: _____ Date: _____

Evaluator Comments:

Name: _____   Date: _____   Score: _____

Procedure 1–1 Steps

Start Time: _____   End Time: _____   Total Time: _____

	Steps	Possible Points	First Attempt	Second Attempt	Third Attempt
1.	*Exhibit dependability and punctuality by being on time and following through with what you say you are going to do.*	15			
2.	*Display a professional appearance.*	15			
3.	*Engage in active listening skills during all encounters.*	15			
4.	*Demonstrate empathy.*	15			
5.	*Exhibit a positive work ethic.*	15			
6.	*Display sensitivity when working with colleagues and patients.*	15			
7.	*Demonstrate courtesy to patients and coworkers.*	15			
8.	*Display tact in dealing with patients and others.*	15			
9.	*Adapt to changes when necessary.*	15			
10.	*Remain confidential at all times.*	15			
11.	*Demonstrate the principles of self-boundaries.*	15			
	Points Awarded / Points Possible	_____/ **165**			

Competency Checklist
Procedure 3–1 Perform Compliance Reporting Based on Public Health Statutes

ABHES Curriculum

MA.A.1.4.a	Follow documentation guidelines
MA.A.1.4.b	Institute federal and state guidelines when releasing medical records or information
MA.A.1.4.f	Comply with federal, state, and local health laws and regulations as they relate to health care settings
MA.A.1.11.b	Demonstrate professional behavior

CAAHEP Core Curriculum

X.C.3	Describe components of the Health Insurance Portability and Accountability Act (HIPAA)
X.P.5	Perform compliance reporting based on public health statutes
X.A.1	Demonstrate sensitivity to patient rights
X.A.2	Protect the integrity of the medical record

Task: Following the steps listed in the procedure, perform compliance reporting based on public health records.

Supplies & Conditions: Paper and pen; computer with Internet access; telephone and fax machine.

Standards: A maximum of three attempts may be used to complete the task. The time limit for each attempt is 10 minutes, with a minimum score of 70 percent. **Scoring:** Determine student's score by dividing points awarded by total points possible and multiplying results by 100.

Forms: Procedure 3–1 Form (optional). Procedure forms can be downloaded from the Student Companion website.

EVALUATION

Evaluator Signature: _____ Date: _____

Evaluator Comments:

399

Name: _____ Date: _____ Score: _____

Procedure 3–1 Steps

Start Time: _____ **End Time:** _____ **Total Time:** _____

	Steps	Possible Points	First Attempt	Second Attempt	Third Attempt
1.	Locate and open the patient's chart (paper or electronic).	10			
2.	Log on to the local public health services website and locate the Disease Reporting link.	10			
3.	Locate the information in the patient's chart to be reported (e.g., tuberculosis).	10			
4.	Following the instructions on the form, accurately complete the confidential report.	20			
5.	Following the reporting criteria, telephone and/or electronically (including fax) report the disease as required.	20			
6.	***Demonstrating sensitivity to patient rights,*** contact the receiving party by telephone to confirm the correct fax number and that the recipient is available to receive PHI. ***Protect the integrity of the medical record.***	20			
7.	Fax a copy of the document (with fax cover sheet) to the public health department.	10			
8.	Remove the fax document(s) and place (or scan) in the patient's chart.	10			
	Points Awarded / Points Possible	_____/ **110**			

Competency Checklist
Procedure 3–2 Report an Illegal Activity in the Health Care Setting Following Proper Protocol

ABHES Curriculum

MA.A.1.4.f   Comply with federal, state, and local health laws and regulations as they relate to health care settings
MA.A.1.11.b   Demonstrate professional behavior

CAAHEP Core Curriculum

X.P.6   Report an illegal activity in the health care setting following proper protocol
X.A.1   Demonstrate sensitivity to patient rights
X.A.2   Protect the integrity of the medical record

Task:	Following the steps listed in the procedure, report an illegal activity in the health care setting following proper protocol.
Supplies & Conditions:	Paper and pen, or computer with word processing or spreadsheet capabilities; telephone.
Standards:	A maximum of three attempts may be used to complete the task. The time limit for each attempt is 10 minutes, with a minimum score of 70 percent. **Scoring:** Determine student's score by dividing points awarded by total points possible and multiplying results by 100.

EVALUATION

Evaluator Signature: _____   Date: _____

Evaluator Comments:

401

Name: _____ Date: _____ Score: _____

Procedure 3–2 Steps

Start Time: _____ End Time: _____ Total Time: _____

	Steps	Possible Points	First Attempt	Second Attempt	Third Attempt
1.	You discover an illegal activity at the medical office where you are working. Document the nature of the activity and the person(s) involved. ***Comply with federal, state, and local health laws and regulations as they relate to health care settings.***	20			
2.	According to the office manual, the proper procedure to report illegal activity is to inform the Quality Assurance (QA) department. Call the QA department. Identify yourself and that you want to report an illegal activity. Obtain and document the name of the person you are speaking with at QA. Ask and confirm that there will be no repercussions for reporting. Ask what steps you are to take if there is any retaliation. Describe the activity and person(s) involved, and what evidence you have. Ask the QA personnel what steps he or she (or the organization) will take to respond to the illegal activity and when to expect an investigation and response.	25			
3.	Document your phone call with the QA department and record the answer to each of your questions.	15			
4.	If no action is taken within the time period noted in Step 2, follow up with QA. Ask for a status report and document the response.	10			
5.	Keep your notes with you as evidence of your reporting. Do NOT under any circumstance violate HIPAA rules in disclosing the illegal activity or by way of written notes or documentation obtained.	10			
	Points Awarded / Points Possible	____/ **80**			

Competency Checklist
Procedure 3–3 Apply HIPAA Rules to Release of Patient Information

ABHES Curriculum

MA.A.1.4.a	Follow documentation guidelines
MA.A.1.4.b	Institute federal and state guidelines when releasing medical records or information
MA.A.1.4.f	Comply with federal, state, and local health laws and regulations as they relate to health care settings
MA.A.1.11.b	Demonstrate professional behavior

CAAHEP Core Curriculum

X.C.3	Describe components of the Health Insurance Portability and Accountability Act (HIPAA)
X.P.2	Apply HIPAA rules in regard to (a) privacy and (b) release of information
X.A.1	Demonstrate sensitivity to patient rights
X.A.2	Protect the integrity of the medical record

Task:	Following the steps listed in the procedure, apply HIPAA rules in regard to privacy and release of information.
Supplies & Conditions:	Paper and pen, or computer with EHR application, or telephone and fax machine.
Standards:	A maximum of three attempts may be used to complete the task. The time limit for each attempt is 10 minutes, with a minimum score of 70 percent. **Scoring:** Determine student's score by dividing points awarded by total points possible and multiplying results by 100.
Forms:	Procedure 3–3 Form (optional). Procedure forms can be downloaded from the Student Companion website.

EVALUATION

Evaluator Signature: _____ Date: _____

Evaluator Comments:

403

Name: _____ Date: _____ Score: _____

Procedure 3–3 Steps

Start Time: _____   **End Time:** _____   **Total Time:** _____

	Steps	Possible Points	First Attempt	Second Attempt	Third Attempt
1.	Locate and open the patient's chart (paper or electronic). Locate the Release of Information form.	10			
2.	Locate the information being requested to be released (e.g., most recent progress note).	10			
3.	Prepare or create fax cover sheet to recipient.	20			
4.	***Demonstrating sensitivity to patient rights,*** contact the receiving party by telephone to confirm the correct fax number and that the recipient is available to receive PHI. ***Protect the integrity of the medical record.***	20			
5.	Fax a copy of the document (with fax cover sheet) to the recipient.	10			
6.	Remove the fax document(s) and place (or scan) in the patient's chart.	10			
	Points Awarded / Points Possible	____/ **80**			

Competency Checklist
Procedure 3–4 Locate a State's Legal Scope of Practice for Medical Assistants

ABHES Curriculum

MA.A.1.1.d	List the general responsibilities of the medical assistant
MA.A.1.4.f	Comply with federal, state, and local health laws and regulations as they relate to health care settings
MA.A.1.4.f(1)	Define scope of practice for the medical assistant within the state where the medical assistant is employed
MA.A.1.11.b	Demonstrate professional behavior

CAAHEP Core Curriculum

X.C.1	Differentiate between scope of practice and standard of care for medical assistants
X.C.2	Compare and contrast provider and medical assistant roles in terms of standard of care
X.P.1	Locate a state's legal scope of practice for medical assistants
X.A.1	Demonstrate sensitivity to patient rights
X.A.2	Protect the integrity of the medical record

Task: Following the steps listed in the procedure, locate a state's legal scope of practice for medical assistants.

Supplies & Conditions: Computer with Internet access, paper, and pen (or computer with word processing or spreadsheet capabilities)

Standards: A maximum of three attempts may be used to complete the task. The time limit for each attempt is 10 minutes, with a minimum score of 70 percent. **Scoring:** Determine student's score by dividing points awarded by total points possible and multiplying results by 100.

EVALUATION

Evaluator Signature: _____   Date: _____

Evaluator Comments:

Name: _____ Date: _____ Score: _____

Procedure 3–4 Steps

Start Time: _____ **End Time:** _____ **Total Time:** _____

	Steps	Possible Points	First Attempt	Second Attempt	Third Attempt
1.	Using a computer, access the Internet and locate the legal scope of practice for the state where you are located.	10			
2.	Using the information obtained in Step 1, click on the *Scope of Practice* link for the state.	10			
3.	Using paper and pen (or computer with word processing application), prepare a written summary of the scope of practice, what you learned from the website, and how you would apply it to your medical assisting duties, ***demonstrating professional behavior***. Cite your sources.	30			
	Points Awarded / Points Possible	_____ / **50**			

Competency Checklist
Procedure 4–1 Develop a Plan for Separation of Personal and Professional Ethics

ABHES Curriculum

MA.A.1.4.b	Institute federal and state guidelines when releasing medical records or information
MA.A.1.4.c	Follow established policies when initiating or terminating medical treatment
MA.A.1.4.g	Display compliance with Code of Ethics of the profession
MA.A.1.5.e	Analyze the effect of hereditary, cultural, and environment influences on behavior

CAAHEP Core Curriculum

XI.C.1	Define (a) ethics and (b) morals
XI.C.2	Differentiate between personal and professional ethics
XI.C.3	Identify the effect of personal morals on professional performance
XI.P.1	Develop a plan for separation of personal and professional ethics
XI.P.2	Demonstrate appropriate response(s) to ethical issues
XI.A.1	Recognize the impact personal ethics and morals have on the delivery of health care

---

Task: Following the steps listed in the procedure, develop a plan for separation of personal and professional ethics.

Supplies & Conditions: Paper and pen, or computer with word processing or spreadsheet capabilities.

Standards: A maximum of three attempts may be used to complete the task. The time limit for each attempt is 10 minutes, with a minimum score of 70 percent. **Scoring:** Determine student's score by dividing points awarded by total points possible and multiplying results by 100.

EVALUATION

Evaluator Signature: _____ Date: _____

Evaluator Comments:

Name: _____ Date: _____ Score: _____

Procedure 4–1 Steps

Start Time: _____ **End Time:** _____ **Total Time:** _____

	Steps	Possible Points	First Attempt	Second Attempt	Third Attempt
1.	Develop a personal plan for yourself to separate personal and professional ethics. You must *differentiate between personal and professional ethics, identify the effect of personal morals on professional performance,* and *display compliance with Codes of Ethics of the profession.*	25			
2.	Verbalize (explain) how you would separate personal and professional ethics, using the information created in Step 1.	25			
3.	Develop a typed plan to separate personal and professional ethics using various ethical issues.	10			
4.	Verbalize (explain) each response to ethical issues.	10			
	Points Awarded / Points Possible	_____/ **70**			

Competency Checklist
Procedure 4–2 Demonstrate Appropriate Responses to Ethical Issues

ABHES Curriculum

MA.A.1.4.b	Institute federal and state guidelines when releasing medical records or information
MA.A.1.4.c	Follow established policies when initiating or terminating medical treatment
MA.A.1.4.g	Display compliance with Code of Ethics of the profession
MA.A.1.5.e	Analyze the effect of hereditary, cultural, and environment influences on behavior

CAAHEP Core Curriculum

XI.C.1	Define (a) ethics and (b) morals
XI.C.2	Differentiate between personal and professional ethics
XI.C.3	Identify the effect of personal morals on professional performance
XI.P.1	Develop a plan for separation of personal and professional ethics
XI.P.2	Demonstrate appropriate response(s) to ethical issues
XI.A.1	Recognize the impact personal ethics and morals have on the delivery of health care

Task:	Following the steps listed in the procedure, demonstrate an appropriate response to ethical issues.
Supplies & Conditions:	Paper and pen, or computer with word processing or spreadsheet capabilities.
Standards:	A maximum of three attempts may be used to complete the task. The time limit for each attempt is 10 minutes, with a minimum score of 70 percent. **Scoring:** Determine student's score by dividing points awarded by total points possible and multiplying results by 100.

EVALUATION

Evaluator Signature: _____ Date: _____

Evaluator Comments:

Name: _____   Date: _____   Score: _____

Procedure 4–2 Steps

Start Time: _____   **End Time:** _____   **Total Time:** _____

	Steps	Possible Points	First Attempt	Second Attempt	Third Attempt
1.	Demonstrate appropriate response(s) to ethical issues in a verbal and written format. Using paper and pen (or your computer), create a two-column document. In column one, select three ethical issues noted in Table 4–1 or the Workbook scenario(s). In column two, list the appropriate response(s) to the ethical issue selected.	25			
2.	Verbalize (explain) how you would demonstrate appropriate responses to ethical issues identified in Step 1.	25			
3.	Develop a typed response to the ethical issues identified in Step 1(from Table 4–1) and your appropriate response to each.	20			
	Points Awarded / Points Possible	____/ **70**			

Name: _____   Date: _____   Score: _____

Competency Checklist
Procedure 5–1 Recognize and Respond to Nonverbal Communication

ABHES Curriculum

MA.A.1.4.a   Follow documentation guidelines
MA.A.1.8.f   Display professionalism through written and verbal communications

CAAHEP Core Curriculum

V.P.2   Respond to nonverbal communication
V.A.1   Demonstrate (a) empathy, (b) active listening, and (c) nonverbal communication
V.A.2   Demonstrate the principles of self-boundaries
V.A.3   Demonstrate respect for individual diversity including: (a) gender, (b) race, (c) religion, (d) age, (e) economic status, and (f) appearance

---

Task: Following the steps listed in the procedure, complete the patient intake, recognizing nonverbal communication and possible barriers to communicating with the patient.

Supplies & Conditions: Patient's chart, pen (if paper chart), computer (if EHR). You need to elicit information about the patient's chief complaint for the provider. Additionally, you notice in the chart that today is the patient's birthday. Optional: Procedure 5–1 form (progress note) can be used to complete this activity.

Standards: A maximum of three attempts may be used to complete the task. The time limit for each attempt is 10 minutes, with a minimum score of 70 percent. **Scoring:** Determine student's score by dividing points awarded by total points possible and multiplying results by 100.

Forms: Procedure 5–1 Scenario and Procedure 5–1 Form (optional). Procedure forms can be downloaded from the Student Companion website; procedure scenarios are provided in the Instructor's Manual.

EVALUATION

Evaluator Signature: _____   Date: _____

Evaluator Comments:

© 2017 Cengage Learning. All Rights Reserved. May not be scanned, copied or duplicated, or posted to a publicly accessible website, in whole or in part.

Name: _____   Date: _____   Score: _____

Procedure 5–1 Steps

Start Time: _____   End Time: _____   Total Time: _____

	Steps	Possible Points	First Attempt	Second Attempt	Third Attempt
1.	Ask the patient the reason for today's office visit, *while demonstrating respect for individual diversity including: gender, race, religion, age, economic status, and appearance.*	5			
2.	Demonstrating perception of nonverbal cues and the patient's level of comprehension, ask the question again.	10			
3.	Ask open-ended questions and use other techniques discussed in this chapter to start a conversation and avoid silence.	5			
4.	During entire contact with patient, *demonstrate empathy, active listening, and nonverbal communication.*	10			
5.	During entire contact with patient, *demonstrate the principles of self-boundaries* by maintaining appropriate distance from patient.	10			
6.	When you have obtained the chief complaint and documented it in the patient's chart, thank the patient and say that the provider will be in shortly.	5			
	Points Awwarded / Points Possible	____ / **45**			

Competency Checklist
Procedure 6–1 Coach Patients Regarding Health Maintenance, Disease Prevention, and Treatment Plans while Considering Cultural Diversity, Developmental Life Stages, and Communication Barriers.

ABHES Curriculum

MA.A.1.5.e	Analyze the effect of hereditary, cultural, and environmental influences on behavior
MA.A.1.8.f	Display professionalism through written and verbal communications

CAAHEP Core Curriculum

V.C.6	Define coaching a patient as it relates to: (a) health maintenance, (b) disease prevention, (c) compliance with treatment plan, (d) community resources, and (e) adaptations relevant to individual patient needs
V.C.14	Relate the following behaviors to professional communication: (a) assertive, (b) aggressive, and (c) passive
V.C.18	Discuss examples of diversity: (a) cultural, (b) social, and (c) ethnic
V.P.4	Coach patients regarding: (a) health maintenance, (b) disease prevention, and (c) treatment plan
V.P.5	Coach patients appropriately considering: (a) cultural diversity, (b) developmental life stages, and (c) communication barriers
V.A.3	Demonstrate respect for individual diversity including: (a) gender, (b) race, (c) religion, (d) age, (e) economic status, and (f) appearance

---

Task:	Following the steps listed in the procedure, coach patients appropriately regarding health maintenance, disease prevention, and treatment plans considering cultural diversity, developmental life stages and communication barriers
Supplies & Conditions:	Paper, pen, computer (if EHR), information ordered by provider for coaching session.
Standards:	A maximum of three attempts may be used to complete the task. The time limit for each attempt is 10 minutes, with a minimum score of 70 percent. **Scoring:** Determine student's score by dividing points awarded by total points possible and multiplying results by 100.
Forms:	Procedure 6–1 Scenario with Procedure 6–1 forms. Procedure forms can be downloaded from the Student Companion website; procedure scenarios are found in the Instructor's Manual.

EVALUATION

Evaluator Signature: _____ Date: _____

Evaluator Comments:

Name: _____ Date: _____ Score: _____

Procedure 6–1 Steps

Start Time: _____ **End Time:** _____ **Total Time:** _____

	Steps	Possible Points	First Attempt	Second Attempt	Third Attempt
1.	Develop a plan of action on how to coach the patient on information ordered by the provider.	15			
2.	Greet the patient and any other person present in the room by name.	5			
3.	Provide a written copy of the instructions and review them one by one verbally with the patient, using language the patient can understand.	15			
4.	Ask the patient to repeat the instructions (act as a verbal mirror) and restate what is said for clarification by all parties.	15			
5.	***Demonstrate empathy, active listening, and nonverbal communication.***	15			
6.	***Demonstrate empathy and respect for individual diversity including gender, race, religion, age, economic status, and appearance during entire contact with patient.***	15			
7.	Provide your name and office phone number if there are additional questions.	10			
8.	Document in the patient's chart what information and instructions were given concerning the procedure.	15			
	Points Awarded / Points Possible	_____/ **105**			

Competency Checklist
Procedure 22–1 Demonstrate Professional Telephone Techniques

ABHES Curriculum

MA.A.1.8f   Display professionalism through written and verbal communications

CAAHEP Core Curriculum

V.P.6   Demonstrate professional telephone techniques
V.A.1   Demonstrate: (a) empathy, (b) active listening, and (c) nonverbal communication
V.A.3   Demonstrate respect for individual diversity including: (a) gender, (b) race, (c) religion, (d) age, (e) economic status, and (f) appearance

Task:	Follow the steps in the procedure and demonstrate professional telephone techniques.
Supplies & Conditions:	Telephone, paper, pen, computer—if available.
Standards:	A maximum of three attempts may be used to complete the task. Students must complete all procedure steps in 10 minutes, with a minimum score of 70 percent. **Scoring:** Determine student's score by dividing points awarded by total points possible and multiplying results by 100.
Forms Needed:	Procedure 22–1 Scenario (optional) with Procedure Form 22–1 (progress note, optional). Procedure forms can be downloaded from the Student Companion website; procedure scenarios are included in the Instructor's Manual.

EVALUATION

Evaluator Signature: _____   Date: _____

Evaluator Comments:

Name: _____ Date: _____ Score: _____

Procedure 22–1 Steps

Start Time: _____ End Time: _____ Total Time: _____

	Steps	Possible Points	First Attempt	Second Attempt	Third Attempt
1.	Answer the telephone promptly (by the third ring) in a polite professional manner. Identify the office and yourself by name.	10			
2.	**Demonstrate empathy, active listening, and professionalism** and correctly record the name and phone number of the caller, the reason for the call, and the date and time of the call.	15			
3.	Before placing a caller on hold, determine whether the call is an emergency situation, and, if so, process the call immediately, using screening (triage) manual, **demonstrating respect for individual diversity**.	15			
4.	Use the telephone screening (triage) manual to ask the appropriate questions and document the patient's responses. Analyze communications in providing appropriate responses and feedback.	15			
5.	If caller must be placed on hold, try to check with him or her periodically to let the caller know you haven't forgotten about him or her, **demonstrating empathy, active listening, and professionalism.**	5			
6.	Accurately document the information in a message (paper or electronic) and route to provider with appropriate level of urgency.	15			
7.	After screening and routing the call, sign-off on message (paper or electronic) with final action taken.	10			
8.	Complete all calls on hold in a timely manner. Screen and complete as many calls as possible before adding names to the provider's callback list, implementing time management principles to maintain effective office function.	10			
	Points Awarded / Points Possible	___ / **95**			

Competency Checklist
Procedure 22–2 Document Telephone Messages Accurately

ABHES Curriculum

MA.A.1.8.f   Display professionalism through written and verbal communications

CAAHEP Core Curriculum

V.P.7   Document telephone messages accurately
V.A.1   Demonstrate: (a) empathy, (b) active listening, and (c) nonverbal communication

---

Task:

Following the steps in the procedure, obtain accurate message(s) from a recording device or answering service, obtaining all necessary information from the caller to process the requests correctly.

Supplies & Conditions:

Telephone message device; pen; paper, phone message log, or computer; appropriate patients' charts.

Standards:

A maximum of three attempts may be used to complete the task. Students must complete all procedure steps in 10 minutes, with a minimum score of 70 percent. **Scoring:** Determine student's score by dividing points awarded by total points possible and multiplying results by 100.

Forms:

Procedure 22–2 Scenario with Procedure 22–2 Form. Procedure forms can be downloaded from the Student Companion website; procedure scenarios are included in the Instructor's Manual.

EVALUATION

Evaluator Signature: _____   Date: _____

Evaluator Comments:

417

Name: _____ Date: _____ Score: _____

Procedure 22–2 Steps

Start Time: _____ End Time: _____ Total Time: _____

	Steps	Possible Points	First Attempt	Second Attempt	Third Attempt
1.	Assemble all necessary items in your work area, avoiding excess noise and distractions.	5			
2.	Check the recording device or call the answering service and, **_using active listening skills_**, write out each message accurately.	15			
3.	Check fax machine and office email for additional messages. Clarify any discrepancies in emails or faxes with the service.	10			
4.	Sign your initials after the message and ensure that you have written the date and time of the message.	15			
5.	List all patients who leave messages so you can access their charts.	5			
6.	Prioritize messages according to the nature of their seriousness and distribute to the appropriate staff member, provider, or department to be processed. **_Display professionalism through written and verbal communications._**	15			
	Points Awarded / Points Possible	_____/ **65**			

Competency Checklist
Procedure 22–3 Telephone a Patient with Test Results

ABHES Curriculum

MA.A.1.8.f   Display professionalism through written and verbal communications

CAAHEP Core Curriculum

V.P.6   Demonstrate professional telephone techniques
V.P.7   Document telephone messages accurately
V.A.1   Demonstrate: (a) empathy, (b) active listening, and (c) nonverbal communication
V.A.3   Demonstrate respect for individual diversity including: (a) gender, (b) race, (c) religion, (d) age,
(e) economic status, and (f) appearance

Task: Using the necessary equipment, follow all the steps in the procedure and inform the patient about laboratory or other test results. Protect PHI (protected health information) according to HIPAA and document the call.

Supplies & Conditions: Patient's chart (paper chart or EMR), telephone, lab results, pen.

Standards: A maximum of three attempts may be used to complete the task. Students must complete all procedure steps in 10 minutes, with a minimum score of 70 percent. **Scoring:** Determine student's score by dividing points awarded by total points possible and multiplying results by 100.

Forms Needed: Procedure 22–3 Scenario with Procedure Form 22–3 (progress note, optional). Procedure forms can be downloaded from the Student Companion website; procedure scenarios are included in the Instructor's Manual.

EVALUATION

Evaluator Signature: _____   Date: _____

Evaluator Comments:

Name: _____ Date: _____ Score: _____

Procedure 22–3 Steps

Start Time: _____ End Time: _____ Total Time: _____

	Steps	Possible Points	First Attempt	Second Attempt	Third Attempt
1.	Obtain the patient's chart, with test results attached, from the provider (with instructions on message to patients).	5			
2.	Check the patient's chart for the signed privacy notice (CCP) to determine who may receive the information.	15			
3.	*Displaying professionalism through verbal communications,* telephone the patient, identifying yourself and the office.	10			
4.	Identify the person you are speaking to.	15			
5.	Inform the patient about test results and any instructions from the provider, *demonstrating empathy and active listening skills.*	15			
6.	Ask the patient to repeat the results to be sure he or she has the correct information, *demonstrating respect for individual diversity.* Instruct the patient to call the office with any questions.	10			
7.	Allow the patient to hang up first.	10			
8.	Document the call in the patient's chart.	15			
	Points Awarded / Points Possible	_____ / **95**			

Competency Checklist
Procedure 22–4 Develop a Current List of Community Resources Related to Patients' Health Care Needs

ABHES Curriculum

MA.A.1.8.f   Display professionalism through written and verbal communications

CAAHEP Core Curriculum

V.P.9   Develop a current list of community resources related to patients' health care needs

---

Task:	Use research tools and techniques to create a list of community resources related to patients' health care needs.
Supplies & Conditions:	Computer with Internet access, telephone directory, and local hospital directory.
Standards:	A maximum of three attempts may be used to complete the task. Students must complete all procedure steps in 60 minutes, with a minimum score of 70 percent. **Scoring:** Determine student's score by dividing points awarded by total points possible and multiplying results by 100.

EVALUATION

Evaluator Signature: _____ Date: _____

Evaluator Comments:

Name: _____ Date: _____ Score: _____

Procedure 22–4 Steps

Start Time: _____ **End Time:** _____ **Total Time:** _____

	Steps	Possible Points	First Attempt	Second Attempt	Third Attempt
1.	Assemble required items (telephone, telephone book, pen, paper, computer with Internet access).	5			
2.	Using the telephone book and Internet, research the community resources available in your area, create a list of available health care resources, and identify the services provided by each.	15			
3.	Verify the information with a follow-up telephone call to the community resource for most current information to be documented. ***Display professionalism through written and verbal communications.***	15			
4.	Create a list in a spreadsheet format (using Microsoft Excel or Word, for instance). In the spreadsheet, identify the communication resource(s), services provided, and contact information.	15			
5.	Print the resource document.	10			
	Points Awarded / Points Possible	_____ / 60			

Competency Checklist
Procedure 22–5 Facilitate Referrals to Community Resources in the Role of a Patient Navigator

ABHES Curriculum

MA.A.1.8.f   Display professionalism through written and verbal communications

CAAHEP Core Curriculum

V.C.6.d   Define coaching a patient as it relates to community resources
V.P.10   Facilitate referrals to community resources in the role of a patient navigator
V.A.1   Demonstrate (a) empathy, (b) active listening, and (c) nonverbal communication
V.A.3   Demonstrate respect for individual diversity including: (a) gender, (b) race, (c) religion, (d) age, (e) economic status, and (f) appearance

---

Task: Use research tools and techniques to facilitate referrals to community resources as a patient navigator.

Supplies & Conditions: Computer with Internet access, telephone directory, and local hospital directory.

Standards: A maximum of three attempts may be used to complete the task. Students must complete all procedure steps in 60 minutes, with a minimum score of 70 percent. **Scoring:** Determine student's score by dividing points awarded by total points possible and multiplying results by 100.

EVALUATION

Evaluator Signature: _____   Date: _____

Evaluator Comments:

Name: _____ Date: _____ Score: _____

Procedure 22–5 Steps

Start Time: _____ End Time: _____ Total Time: _____

	Steps	Possible Points	First Attempt	Second Attempt	Third Attempt
1.	Assemble required items (telephone, telephone book, pen, paper, computer with Internet access, patient's chart).	5			
2.	Using the telephone book, Internet, and current list of community resources created in Procedure 22-4, facilitate referrals in the role as a patient navigator (coaching the patient during the referral process). ***Demonstrate respect for individual diversity.***	15			
3.	***Displaying professionalism through verbal communications***, verify the information with the patient on the telephone. Then place a follow-up call to the patient (or caller) following HIPAA guidelines within 48 hours, ***demonstrating empathy and active listening skills***.	15			
4.	Print the referral information and document in the patient chart.	15			
	Points Awarded / Points Possible	____ / **50**			

Competency Checklist
Procedure 23–1 Compose Professional Correspondence Utilizing Electronic Technology

ABHES Curriculum

MA.A.1.8.f   Display professionalism through written and verbal communications

CAAHEP Core Curriculum

V.C.7	Recognize elements of fundamental writing skills
V.C.8	Discuss applications of electronic technology in professional communication
V.P.8	Compose professional correspondence utilizing electronic technology
V.A.1.a	Demonstrate empathy
V.A.3	Demonstrate respect for individual diversity including: (a) gender, (b) race, (c) religion, (d) age, (e) economic status, and (f) appearance

---

Task:	Following the steps in the procedure, respond to written communication, and compose professional correspondence utilizing electronic technology.
Supplies & Conditions:	Computer, paper (letterhead), received correspondence.
Standards:	A maximum of three attempts may be used to complete the task. Students must complete all procedure steps in 30 minutes, with a minimum score of 70 percent. **Scoring:** Determine student's score by dividing points awarded by total points possible and multiplying results by 100.
Forms:	Procedure 23–1 Scenario with Procedure 23–1 Form. Procedure forms can be downloaded from the Student Companion website; procedure scenarios are included in the Instructor's Manual.

EVALUATION

Evaluator Signature: _____   Date: _____

Evaluator Comments:

Name: _____ Date: _____ Score: _____

Procedure 23–1 Steps

Start Time:_____ End Time: _____ Total Time: _____

	Steps	Possible Points	First Attempt	Second Attempt	Third Attempt
1.	Assemble equipment and supplies; bring up the word processing screen. Select your letter style.	5			
2.	Correctly type the date, inside address, appropriate salutation, and reference line.	15			
3.	*Displaying professionalism through written and verbal communications,* correctly type or enter the body (content) of the letter. *Demonstrate empathy and respect for individual diversity.*	15			
4.	Correctly enter the closing elements: a complimentary closing, sender's name and official title, typist's initials, enclosures, cc or bcc recipients, and postscript.	15			
5.	Print a draft copy (or use the Print Preview feature in Word) and proofread the letter, making any necessary corrections.	10			
6.	Print the letter on letterhead and prepare an envelope.	5			
7.	Present the letter with envelope to the person (provider) for signature.	5			
8.	Make a copy and file it in the patient's chart (or scan into the EHR), if it concerns a patient, or in the appropriate business folder. *Note:* If using a letter template from the EHR, it will be automatically saved in the correspondence tab.	15			
	Points Awarded / Points Possible	____ / **85**			

Competency Checklist
Procedure 24–1 Open the Office and Evaluate the Work Environment to Identify Unsafe Working Conditions

ABHES Curriculum

MA.A.1.11.b   Demonstrate professional behavior

CAAHEP Core Curriculum

XII.P.5   Evaluate the work environment to identify unsafe working conditions

---

Task:	Following the steps listed in the procedure, role-play the actions necessary to prepare a medical office to receive patients.
Supplies & Conditions:	A simulated office if available; in a classroom or lab setting, role-play, describing actions verbally while performing.
Standards:	A maximum of three attempts may be used to complete the task. The time limit for each attempt is 20 minutes, with a minimum score of 70 percent. **Scoring:** Determine student's score by dividing points awarded by total points possible and multiplying results by 100.

EVALUATION

Evaluator Signature: _____   Date: _____

Evaluator Comments:

Name: _____ Date: _____ Score: _____

Procedure 24–1 Steps

Start Time: _____ End Time: _____ Total Time: _____

	Steps	Possible Points	First Attempt	Second Attempt	Third Attempt
1.	Unlock the reception room door.	5			
2.	Evaluate and prepare the reception room for cleanliness, comfort, and safety.	15			
3.	Prepare the front desk area.	15			
4.	*If working in a paper-based office*: Pull the charts of patients to be seen. Check each patient's previous visit to see whether any studies were ordered and place results into chart. *If working in an EHR office*: Review the patient schedule, check for previously ordered studies, and scan to chart. (Provide original copy to provider for review and validation prior to scanning.)	15			
5.	If it is the policy of the office, prepare a list (or print from the practice management system) of the patients to be seen by provider and the times of their appointments. Place copies in designated areas.	5			
6.	Inspect and prepare exam and lab rooms for cleanliness and safety.	15			
7.	List three to five safe working conditions identified: 1. _____ 2. _____ 3. _____ 4. _____ 5. _____	15			
8.	List three to five unsafe working conditions identified: 1. _____ 2. _____ 3. _____ 4. _____ 5. _____	15			
	Points Awarded / Points Possible	_____/ **100**			

Competency Checklist
Procedure 24–2 Perform an Inventory of Equipment and Supplies with Documentation

ABHES Curriculum

    MA.A.1.8.e   Maintain inventory of equipment and supplies

CAAHEP Core Curriculum

    VI.C.10   List steps involved in completing an inventory
    VI.P.9   Perform an inventory with documentation

Task: Following the steps listed in the procedure, perform a supply inventory; arrange any items that are time sensitive in front; count the number of items in storage and accurately record on the list.

Supplies & Conditions: Clipboard, supply inventory checklist, pen, and paper, in a simulated medical office situation. Procedure Form 24–2 can be used to complete this activity.

Standards: A maximum of three attempts may be used to complete the task. The time limit for each attempt is 30 minutes, with a minimum score of 70 percent. **Scoring:** Determine student's score by dividing points awarded by total points possible and multiplying results by 100.

Forms: Procedure Form 24–2. Procedure forms can be downloaded from the Student Companion website.

EVALUATION

Evaluator Signature: _____ Date: _____

Evaluator Comments:

Name: _____ Date: _____ Score: _____

Procedure 24–2 Steps

Start Time: _____ **End Time:** _____ **Total Time:** _____

	Steps	Possible Points	First Attempt	Second Attempt	Third Attempt
1.	Enter the date on the form.	5			
2.	Check the package dates on time-sensitive materials. Arrange the supplies with the first to expire in front.	10			
3.	Count each category of items on the inventory list and complete the form.	15			
4.	Give the completed form to the appropriate person to order supplies (if you are not the designated person).	10			
	Points Awarded / Points Possible	____/ **40**			

Competency Checklist
Procedure 24–3 Close the Office and Evaluate the Work Environment to Identify Unsafe Working Conditions

ABHES Curriculum

MA.A.1.11.b   Demonstrate professional behavior

CAAHEP Core Curriculum

XII.P.5   Evaluate the work environment to identify unsafe working conditions
XII.A.2   Demonstrate self-awareness in responding to an emergency situation

---

Task:	Following the steps listed in the procedure, role-play the actions required to close the office and evaluate the work environment to identify unsafe working conditions. Actions must be verbally described while performing the procedure.
Supplies & Conditions:	A simulated office if available; otherwise, role-play, explaining the procedure.
Standards:	A maximum of three attempts may be used to complete the task. The time limit for each attempt is 20 minutes, with a minimum score of 70 percent. **Scoring:** Determine student's score by dividing points awarded by total points possible and multiplying results by 100.

EVALUATION

Evaluator Signature: _____   Date: _____

Evaluator Comments:

Name: _____   Date: _____   Score: _____

Procedure 24–3 Steps

Start Time: _____   End Time: _____   Total Time: _____

	Steps	Possible Points	First Attempt	Second Attempt	Third Attempt
1.	Verify that all patients for the day have completed their visit and left the office.	15			
2.	Check to see that records are collected and filed in locked cabinets.	10			
3.	**Demonstrating professional behavior**, place any money in the safe or take to the bank to be deposited.	15			
4.	Turn off all electrical appliances and computers.	5			
5.	Check that rooms are cleaned and supplied for the next day. Straighten reception room if time allows.	10			
6.	*For paper offices*: Pull charts for the next day if time allows and prep with lab reports, consults, or available hospital reports. *For paperless offices (EHR)*: Review the next day's schedule for previously ordered studies. Scan to patient EHR chart; provide original to provider for review and validation prior to scanning.	5			
7.	Activate the answering device on the phone or notify the answering service and indicate when you will be back in the office.	10			
8.	Close and lock all access doors to office. Check that all windows are closed and locked and blinds shut. Turn off lights. Activate alarm system if available. If necessary, **demonstrate self-awareness to an emergency situation.**	15			
9.	Set the lock and close the door; check to confirm that it is locked. If necessary, **demonstrate self-awareness to an emergency situation.**	15			
	Points Awarded / Points Possible	_____/ **100**			

Competency Checklist
Procedure 24–4 Use Proper Ergonomics

CAAHEP Core Curriculum

XII.C.7.b   Identify principles of ergonomics

Task:	Evaluate your workstation for proper ergonomics and role-play the actions required to demonstrate proper ergonomics.
Supplies & Conditions:	Computer with Internet access and printer. A simulated office if available; otherwise, role-play, evaluating your workstation for proper ergonomics.
Standards:	A maximum of three attempts may be used to complete the task. Students must complete all procedure steps in 5 minutes, with a minimum score of 70 percent. **Scoring:** Determine student's score by dividing points awarded by total points possible and multiplying results by 100.

EVALUATION

Evaluator Signature: _____   Date: _____

Evaluator Comments:

Name: _____ Date: _____ Score: _____

Procedure 24–4 Steps

Start Time: _____ End Time: _____ Total Time: _____

	Steps	Possible Points	First Attempt	Second Attempt	Third Attempt
1.	Using a computer, access the OSHA website and download and print the etools: Computer Workstation checklist.	15			
2.	Using the form printed in Step 1, evaluate your workstation for proper ergonomics. Document your findings on the checklist form.	25			
3.	After evaluation of the workstation, demonstrate use of proper ergonomics.	25			
	Points Awarded / Points Possible	_____ / **65**			

Competency Checklist
Procedure 24–5 Perform Routine Maintenance of Administrative or Clinical Equipment

ABHES Curriculum

MA.A.1.8.e(1) Perform routine maintenance of administrative equipment

CAAHEP Core Curriculum

VI.C.9   Explain the purpose of routine maintenance of administrative and clinical equipment
VI.P.8   Perform routine maintenance of administrative or clinical equipment
XII.A.2   Demonstrate self-awareness in responding to an emergency situation

---

Task: Perform routine maintenance of administrative and clinical equipment.

Supplies & Conditions: Equipment list, clipboard, pen, and access to any necessary maintenance supplies.

Standards: A maximum of three attempts may be used to complete the task. Students must complete all procedure steps in 30 minutes, with a minimum score of 70 percent. **Scoring:** Determine student's score by dividing points awarded by total points possible and multiplying results by 100.

Forms: Procedure Form 24–5. Procedure forms can be downloaded from the Student Companion website.

EVALUATION

Evaluator Signature: _____ Date: _____

Evaluator Comments:

Name: _____ Date: _____ Score: _____

Procedure 24–5 Steps

Start Time: _____ End Time: _____ Total Time: _____

	Steps	Possible Points	First Attempt	Second Attempt	Third Attempt
1.	Assemble equipment and supplies.	5			
2.	Inspect each item on the list for cleanliness and record findings. If not clean, clean the item appropriately.	15			
3.	***Demonstrating self-awareness to an emergency situation***, check the equipment for safety factors: a. Electric cord and plugs b. Loose screws or bolts	15			
4.	Check for operability: a. Test any light source; replace burned-out bulbs. b. Inspect items for wear; order replacement parts. c. Briefly operate seldom-used equipment.	15			
5.	Check required operational standards: a. Freezer temperature b. Refrigerator temperature c. Autoclave test strip	15			
6.	Correctly fill out the equipment maintenance checklist, sign it, and submit it to the appropriate person for action. a. Write the date on the maintenance checklist. b. Note and report equipment that requires repairs.	15			
	Points Awarded / Points Possible	_____ / **80**			

Competency Checklist
Procedure 25–1 Manage the Appointment Schedule Using Established Priorities

ABHES Curriculum

MA.A.1.7.a	Perform basic keyboarding skills
MA.A.1.8.d	Apply scheduling principles: (1) Schedule of in- and outpatient procedures, and (2) Admission or hospital procedures

CAAHEP Core Curriculum

VI.C.1	Identify different types of appointment scheduling methods
VI.C.2	Identify advantages and disadvantages of the following appointment systems: (a) manual, and (b) electronic
VI.C.3	Identify critical information required for scheduling patient procedures
VI.P.1	Manage appointment schedule using established priorities
VI.P.2	Schedule a patient procedure
VI.A.1	Display sensitivity when managing appointments

Task:	In a simulated situation, schedule an appointment for a patient procedure by either appointment book or computer, remembering to follow HIPAA guidelines for safeguarding protected health information (PHI).
Supplies & Conditions:	Appointment book, appointment cards, or computer with practice management scheduling program.
Standards:	A maximum of three attempts may be used to complete the task. The time limit for each attempt is 15 minutes, with a minimum score of 70 percent. **Scoring:** Determine student's score by dividing points awarded by total points possible and multiplying results by 100.
Forms:	Procedure 25–1 Scenario with Procedure 25–1 Forms. Procedure forms can be downloaded from the Student Companion website; procedure scenarios are included in the Instructor's Manual.

EVALUATION

Evaluator Signature: _____   Date: _____

Evaluator Comments:

Name: _____   Date: _____   Score: _____

Procedure 25–1 Steps

	Steps	Possible Points	First Attempt	Second Attempt	Third Attempt
1.	Determine which method will be used for scheduling: manual appointment book or computer PM entry. ***Display sensitivity when managing appointments.*** a. If using a paper scheduling system, mark off the hours when the provider will be unable to see patients. b. If using an electronic PM scheduling system, open the scheduling module and navigate to the correct date.	20			
2.	*Applying scheduling principles*, manage the schedule using the Wave method, creating appointment slot/types where patients are scheduled during the first 30 minutes of each hour, leaving the last 30 minutes for same-day appointments. Record the Wave template schedule in the paper appointment book or electronic practice management system performing basic keyboarding skills.	25			
	Points Awarded / Points Possible	_____ / **45**			

Competency Checklist
Procedure 25–2 Schedule a Patient Procedure

ABHES Curriculum

MA.A.1.7.a	Perform basic keyboarding skills
MA.A.1.8.d	Apply scheduling principles: (1) Schedule of in- and outpatient procedures, and (2) Admission or hospital procedures

CAAHEP Core Curriculum

VI.C.3	Identify critical information required for scheduling patient procedures
VI.P.1	Manage appointment schedule using established priorities
VI.P.2	Schedule a patient procedure
VI.A.1	Display sensitivity when managing appointments
X.A.1	Demonstrate sensitivity to patient rights

Task:	In a simulated situation and in a professional manner, schedule appointment(s) for a patient procedure by either appointment book or computer, remembering to follow HIPAA guidelines for safeguarding protected health information (PHI).
Supplies & Conditions:	Patient's chart with procedure request, appointment book (or computer with PM scheduling program), phone directory, phone, pen, and paper.
Standards:	A maximum of three attempts may be used to complete the task. The time limit for each attempt is 15 minutes, with a minimum score of 70 percent. **Scoring:** Determine student's score by dividing points awarded by total points possible and multiplying results by 100.
Forms:	Procedure 25–2 Scenario. Procedure scenarios are included in the Instructor's Manual.

EVALUATION

Evaluator Signature: _____   Date: _____

Evaluator Comments:

Name: _____ Date: _____ Score: _____

Procedure 25–2 Steps

Start Time: _____ End Time: _____ Total Time: _____

	Steps	Possible Points	First Attempt	Second Attempt	Third Attempt
1.	Determine which method will be used for scheduling: manual appointment book or computer PM entry. ***Display sensitivity when managing appointments.*** a. If using a paper scheduling system, mark off the hours when the provider will be unable to see patients. b. If using an electronic PM scheduling system, open the scheduling module and navigate to the correct date.	20			
2.	***Applying scheduling principles,*** schedule appointments for new and existing patients, using established priorities for a procedure (e.g., bone density screening). Write patients' names in the schedule book or enter them in the appropriate time slot on the PM appointment screen.	30			
3.	Complete an appointment card and give it to the patient or print out an appointment reminder slip, using the PM scheduling software. If the patient is enrolled in a patient portal (e.g., the one in Harris CareTracker), confirm the type of appointment reminder. ***Demonstrating sensitivity to patient rights***, place appointment reminder as indicated (e.g., patient portal message; phone call to home or cell phone; or automated appointment reminder, e.g., TeleVox).	30			
	Points Awarded / Points Possible	_____/ **80**			

Competency Checklist
Procedure 25–3 Apply HIPAA Rules in Regard to Patient Privacy and Release of Information When Scheduling a Patient Procedure

ABHES Curriculum

MA.A.1.8.d   Apply scheduling principles: (1) Schedule of in- and outpatient procedures, and (2) Admission or hospital procedures

CAAHEP Core Curriculum

VI.C.3   Identify critical information required for scheduling patient procedures
VI.P.1   Manage appointment schedule using established priorities
VI.A.1   Display sensitivity when managing appointments
X.C.4   Summarize the Patient Bill of Rights
X.P.2   Apply HIPAA rules in regard to: (a) privacy, and (b) release of information
X.P.4   Apply the Patient's Bill of Rights as it relates to: (a) choice of treatment, (b) consent for treatment, and (c) refusal of treatment
X.A.1   Demonstrate sensitivity to patient rights
X.A.2   Protect the integrity of the medical record

Task:	Complete the steps in the procedure n a professional manner, schedule appointment patient procedure, and apply HIPAA rules in regard to patient privacy and release of information. Apply the Patient's Bill of Rights as it relates to choice of treatment, consent for treatment, or refusal of treatment.
Supplies & Conditions:	Patient's chart (paper or electronic) with referral request, phone directory, phone, pen, and paper. Computer with EMR and practice management (PM) systems.
Standards:	A maximum of three attempts may be used to complete the task. The time limit for each attempt is 30 minutes, with a minimum score of 70 percent. **Scoring:** Determine student's score by dividing points awarded by total points possible and multiplying results by 100.
Forms Needed:	Procedure 25-3 Scenario. Procedure scenarios are included in the Instructor's Manual.

EVALUATION

Evaluator Signature: _____   Date: _____

Evaluator Comments:

441

Name: _____ Date: _____ Score: _____

Procedure 25–3 Steps

Start Time: _____ End Time: _____ Total Time: _____

	Steps	Possible Points	First Attempt	Second Attempt	Third Attempt
1.	*Displaying sensitivity when managing appointments*, obtain or access the patient's chart with request for referral to another facility for surgical consult. Review patient's insurance information and determine whether preauthorization is required.	15			
2.	Apply the Patient's Bill of Rights as it relates to the choice of and consent for treatment. *Demonstrate sensitivity to patient's rights.*	15			
3.	Locate and record correct phone number and address of referral's facility.	10			
4.	Place the call to the referral office and provide the administrative medical assistant with all appropriate information. *Protecting the integrity of the medical record*, apply HIPAA rules in regard to privacy and release of information.	15			
5.	*Applying scheduling principles*, prepare a copy of all information pertinent to the appointment to give to the patient, including the time, day, date, name, address, and directions to the facility if needed. If the patient is not present when the appointment is made, phone the patient to provide the necessary information.	15			
6.	Fax, mail or send electronically via the provider portal the procedure appointment information, *protecting the integrity of the medical record.*	10			
7.	Send a follow-up letter or message via the patient portal to the patient with printed instructions, referral's contact information, directions, and appointment time.	10			
8.	Record all actions in the patient's chart and initial the patient's chart with date and time, signifying that the request was completed.	10			
	Points Awarded / Points Possible	____/ **100**			

Competency Checklist
Procedure 25–4 Explain General Office Policies to the Patient

CAAHEP Core Curriculum

V.P.4(a)	Coach patients regarding: office policies
X.C.4	Summarize the Patient Bill of Rights
X.P.2	Apply HIPAA rules in regard to: (a) privacy, and (b) release of information
X.P.4	Apply the Patient's Bill of Rights as it relates to: (a) choice of treatment, (b) consent for treatment, and (c) refusal of treatment
X.A.1	Demonstrate sensitivity to patient rights
X.A.2	Protect the integrity of the medical record

Task:	Explain both the practice's expectations for patients as well as what legal and ethical rights the patient can expect. Apply HIPAA rules regarding privacy and release of information.
Supplies & Conditions:	Quiet room, free from distraction, printed patient education materials.
Standards:	A maximum of three attempts may be used to complete the task. The time limit for each attempt is 15 minutes, with a minimum score of 70 percent. **Scoring:** Determine student's score by dividing points awarded by total points possible and multiplying results by 100.

EVALUATION

Evaluator Signature: _____ Date: _____

Evaluator Comments:

Name: _____ Date: _____ Score: _____

Procedure 25–4 Steps

Start Time: _____ End Time: _____ Total Time: _____

	Steps	Possible Points	First Attempt	Second Attempt	Third Attempt
1.	Identify patient.	15			
2.	Invite the patient into a room free of distractions and demonstrate sensitivity to patient's privacy by closing the door to **maintain and protect the patient's privacy and integrity of the medical record**.	15			
3.	Introduce yourself, identify your role in the practice, and tell the patient what to expect from the conversation, using language the patient can understand and making the patient feel at ease.	15			
4.	Provide preprinted information and policies, preferably in the patient's native language (or with verification through a translator followed by documentation of patient's response to explanations).	15			
5.	Provide the patient with an opportunity to ask questions.	15			
6.	Refer questions to appropriate others for further explanation or clarification.	5			
7.	Document time, date, patient response, and any materials provided in the patient record.	15			
	Points Awarded / Points Possible	____/ 95			

444

Competency Checklist
Procedure 26–1 Create and Organize a Patient's Medical Record

ABHES Curriculum

MA.A.1.8.a   Gather and process documents

CAAHEP Core Curriculum

VI.C.4   Define types of information contained in the patient's medical record
VI.C.5   Identify methods of organizing the patient's medical record based on: (a) problem-oriented medical record (POMR) and (b) source-oriented medical record (SOMR)
VI.C.6   Identify equipment and supplies needed for medical records in order to: (a) Create, (b) Maintain, and (c) Store
VI.C.7   Describe filing indexing rules
VI.P.3   Create a patient's medical record
VI.P.4   Organize a patient's medical record
VI.P.6   Utilize an EMR
VI.P.7   Input patient data utilizing a practice management system

---

Task: Following the steps listed in the procedure, prepare an accurate and complete patient chart to submit to the provider for final review.

Supplies & Conditions: Chart or folder, patient records, privacy forms, tabs (if using electronic records: computer and EHR program).

Standards: A maximum of three attempts may be used to complete the task. The time limit for each attempt is 10 minutes, with a minimum score of 70 percent. **Scoring:** Determine student's score by dividing points awarded by total points possible and multiplying results by 100.

EVALUATION

Evaluator Signature: _____   Date: _____

Evaluator Comments:

Name: _____   Date: _____   Score: _____

Procedure 26–1 Steps

Start Time: _____   **End Time:** _____   **Total Time:** _____

	Steps	Possible Points	First Attempt	Second Attempt	Third Attempt
1.	Prepare chart or folder for patient (electronic or paper). Verify accurate spelling of name. Include demographics, insurance information, privacy forms, and emergency contact information.	15			
2.	Retrieve and compile available reports and information. Verify that all records are for the correct patient before including in the record.	15			
3.	Sort and organize records by type: operative notes, progress notes from various providers, laboratory reports, radiology, medication flow sheets, immunization records, and so on. (If using electronic records, organize the documents and enter information or scan to correct tab in the EHR.)	15			
4.	Verify accuracy and completeness and submit to provider for final review.	15			
	Points Awarded / Points Possible	_____/ **60**			

Competency Checklist
Procedure 26–2 Use an Alphabetic Filing System

ABHES Curriculum

MA.A.1.4.a   Follow documentation guidelines

CAAHEP Core Curriculum

VI.P.5   File patient medical records

Task: Following the steps listed in the procedure, within an alphabetic filing system, accurately file and store a new file and then prepare an OUTguide and pull an existing file.

Supplies & Conditions: Items to be filed, cabinet for files, name of patient file to be pulled, OUTguide (card).

Standards: A maximum of three attempts may be used to complete the task. The time limit for each attempt is 10 minutes, with a minimum score of 70 percent. **Scoring:** Determine student's score by dividing points awarded by total points possible and multiplying results by 100.

EVALUATION

Evaluator Signature: _____   Date: _____

Evaluator Comments:

Name: _____ Date: _____ Score: _____

Procedure 26–2 Steps

Start Time: _____ End Time: _____ Total Time: _____

	Steps	Possible Points	First Attempt	Second Attempt	Third Attempt
	File a New Item				
1.	Use the rules for filing items alphabetically.	15			
2.	Determine the appropriate storage file.	15			
3.	When filing new material, scan the guides for the area nearest the letters of the name on the items you have to file.	15			
4.	Place the folder in the correct alphabetic order between two files.	15			
	Pull an Item from Existing Files				
5.	Find the name of the patient in the alphabetic file. Double-check the spelling of the name for accuracy.	15			
6.	Complete the OUTguide with the date and your name or with the name of the person requesting the chart.	15			
7.	Pull the file needed and replace with the OUTguide.	15			
	Points Awarded / Points Possible	____/ **105**			

Competency Checklist
Procedure 26–3 Use a Numeric Filing System

ABHES Curriculum

MA.A.1.4.a   Follow documentation guidelines

CAAHEP Core Curriculum

VI.P.5   File patient medical records

Task: Following the steps listed in the procedure, within a numeric filing system, accurately file and store a new file and then prepare an OUTguide and pull an existing file.

Supplies & Conditions: Items to be filed, cabinet for files, name of patient file to be pulled, OUTguide (card).

Standards: A maximum of three attempts may be used to complete the task. The time limit for each attempt is 10 minutes, with a minimum score of 70 percent. **Scoring:** Determine student's score by dividing points awarded by total points possible and multiplying results by 100.

EVALUATION

Evaluator Signature: _____ Date: _____

Evaluator Comments:

Name: _____ Date: _____ Score: _____

Procedure 26–3 Steps

Start Time: _____ End Time: _____ Total Time: _____

	Steps	Possible Points	First Attempt	Second Attempt	Third Attempt
	File a New Item				
1.	Use the rules for numerical filing.	15			
2.	Determine the appropriate storage file.	15			
3.	Match the first two or three numbers with those already in the file. If using terminal digits, match the last two numbers.	15			
4.	Match the remaining numbers with those in the file.	15			
	Pull an Item from Existing Files				
5.	Find the name of the patient in the card file to obtain the account number. Double-check the spelling of the name for accuracy.	15			
6.	Complete the OUTguide with the date, name of person pulling file, or name of requestor.	15			
7.	Locate the file.	15			
8.	Pull the requested file and replace with the prepared OUTguide.	15			
	Points Awarded / Points Possible	_____/ **120**			

Competency Checklist
Procedure 27–1 Verify Insurance Coverage and Eligibility for Services

ABHES Curriculum

MA.A.1.8.c(2)   Differentiate managed care; i.e., HMO, PPO, EPO, IPA including referrals and pre-certification

CAAHEP Core Curriculum

VI.P.7	Input patient data utilizing a practice management system
VII.C.5	Identify types of information contained in the patient's billing record
VII.C.6	Explain patient financial obligations for services rendered
VII.P.4	Inform a patient of financial obligations for services rendered
VII.A.1	Demonstrate professionalism when discussing patient's billing record
VII.A 2	Display sensitivity when requesting payment for services rendered
VIII.C.1	Identify: (a) types of third party plans, (b) information required to file a third party claim, and (c) the steps for filing a third party claim
VIII.C.2	Outline managed care requirements for patient referral
VIII.C.3	Describe processes for: (a) verification of eligibility for services, (b) precertification, and (c) preauthorization
VIII.P.1	Interpret information on an insurance card
VIII.P.2	Verify eligibility for services including documentation
VIII.A.1	Interact professionally with third party representatives
VIII.A.3	Show sensitivity when communicating with patients regarding third party requirements

---

Task:	Interpret information on a patient's insurance card and verify the patient's insurance coverage and accurate billing information prior to rendering service to prevent claim rejection due to patient ineligibility for coverage.
Supplies & Conditions:	Computer, patient insurance identification card, insurance website address, individual password for access on website, and telephone.
Standards:	A maximum of three attempts may be used to complete the task. The time limit for each attempt is 15 minutes, with a minimum score of 70 percent. **Scoring:** Determine student's score by dividing points awarded by total points possible and multiplying results by 100.

EVALUATION

Evaluator Signature: _____   Date: _____

Evaluator Comments:

Name: _____ Date: _____ Score: _____

Procedure 27–1 Steps

Start Time: _____ End Time: _____ Total Time: _____

	Steps	Possible Points	First Attempt	Second Attempt	Third Attempt
1.	Interpret the information on the patient's insurance card. Determine if the insurance is managed care (HMO, PPO, EPO, IPA). Access website for patient's insurance carrier or the EHR application with electronic eligibility features. If website is not available, call the insurance company. ***Interact professionally with third-party representatives.***	15			
2.	Locate the section of the website for Provider Information.	10			
3.	Enter protected area of website.	10			
4.	Access area of website for verifying eligibility.	10			
5.	Complete all required fields on the screen.	15			
6.	Verify on screen that you have the correct patient information and that the patient is eligible for services.	15			
7.	Print results for inclusion in the patient's record either on paper or enter or scan the results in a practice management system of an EHR.	15			
8.	Notify the patient if the insurer indicates that he or she is not eligible for services. ***Demonstrating professionalism when discussing the patient's billing record, ensure that you show sensitivity when communicating with patients regarding third-party requirements. Display sensitivity when requesting payment for services rendered.***	15			
	Points Awarded / Points Possible	_____ / **105**			

Competency Checklist
Procedure 27–2 Obtain Precertification or Preauthorization (Predetermination) and Inform a Patient of Financial Obligations for Services Rendered

ABHES Curriculum

MA.A.1.8.c(2) Differentiate managed care; i.e., HMO, PPO, EPO, IPA including referrals and pre-certification

CAAHEP Core Curriculum

VI.P.7	Input patient data utilizing a practice management system
VII.C.5	Identify types of information contained in the patient's billing record
VII.C.6	Explain patient financial obligations for services rendered
VII.P.4	Inform a patient of financial obligations for services rendered
VII.A.1	Demonstrate professionalism when discussing patient's billing record
VII.A.2	Display sensitivity when requesting payment for services rendered
VIII.C.1	Identify: (a) types of third party plans, (b) information required to file a third party claim, and (c) the steps for filing a third party claim
VIII.C.3	Describe processes for: (a) verification of eligibility for services, (b) precertification, and (c) preauthorization
VIII.P.3	Obtain precertification or preauthorization including documentation
VIII.A.1	Interact professionally with third party representatives
VIII.A.2	Display tactful behavior when communicating with medical providers regarding third party requirements

Task:	Following the steps listed in the procedure, obtain precertification or preauthorization (predetermination) for a procedure to avoid claim rejection, and inform patient of financial obligations for services rendered.
Supplies & Conditions:	Access to computer and Internet, precertification or preauthorization (predetermination) form for patient's insurance carrier, and patient information for completion of form, telephone, and fax machine.
Standards:	A maximum of three attempts may be used to complete the task. The time limit for each attempt is 15 minutes, with a minimum score of 70 percent. **Scoring:** Determine student's score by dividing points awarded by total points possible and multiplying results by 100.

EVALUATION

Evaluator Signature: _____ Date: _____

Evaluator Comments:

Name: _____ Date: _____ Score: _____

Procedure 27–2 Steps

Start Time: _____ End Time: _____ Total Time: _____

	Steps	Possible Points	First Attempt	Second Attempt	Third Attempt
1.	Research procedure to determine whether precertification or preauthorization is required. Differentiate managed care (HMO, PPO, EPO, IPA), including referrals and precertification. ***Display tactful behavior when communicating with medical providers regarding third-party requirements.***	15			
2.	Locate the precertification or preauthorization (predetermination) form on the website. Call the insurance company directly if you have questions or cannot locate the form(s). ***Interact professionally with third-party representatives.***	15			
3.	Complete the precertification or preauthorization (predetermination) form correctly.	25			
4.	Fax the form to the patient's insurance organization, then file in patient's chart (or scan to patient's EHR using a practice management system).	15			
5.	Contact the patient and inform him or her of any financial obligations that will be due for services rendered. ***Demonstrate professionalism when discussing the patient's billing record, and display sensitivity when requesting payment for services rendered.***	15			
	Points Awarded / Points Possible	_____/ 85			

Competency Checklist
Procedure 28–1 Perform Procedural Coding

ABHES Curriculum

MA.A.1.8.c(3)   Perform diagnostic and procedural coding

CAAHEP Core Curriculum

IX.P.1   Perform procedural coding
IX.A.1   Utilize tactful communication skills with medical providers to ensure accurate code selection

---

Task: Accurately locate and assign the correct CPT code from information indicated on a patient
                             encounter form (paper form).

Supplies & Conditions: Patient encounter form (paper) and current CPT manual

Standards: A maximum of three attempts may be used to complete the task. The time limit for each attempt
                             is five minutes, with a minimum score of 80 percent. **Scoring:** Determine student's score by
                             dividing points awarded by total points possible and multiplying results by 100.

Forms: Procedure Form 28–1. Procedure forms can be downloaded from the Student Companion
                             website.

EVALUATION

Evaluator Signature: _____   Date: _____

Evaluator Comments:

Name: _____ Date: _____ Score: _____

Procedure 28–1 Steps

Start Time: _____ End Time: _____ Total Time: _____

	Steps	Possible Points	First Attempt	Second Attempt	Third Attempt
1.	Review the encounter form. *Utilize tactful communication skills with medical providers to ensure accurate code selection.*	15			
2.	Identify the procedure indicated on the encounter form. Determine the main term for the procedure performed. Read the description of the procedure and isolate the main term.	15			
3.	Turn to the alphabetic index in the CPT manual. Turn to the letter that the main term begins with and then locate the main term.	15			
4.	Search through any subterms listed under the main term. Look for the subterm that further narrows the code options; research each code listed.	15			
5.	Indicate the correct code on the encounter form next to the narrative for the procedure.	15			
	Points Awarded / Points Possible	_____/ **75**			

Competency Checklist
Procedure 28–2 Utilize Medical Necessity Guidelines

ABHES Curriculum

MA.A.1.8.c(3)   Perform diagnostic and procedural coding

CAAHEP Core Curriculum

IX.C.5   Define medical necessity as it applies to procedural and diagnostic coding
IX.P.3   Utilize medical necessity guidelines
IX.A.1   Utilize tactful communication skills with medical providers to ensure accurate code selection

---

Task: Accurately locate the order and correct CPT and ICD codes from information indicated on a patient encounter form utilizing medical necessity guidelines.

Supplies & Conditions: Patient encounter form (paper) and current ICD-9 or 10-CM manual; computer with Internet access.

Standards: A maximum of three attempts may be used to complete the task. The time limit for each attempt is five minutes, with a minimum score of 80 percent. **Scoring:** Determine student's score by dividing points awarded by total points possible and multiplying results by 100.

Forms: Procedure Forms 28–3A and 28–3B (Optional CMS-849 Form). Procedure forms can be downloaded from the Student Companion website.

EVALUATION

Evaluator Signature: _____   Date: _____

Evaluator Comments:

Name: _____ Date: _____ Score: _____

Procedure 28–2 Steps

Start Time: _____ End Time: _____ Total Time: _____

	Steps	Possible Points	First Attempt	Second Attempt	Third Attempt
1.	Review the encounter form and progress note documentation. Review the narrative diagnostic finding(s) indicated on the encounter form and either underline or highlight the documentation and procedure and diagnosis code(s) regarding a seat lift mechanism. ***Utilize tactful communication skills with medical providers to ensure accurate code selection.***	15			
2.	Identify the section of the progress note or the actual order for the seat lift mechanism.	15			
3.	Using a computer, access the Internet and the CMS website. Locate the Medical Necessity form as indicated.	15			
4.	Complete the Medical Necessity form using information from the patient's chart, progress note, and order for the seat lift mechanism. Follow the medical necessity guidelines provided by CMS.	15			
5.	Submit the completed form to your provider for signature and date.	15			
6.	Submit the claim.	15			
	Points Awarded / Points Possible	_____/ 90			

Competency Checklist
Procedure 28–3 Perform Diagnostic Coding

ABHES Curriculum

MA.A.1.8.c(3)   Perform diagnostic and procedural coding

CAAHEP Core Curriculum

IX.P.2   Perform diagnostic coding
IX.A.1   Utilize tactful communication skills with medical providers to ensure accurate code selection

---

Task:	Accurately locate and assign the correct ICD-9 or 10-CM code from information indicated on a patient encounter form.
Supplies & Conditions:	Patient encounter form (paper) and current ICD-9 or 10-CM manual
Standards:	A maximum of three attempts may be used to complete the task. The time limit for each attempt is five minutes, with a minimum score of 80 percent. **Scoring:** Determine student's score by dividing points awarded by total points possible and multiplying results by 100.
Forms:	Procedure Form 28–3. Procedure forms can be downloaded from the Student Companion website.

EVALUATION

Evaluator Signature: _____   Date: _____

Evaluator Comments:

Name: _____ Date: _____ Score: _____

Procedure 28–3 Steps

Start Time: _____ End Time: _____ Total Time: _____

	Steps	Possible Points	First Attempt	Second Attempt	Third Attempt
1.	Review the narrative diagnostic finding(s) indicated on the encounter form and either underline or highlight them. ***Utilize tactful communication skills with medical providers to ensure accurate code selection.***	15			
2.	Identify the main terms in the diagnostic statement(s). Read each diagnosis and identify the correct term to be looking up in the index.	15			
3.	Locate the alphabetic index of the ICD-9 or 10-CM manual and the correct main term.	15			
4.	After locating the main term, review any subterms listed.	15			
5.	Turn to the tabular list of the ICD-9 or 10-CM manual and locate the code listed beside the subterm in the index.	15			
6.	Read the description of the code and any coding conventions related to the code. Continue the process until you have found the correct code.	15			
7.	On the encounter form, write down the code you have determined best describes the condition that is reported.	15			
	Points Awarded / Points Possible	_____/ **105**			

Competency Checklist
Procedure 29–1 Perform Accounts Receivable Procedures to Patient Accounts, Including Posting Charges, Payments, and Adjustments

ABHES Curriculum

MA.A.1.8.b   Perform billing and collections procedures: (1) Accounts payable and accounts receivable, and (2) Post adjustments

CAAHEP Core Curriculum

VII.C.5   Identify types of information contained in the patient's billing record
VII.C.6   Explain patient financial obligations for services rendered
VII.P.1   Perform accounts receivable procedures to patient accounts including posting: (a) charges, (b) payments, and (c) adjustments

---

Task:	Following the steps listed in the procedure, accurately record charges, payments, and adjustments on a patient ledger or computer accounting program.
Supplies & Conditions:	In a simulated medical office situation, students will be placed in a quiet setting and provided with a computerized system or pegboard system with ledger cards, day sheet, and black and red ink pens.
Standards:	A maximum of three attempts may be used to complete the task. The time limit for each attempt is 30 minutes, with a minimum score of 85 percent. **Scoring:** Determine student's score by dividing points awarded by total points possible and multiplying results by 100.
Forms:	Procedure 29–1 scenario with Procedure Form 29–1. Procedure forms can be downloaded from the Student Companion website; procedure scenarios are provided in the Instructor's Manual.

EVALUATION

Evaluator Signature: _____   Date: _____

Evaluator Comments:

Name: _____ Date: _____ Score: _____

Procedure 29–1 Steps

Start Time: _____ **End Time:** _____ **Total Time:** _____

	Steps	Possible Points	First Attempt	Second Attempt	Third Attempt
1.	Pull patient ledger card or pull up patient account on the computerized program.	5			
2.	Post charges with descriptions. Add charges for a new total.	10			
3.	Post insurance payments with descriptions. Add payments for a new total.	10			
4.	Post insurance adjustments with descriptions. Add adjustments for a new total.	10			
5.	Post patient payments with descriptions. Add payments for a new total.	10			
6.	Post and calculate total charges.	15			
7.	Post and calculate total payments.	15			
8.	Post and calculate amount due.	15			
9.	Check off each posted item on the encounter form.	5			
	Points Awarded / Points Possible	_____ / **95**			

Competency Checklist
Procedure 29–2 Inform a Patient of Financial Obligations for Services Rendered

ABHES Curriculum

MA.A.1.8.b   Perform billing and collection procedures

CAAHEP Core Curriculum

VII.C.5   Identify types of information contained in the patient's billing record
VII.C.6   Explain patient financial obligations for services rendered
VII.P.1   Perform accounts receivable procedures to patient accounts including posting: (a) charges, (b) payments, and (c) adjustments
VII.P.4   Inform a patient of financial obligations for services rendered
VII.A.1   Demonstrate professionalism when discussing patient's billing record
VII.A.2   Display sensitivity when requesting payment for services rendered

---

Task: Explain patient financial obligations for services rendered in a professional manner and displaying sensitivity.

Supplies & Conditions: Procedure cost estimate form (example Figure 29–11), pen, paper, telephone, patient chart (paper or electronic).

Standards: A maximum of three attempts may be used to complete the task. The time limit for each attempt is 30 minutes, with a minimum score of 85 percent. **Scoring:** Determine student's score by dividing points awarded by total points possible and multiplying results by 100.

Forms: Procedure Form 29–2. Procedure forms can be downloaded from the Student Companion website.

EVALUATION

Evaluator Signature: _____   Date: _____

Evaluator Comments:

Name: _____ Date: _____ Score: _____

Procedure 29–2 Steps

Start Time: _____ End Time: _____ Total Time: _____

	Steps	Possible Points	First Attempt	Second Attempt	Third Attempt
1.	Access patient chart. Refer to procedure/services.	5			
2.	Identify charge for procedure/services on the encounter or referral form.	10			
3.	Complete a procedure/service cost estimate.	15			
4.	Review the cost estimate with the patient (in person or by telephone). Provide a copy of the cost estimate to the patient (in person or via mail). ***Demonstrate professionalism when discussing patient's billing record. Display sensitivity when requesting payment for services rendered.***	35			
5.	Confirm that patient understands the financial obligation. Document the discussion in the patient's chart. Have patient sign any appropriate documents reflecting financial policy.	15			
	Points Awarded / Points Possible	_____/ **80**			

Competency Checklist
Procedure 30–1 Complete an Insurance Claim Form

CAAHEP Core Curriculum

VIII.C.1	Identify: (a) types of third party plans, (b) information required to file a third party claim, and (c) the steps for filing a third party claim
VIII.P.4	Complete an insurance claim form

Task:	Following the steps listed in the procedure, accurately complete a claim form for processing.
Supplies & Conditions:	CMS-1500 form, patient record, account ledger or information, computer, and software.
Standards:	A maximum of three attempts may be used to complete the task. The time limit for each attempt is 30 minutes, with a minimum score of 100 percent. **Scoring:** Determine student's score by dividing points awarded by total points possible and multiplying results by 100.
Forms:	Procedure Form 30-1 (CMS-1500 form). Procedure forms can be downloaded from the Student Companion website.

EVALUATION

Evaluator Signature: _____ Date: _____

Evaluator Comments:

465

Name: _____   Date: _____   Score: _____

Procedure 30–1 Steps

Start Time: _____   End Time: _____   Total Time: _____

	Steps	Possible Points	First Attempt	Second Attempt	Third Attempt
1.	Check for a photocopy of the patient's insurance card.	5			
2.	Check the chart to see whether the patient signature is on file for release of information and assignment of benefits.	15			
3.	Correctly complete boxes 1 to 3. **(The remaining steps of the procedure correspond to the box numbers on the CMS-1500 form.)**	15			
4.	Enter the insured's name.	5			
5.	Enter the patient's full address and telephone number.	5			
6.	Enter the patient's relationship to the insured.	5			
7.	Enter the insured's full address and telephone number.	5			
8.	[Reserved for NUCC use]. *Leave blank.*	5			
9.	Enter the other insured's name and necessary information.	5			
10.	Check the appropriate box regarding patient's condition related to: (Employment, Auto Accident, Other Accident, Claim Codes).	5			
11.	Enter the insured's policy or FECA number (and other necessary information).	5			
12.	Obtain the patient's or authorized person's signature.	5			
13.	Obtain the insured's or authorized person's signature, or stamp "signature on file" if you have the record to prove it.	5			
14.	Record the date of the current illness, injury, or pregnancy (LMP).	5			
15.	Record the "Other Date" the patient was first treated for the same or similar illness.	5			
16.	Enter the dates the patient is unable to work (from/to) *or leave blank.*	5			
17.	Complete with the name of the referring provider or other source if different than treating provider. *If same as treating provider, leave blank.*	5			
18.	Complete with dates of hospitalization if applicable. *If not, leave blank.*	5			
19.	Accidental Claim information (designated by NUCC). *Leave blank.*	5			
20.	Mark the appropriate box regarding outside lab services [Yes] or [No] and the $Charges. *If [No], leave $Charges blank.*	5			

466

Name: _____ Date: _____ Score: _____

21.	Enter the ICD code(s) on a separate line for each diagnosis or nature of illness or injury.	5			
22.	Resubmission code. *Leave blank.*	5			
23.	Complete *if applicable* with prior authorization number.	5			
24.	Complete A through J with appropriate CPT or HCPCS codes for services.	5			
25.	Add the provider's federal tax ID number: Social Security number [SSN] or practice tax identification number [EIN] and mark the appropriate box.	5			
26.	Add the patient's account number if applicable.	5			
27.	Check one box regarding assignment.	5			
28.	Enter the total charged.	5			
29.	Enter the amount paid.	5			
30.	Reserved for NUCC use. *Leave blank.*	5			
31.	Obtain provider's signature (including degree or credentials) and date.	5			
32.	Enter the name and address of the facility where services were rendered.	5			
33.	Enter the billing provider's name, address, and telephone number, and NPI number.	5			
	Points Awarded / Points Possible	____/ **185**			

Competency Checklist
Procedure 30–2 Process Insurance Claims

ABHES Core Curriculum

MA.A.1.8.c   Process insurance claims

CAAHEP Core Curriculum

VIII.C.1   Identify: (a) types of third party plans, (b) information required to file a third party claim, and (c) the steps for filing a third party claim

---

Purpose:	Process insurance claims. Accurately record payments and adjustments on patient ledgers (accounts) or enter this information in a computerized system.
Equipment:	Ledger card (account), checks amount(s), black and red ink pens, or a computer system.
Standards:	A maximum of three attempts may be used to complete the task. The time limit for each attempt is 30 minutes, with a minimum score of 100 percent. **Scoring:** Determine student's score by dividing points awarded by total points possible and multiplying results by 100.
Forms:	Procedure Form 30-2 (Patient Ledger). Procedure forms can be downloaded from the Student Companion website.

EVALUATION

Evaluator Signature: _____   Date: _____

Evaluator Comments:

Procedure 30–2 Steps

Start Time: _____ End Time: _____ Total Time: _____

	Steps	Possible Points	First Attempt	Second Attempt	Third Attempt
1.	Pull the patient ledger or pull up the patient account from the computerized practice management or accounting program.	5			
2.	Post the amount of the insurance payment in the credit column.	15			
3.	Post the amount of the insurance adjustment in the credit column.	15			
4.	Note on the patient ledger or within the computerized program the name of the insurance company making the payment and adjustment.	5			
5.	Note on the patient ledger or within the computerized program the date the insurance payment and adjustment are processed.	5			
6.	Note on the patient ledger or within the computerized program the check number of each insurance payment and adjustment processed.	5			
7.	Check that the balance reflects the current status of the account.	5			
8.	Check all entries for accuracy and compare the amount of the checks with the amount of the payment and adjustment indicated on the patient ledger (account) or computerized program.	15			
9.	Make a photocopy of the checks for the accounts receivable record.	5			
10.	Return the ledger (account) to the file or save and close the account on the computerized program.	5			
	Points Awarded / Points Possible	_____/ 80			

Competency Checklist
Procedure 31–1 Post Nonsufficient Funds (NSF) Checks and Collection Agency Payments Utilizing EMR and Practice Management Systems

ABHES Curriculum

MA.A.1.7.b	Utilize Electronic Medical Records (EMR) and Practice Management Systems
MA.A.1.7.c	Comply with federal, state, and local laws relating to exchange of information
MA.A.1.8.b	Perform billing and collection procedures: (1) Accounts payable and accounts receivable, (2) Post adjustments, and (3) Payment procedures: i.e., credit balance, non-sufficient funds, refunds

CAAHEP Core Curriculum

VII.C.4	Describe types of adjustments made to patient accounts including: (a) non-sufficient funds (NSF) check, (b) collection agency transaction, (c) credit balance, and (d) third party
VII.P.3	Obtain accurate patient billing information

Task:	Following the steps listed in the procedure, obtain accurate patient billing information, post NSF checks and collection agency payments on the patient ledger or in a computerized (practice management) system.
Supplies & Conditions:	Patient ledger (account history), returned NSF checks from the bank, checks from the collection agency, pen with black ink, calculator, or practice management software.
Standards:	A maximum of three attempts may be used to complete the task. The time limit for each attempt is 30 minutes, with a minimum score of 85 percent. **Scoring:** Determine student's score by dividing points awarded by total points possible and multiplying results by 100.
Forms:	Procedure Form 31–1. Procedure forms can be downloaded from the Student Companion website.

EVALUATION
Evaluator Signature: _____ Date: _____
Evaluator Comments:

Name: _____ Date: _____ Score: _____

Procedure 31–1 Steps

Start Time: _____ End Time: _____ Total Time: _____

	Steps	Possible Points	First Attempt	Second Attempt	Third Attempt
1.	Pull patient ledger or bring up the patient account history in the practice management software.	10			
2.	Obtain the patient's correct billing information by checking the demographic information contained in the patient's chart.	10			
3.	Post the NSF check in the debit/charges column, adding back into the account the amount the check was originally issued for.	15			
4.	Date the entry, noting NSF on the description portion of the patient ledger or account history.	15			
5.	Review the check sent from the collection agency.	10			
6	Post the amount of the check received in the credit column on the patient ledger or account history. Compute the new balance.	15			
	Points Awarded / Points Possible	____/ **75**			

Competency Checklist
Procedure 31–2 Process a Credit Balance and Refund

ABHES Curriculum

MA.A.1.7.c	Comply with federal, state, and local laws relating to exchange of information
MA.A.1.8.b	Perform billing and collection procedures: (1) Accounts payable and accounts receivable, (2) Post adjustments, and (3) Payment procedures: i.e. credit balance, non-sufficient funds, refunds

CAAHEP Core Curriculum

VII.P.1	Perform accounts receivable procedures to patient accounts including posting: (a) charges, (b) payments, and (c) adjustments
VII.C.4	Describe types of adjustments made to patient accounts including: (a) non-sufficient funds (NSF) check, (b) collection agency transaction, (c) credit balance, and (d) third party

---

Task:	Following the steps in the procedures, accurately process a credit balance and refund on a patient ledger or in a computerized (practice management) system.
Supplies & Conditions:	Patient ledger (account history), company check, envelope, pen with black ink, or a computerized (practice management) accounting system.
Standards:	A maximum of three attempts may be used to complete the task. The time limit for each attempt is 30 minutes, with a minimum score of 85 percent. **Scoring:** Determine student's score by dividing points awarded by total points possible and multiplying results by 100.
Forms:	Procedure Forms 31–2A and 31-2B. Procedure forms can be downloaded from the Student Companion website.

EVALUATION

Evaluator Signature: _____   Date: _____

Evaluator Comments:

Name: _____ Date: _____ Score: _____

Procedure 31–2 Steps

Start Time: _____ **End Time:** _____ **Total Time:** _____

	Steps	Possible Points	First Attempt	Second Attempt	Third Attempt
1.	Pull patient ledger or bring up the patient's account history in the practice management software.	10			
2.	Post the amount of the overpayment in the credit column, preceded by a negative (–) sign.	15			
3.	Indicate on the patient ledger (account history) the date the refund is being processed and to whom the refund is being issued.	15			
4.	Correctly complete the refund check to the patient.	15			
5.	Check all entries for accuracy and compare the refund amount with the amount indicated on the patient ledger or account history.	5			
6.	Obtain the proper signature(s) on the check.	15			
7.	Make a copy of the check for the accounts payable record.	10			
8.	Address an envelope to the payee and mail the check.	10			
9.	Return the patient ledger to the file or save and close the account in the PM software.	15			
	Points Awarded / Points Possible	_____/ **110**			

Name: _____ Date: _____ Score: _____

Competency Checklist
Procedure 32–1 Prepare a Check

CAAHEP Core Curriculum

VII.C.2   Describe banking procedures as related to the ambulatory care setting
VII.C.3   Identify precautions for accepting the following types of payments: (a) cash, (b) check, (c) credit card, (d) debit card

---

Task: Following the steps listed in the procedure, prepare a check and corresponding check stub.

Supplies & Conditions: In a simulated medical office situation, given the necessary equipment, a payee, the amount due, a signature name, and a previous balance, prepare a check and stub following the steps of the procedure. The check must be without error and contain the five essential factors, and the stub entries must agree with the check information, with the balance accurately figured. Procedure Form 32–1 can be used to complete this activity.

Standards: A maximum of three attempts may be used to complete the task. The time limit for each attempt is 10 minutes, with a minimum score of 85 percent. **Scoring:** Determine student's score by dividing points awarded by total points possible and multiplying results by 100.

Forms Needed: Procedure 32–1 Scenario with Procedure 32–1 Form. Procedure forms can be downloaded from the Student Companion website; procedure scenarios are included in the Instructor's Manual.

EVALUATION

Evaluator Signature: _____   Date: _____

Evaluator Comments:

Name: _____ Date: _____ Score: _____

Procedure 32–1 Steps

Start Time: _____ End Time: _____ Total Time: _____

	Steps	Possible Points	First Attempt	Second Attempt	Third Attempt
1.	Assemble equipment and supplies.	5			
2.	Correctly complete the check stub with all appropriate components and then calculate the new balance.	15			
3.	Correctly complete the check with all appropriate components.	15			
4.	Obtain authorized signature on check.	10			
	Points Awarded / Points Possible	____/ **45**			

Competency Checklist
Procedure 32–2 Prepare a Deposit Slip

CAAHEP Core Curriculum

| VII.C.2 | Describe banking procedures as related to the ambulatory care setting |
| VII.P.2 | Prepare a bank deposit |

Task: Following the steps listed in the procedure, prepare coin and currency and list checks accurately, entering and totaling amounts on the deposit slip.

Supplies & Conditions: In a simulated medical office situation, students will be placed in a quiet setting and provided a deposit slip, pen with black or blue ink, calculator, cash, currency, checks, and coin wraps to be deposited. Procedure Form 32–2 can be used to complete this activity.

Standards: A maximum of three attempts may be used to complete the task. The time limit for each attempt is 10 minutes, with a minimum score of 85 percent. **Scoring:** Determine student's score by dividing points awarded by total points possible and multiplying results by 100.

Forms Needed: Procedure 32–2 Scenario with Procedure 32–2 Form. Procedure forms can be downloaded from the Student Companion website; procedure scenarios are included in the Instructor's Manual.

EVALUATION

Evaluator Signature: _____ Date: _____

Evaluator Comments:

Name: _____ Date: _____ Score: _____

Procedure 32–2 Steps

Start Time: _____ **End Time:** _____ **Total Time:** _____

	Steps	Possible Points	First Attempt	Second Attempt	Third Attempt
1.	Assemble equipment and supplies.	5			
2.	Separate money to be deposited by coin, bills, and check.	5			
3.	Arrange dollar currency by denomination, portrait, and direction. Total the currency and record it on the deposit slip.	15			
4.	Count the coins; wrap large amounts. Enter the amount of coins on the deposit slip.	15			
5.	Check to ensure that all checks are endorsed. Arrange checks face up from greatest to least. Enter checks by number, maker, and amount on the deposit slip.	15			
6.	Total all checks listed on the back of the deposit slip and enter the total in the appropriate space on the back of the deposit slip; bring the total to the front of the deposit slip, writing in the appropriate space.	15			
7.	Total the currency, coin, and checks and enter it on the deposit slip.	15			
8.	Make a copy of deposit slip for your office files.	10			
9.	Enter the deposit total on the check stub in the checkbook.	15			
10.	Deposit at the bank and obtain a receipt for records.	15			
	Points Awarded / Points Possible	____/ **125**			

Competency Checklist
Procedure 32–3 Reconcile a Bank Statement

CAAHEP Core Curriculum

VII.C.2	Describe banking procedures as related to the ambulatory care setting
VII.C.3	Identify precautions for accepting the following types of payments: (a) cash, (b) check, (c) credit card, (d) debit card

---

Task: Follow the procedure steps to reconcile a bank statement so that the checkbook balance equals the bank statement balance.

Supplies & Conditions: In a simulated medical office situation, students will be placed in a quiet setting and provided with a bank statement and canceled checks or photocopies, reconciliation worksheet, pen or pencil, and calculator or adding machine. Procedure Form 32–3 can be used to complete this activity.

Standards: A maximum of three attempts may be used to complete the task. The time limit for each attempt is 20 minutes, with a minimum score of 85 percent. **Scoring:** Determine student's score by dividing points awarded by total points possible and multiplying results by 100.

Forms Needed: Procedure 32–3 Scenario with Procedure 32–3 Form. Procedure forms can be downloaded from the Student Companion Website; procedure scenarios are included in the Instructor's Manual.

EVALUATION

Evaluator Signature: _____ Date: _____

Evaluator Comments:

Name: _____ Date: _____ Score: _____

Procedure 32–3 Steps

Start Time: _____ **End Time:** _____ **Total Time:** _____

	Steps	Possible Points	First Attempt	Second Attempt	Third Attempt
1.	Assemble equipment and supplies.	5			
2.	Compare the opening balance on the new statement with the closing balance on the previous statement. List the bank balance in the appropriate space on the reconciliation worksheet.	10			
3.	In the checkbook, check off all deposits credited to the account. Add to the bank statement balance any deposits not shown on the bank statement.	15			
4.	Put checks in numeric order and compare the check entries on the statement with the returned checks. Check off all returned checks in the checkbook. Determine whether you have any outstanding checks and, if so, list them on the reconciliation worksheet and total them.	15			
5.	Subtract from your checkbook balance items such as withdrawals, automatic payments, or service charges that appear on the statement but not in the checkbook.	15			
6.	Add to your checkbook balance any interest earned as indicated on your statement.	15			
7.	Make sure the balance in your checkbook and the balance on the bank statement agree.	15			
	Points Awarded / Points Possible	____/ 90			

Competency Checklist
Procedure 33–1 Establish and Maintain a Petty Cash Fund

Task:	Following the steps listed in the procedure, prepare a check and corresponding check stub.
Supplies & Conditions:	In a simulated medical office situation, students will be placed in a quiet setting and provided with a pen with black or blue ink, calculator, vouchers, receipts, petty cash form, and computer. Procedure Form 33–1 can be used to complete this activity.
Standards:	A maximum of three attempts may be used to complete the task. The time limit for each attempt is 15 minutes, with a minimum score of 85 percent. **Scoring:** Determine student's score by dividing points awarded by total points possible and multiplying results by 100.
Forms Needed:	Procedure 33–1 Form with Procedure 33–1 Scenario(s). Procedure forms can be downloaded from the Student Companion website; procedure scenarios are included in the Instructor's Manual.

EVALUATION

Evaluator Signature: _____ Date: _____

Evaluator Comments:

Name: _____ Date: _____ Score: _____

Procedure 33–1 Steps

Start Time: _____ **End Time:** _____ **Total Time:** _____

	Steps	Possible Points	First Attempt	Second Attempt	Third Attempt
1.	Assemble equipment and supplies.	5			
2.	Enter the opening balance on the petty cash form.	15			
3.	Refer to a voucher and enter the description, number, and amount disbursed and compute the balance.	15			
4.	Refer to a bill and enter the description and amount disbursed and compute the balance.	15			
5.	Continue until all items are listed and the remaining balance is computed.	15			
6.	Notify the provider or manager to write a new check for the difference between the balance and the established fund amount when it reaches the agreed-upon level.	15			
	Points Awarded / Points Possible	_____/ **80**			

Competency Checklist
Procedure 34–1: Participate in a Mock Exposure Event with Documentation of Specific Steps

ABHES Curriculum

MA.A.1.4.e	Perform risk management procedures
MA.A.1.4.f	Comply with federal, state, and local health laws and regulations as they relate to health care settings

CAAHEP Core Curriculum

III.P.1	Participate in blood-borne pathogen training
XII.P.4	Participate in a mock exposure event with documentation of specific steps

---

Task: To provide documentation required by OSHA in the event an employee becomes injured or is exposed to blood or body fluids. A postexposure plan must be followed, and an incident report must be filled out.

Supplies & Conditions: OSHA Form 301 (Injury and Illness Incident Report), pen.

Standards: A maximum of three attempts may be used to complete the task. The time limit for each attempt is 15 minutes, with a minimum score of 70 percent. **Scoring:** Determine student's score by dividing points awarded by total points possible and multiplying results by 100.

Forms: Procedure 34–1 Scenario with Procedure 34–1 Form. Procedure forms can be downloaded from the Student Companion website; procedure scenarios are included in the Instructor's Manual.

EVALUATION

Evaluator Signature: _____ Date: _____

Evaluator Comments:

Name: _____ Date: _____ Score: _____

Procedure 34–1 Steps

Start Time: _____ End Time: _____ Total Time: _____

	Steps	Possible Points	First Attempt	Second Attempt	Third Attempt
1.	Report the incident to a supervisor immediately for documentation.	15			
2.	Assemble equipment.	15			
3.	Fill in the demographic information about the employee.	15			
4.	Fill in the information about the physician or other health care professional.	15			
5.	Complete the section regarding information about the case.	15			
6.	Fill in what the employee was doing just before the incident occurred.	15			
7.	In the space provided, explain what happened.	15			
8.	Explain what the injury or illness was.	15			
9.	Explain what object or substance directly harmed the employee.	15			
10.	If the employee died, fill in the section concerned with when the death occurred.	15			
	Points Awarded / Points Possible	_____ / **150**			

Competency Checklist
Procedure 34–2: Hand Washing for Medical Asepsis

ABHES Curriculum

MA.A.1.9.a   Practice standard precautions

CAAHEP Core Curriculum

III.P.3   Perform handwashing

Task:	To reduce pathogens on the hands and wrists, thereby decreasing direct and indirect transmission of infectious microorganisms. Average duration is a vigorous 15-second scrub following each patient contact. (Some facilities may recommend two minutes at the start of your workday, before beginning to work with patients.) Standard precautions recommend proper hand washing to be performed to avoid the transfer of microorganisms to other patients, yourself, or the environment.
Supplies & Conditions:	Sink (preferably with a foot-operated lid), antimicrobial liquid soap, nail stick or brush, disposable paper towels, lotion, and a waste receptacle.
Standards:	A maximum of three attempts may be used to complete the task. The time limit for each attempt is 5 minutes, with a minimum score of 70 percent. **Scoring:** Determine student's score by dividing points awarded by total points possible and multiplying results by 100.

EVALUATION

Evaluator Signature: _____   Date: _____

Evaluator Comments:

Name: _____   Date: _____   Score: _____

Procedure 34–2 Steps

Start Time: _____   End Time: _____   Total Time: _____

	Steps	Possible Points	First Attempt	Second Attempt	Third Attempt
1.	Assemble equipment.	15			
2.	Remove all jewelry.	15			
3.	Use a paper towel to turn on faucet and adjust water temperature to lukewarm.	15			
4.	Discard paper towel.	5			
5.	Wet hands and apply soap; use friction, and work into lather, being sure to cover all parts of the hands, including the wrists.	15			
6.	Rinse well, hands pointed down; be sure not to touch the inside of the sink.	15			
7.	If the first hand cleansing of the day, use a nail stick or a nail brush on the nails and cuticles and repeat steps 5 and 6.	15			
8.	Use paper towels to dry hands with a blotting method from hands to elbows, discarding each towel after one use.	15			
9.	Turn faucet off with a clean paper towel and discard the towel.	15			
10.	Apply lotion.	15			
	Points Awarded / Points Possible	____/ **140**			

486

Competency Checklist
Procedure 34–3: Remove Nonsterile Gloves

ABHES Curriculum

MA.A.1.9.a   Practice standard precautions

CAAHEP Core Curriculum

III.P.10.b   Demonstrate proper disposal of biohazardous material: regulated wastes
III.A.1   Recognize the implications for failure to comply with Centers for Disease Control (CDC) regulations in health care settings

---

Task: To remove and dispose of contaminated gloves without exposing surroundings to contamination.

Supplies & Conditions: Biohazard waste container, contaminated gloves, hand-washing equipment

Standards: A maximum of three attempts may be used to complete the task. The time limit for each attempt is 5 minutes, with a minimum score of 70 percent. **Scoring:** Determine student's score by dividing points awarded by total points possible and multiplying results by 100.

EVALUATION

Evaluator Signature: _____   Date: _____

Evaluator Comments:

Name: _____ Date: _____ Score: _____

Procedure 34–3 Steps

Start Time: _____ End Time: _____ Total Time: _____

	Steps	Possible Points	First Attempt	Second Attempt	Third Attempt
1.	Hold hands down and away from the body. ***Recognize the implications for failure to comply with Centers for Disease Control (CDC) regulations in health care settings.***	10			
2.	Grasp the used glove by the palm of the nondominant hand with the dominant hand and remove it by turning the glove inside out.	15			
3.	Holding the glove that has been removed in the dominant gloved hand, insert two to three fingers inside the back of the contaminated glove and turn it inside out over the other.	15			
4.	Dispose of gloves into biohazard waste container.	10			
5.	Wash hands thoroughly.	15			
	Points Awarded / Points Possible	____/ 65			

Competency Checklist
Procedure 34–4: Choose, Apply, and Remove Appropriate Personal Protective Equipment (PPE)

ABHES Curriculum

MA.A.1.9.a   Practice standard precautions

CAAHEP Core Curriculum

III.P.1   Participate in blood-borne pathogen training
III.P.2   Select appropriate barrier/personal protective equipment (PPE)
III.P.10.b   Demonstrate proper disposal of biohazardous material: regulated wastes
III.A.1   Recognize the implications for failure to comply with Centers for Disease Control (CDC) regulations in health care settings

---

Task: To provide protection from infectious contamination.

Supplies & Conditions: Disposable gown, cap, mask, gloves, safety glasses, hand-washing equipment, and biohazard waste receptacle and/or laundry bag.

Standards: A maximum of three attempts may be used to complete the task. The time limit for each attempt is 15 minutes, with a minimum score of 70 percent. **Scoring:** Determine student's score by dividing points awarded by total points possible and multiplying results by 100.

EVALUATION

Evaluator Signature: _____   Date: _____

Evaluator Comments:

Name: _____ Date: _____ Score: _____

Procedure 34–4 Steps

Start Time: _____ End Time: _____ Total Time: _____

	Steps	Possible Points	First Attempt	Second Attempt	Third Attempt
1.	Review provider orders and facility protocols relative to the type of infectious exposure.	15			
2.	Choose and place appropriate PPE to be applied in a designated area for application.	15			
3.	Remove jewelry, lab coat, and other items not necessary in providing patient care or cleanup process.	10			
4.	Wash hands; apply gown and tie securely to cover outer garments completely. ***Recognize the implications for failure to comply with Centers for Disease Control (CDC) regulations in health care settings.***	15			
5.	Apply mask.	15			
6.	Apply safety glasses.	15			
7.	Apply cap if necessary to cover hair and ears completely.	15			
8.	Apply gloves and pull over the cuff of the gown to ensure no skin is exposed.	15			
9.	Enter exposure area and clean up the contaminants following facility protocol.	15			
10.	Dispose of contaminated articles into biohazard bag. If any reusable equipment is involved, transport to appropriate area, following protocol for proper cleaning.	15			
11.	Remove contaminated gloves, place in biohazard bag, and wash hands.	15			
12.	Remove mask, safety glasses, and hair covering; dispose of properly. (If they are contaminated, you must reapply new gloves first before removing.)	15			
13.	Remove contaminated gown.	15			
14.	Wash hands.	15			
	Points Awarded / Points Possible	_____ / **205**			

Competency Checklist
Procedure 34–5: Sanitize Instruments

ABHES Curriculum

MA.A.1.9.a   Practice standard precautions

CAAHEP Core Curriculum

III.P.2   Select appropriate barrier/personal protective equipment (PPE)
III.P.4   Prepare items for autoclaving
III.A.1   Recognize the implications for failure to comply with Centers for Disease Control (CDC) regulations in
               health care settings

Task:	To clean instruments properly to remove all tissue and debris.
Supplies & Conditions:	Sink with running water, sanitizing agent with enzymatic action, soft brush, towels, disposable paper towels, protective plastic apron, heavy-duty gloves, and goggles.
Standards:	A maximum of three attempts may be used to complete the task. The time limit for each attempt is 15 minutes, with a minimum score of 70 percent. **Scoring:** Determine student's score by dividing points awarded by total points possible and multiplying results by 100.

EVALUATION

Evaluator Signature: _____   Date: _____

Evaluator Comments:

Name: _____ Date: _____ Score: _____

Procedure 34–5 Steps

Start Time: _____ End Time: _____ Total Time: _____

	Steps	Possible Points	First Attempt	Second Attempt	Third Attempt
1.	Apply PPE: goggles, apron, and heavy-duty gloves. *Recognize the implications for failure to comply with Centers for Disease Control (CDC) regulations in health care settings.*	15			
2.	If instruments need to be transported from one place to another, place the instrument in a container labeled "Biohazard."	15			
3.	Rinse instruments in cool water and place in disinfectant solution.	15			
4.	Scrub each instrument well with detergent and water (be sure to include inside edges, serrations, grooves, hinges, and all surfaces); scrub under running water.	15			
5.	Rinse instruments with hot water.	15			
6.	Place instruments on a clean towel and dry thoroughly with disposable paper towels.	15			
7.	Remove PPE and wash hands.	15			
	Points Awarded / Points Possible	_____/ **105**			

Name: _____ Date: _____ Score: _____

Competency Checklist
Procedure 34–6: Disinfect (Chemical "Cold" Sterilization) Endoscopes

ABHES Curriculum

MA.A.1.9.a   Practice standard precautions and perform disinfection/sterilization techniques

CAAHEP Core Curriculum

III.P.2   Select appropriate barrier/personal protective equipment (PPE)
III.P.5   Perform sterilization procedures
III.A.1   Recognize the implications for failure to comply with Centers for Disease Control (CDC) regulations in health care settings

---

Task: To sterilize heat-sensitive items such as endoscopes, using appropriate chemical disinfectant (glutaraldehyde-based) solution. (This procedure may also be used for delicate cutting instruments.)

Supplies & Conditions: Chemical disinfectant, timer, sterile water, airtight container, heavy-duty gloves, sterile gloves, poly-lined towels, and sterile towels.

Standards: A maximum of three attempts may be used to complete the task. The time limit for each attempt is 20 minutes, with a minimum score of 70 percent. **Scoring:** Determine student's score by dividing points awarded by total points possible and multiplying results by 100.

EVALUATION

Evaluator Signature: _____   Date: _____

Evaluator Comments:

493

Name: _____ Date: _____ Score: _____

Procedure 34–6 Steps

Start Time: _____ End Time: _____ Total Time: _____

	Steps	Possible Points	First Attempt	Second Attempt	Third Attempt
1.	Ensure that the endoscope has been sanitized thoroughly and dried prior to chemical disinfecting (sterilization). ***Recognize the implications for failure to comply with Centers for Disease Control (CDC) regulations in health care settings.***	15			
2.	Read manufacturer's instructions for preparation of solution.	15			
3.	Apply PPE.	15			
4.	Prepare solution and pour into a container with an airtight lid, being careful not to splash the chemical.	15			
5.	Place items into solution and completely submerge.	15			
6.	Close the lid securely and label the outside of the container with the name of solution, date, and time required according to the manufacturer for sterilization procedure.	15			
7.	When required processing time is completed, lift lid and remove endoscope, using sterile gloves.	15			
8.	Rinse scope thoroughly inside and out with sterile water and drain remainder water from scope by holding in an upright position.	15			
9.	Place scope on sterile poly-lined towels and dry completely, using sterile towels.	15			
10.	Place scope in storage container or area until next use.	15			
11.	Remove PPE and dispose of properly.	15			
12.	Wash hands.	15			
	Points Awarded / Points Possible	_____/ **180**			

Competency Checklist
Procedure 34–7: Wrap Items for Autoclaving

ABHES Curriculum

MA.A.1.9.a   Practice standard precautions and perform disinfection/sterilization techniques

CAAHEP Core Curriculum

III.P.4   Prepare items for autoclaving

Task: To wrap items to be autoclaved so that they will be protected from contamination after the sterilization process is completed for storage and handling.

Supplies & Conditions: Autoclave paper or cloth, disposable plastic sealed pouches, autoclave tape, items to be sterilized or autoclaved, sterilization indicators, gauze, tip protectors, indelible pen.

Standards: A maximum of three attempts may be used to complete the task. The time limit for each attempt is 15 minutes, with a minimum score of 70 percent. **Scoring:** Determine student's score by dividing points awarded by total points possible and multiplying results by 100.

EVALUATION

Evaluator Signature: _____   Date: _____

Evaluator Comments:

Name: _____ Date: _____ Score: _____

Procedure 34–7 Steps

Start Time: _____ End Time: _____ Total Time: _____

	Steps	Possible Points	First Attempt	Second Attempt	Third Attempt
1.	Wash hands and assemble all necessary items.	15			
2.	Ensure that items have been sanitized before wrapping for autoclave process.	15			
3.	Check items for flaws and make sure they function properly.	10			
4.	Place two squares of autoclave paper adequate in size to wrap item(s) on a clean, flat surface in a diamond shape with one corner of the paper facing toward you; place item(s) as well as a sterilization indicator in the center of the paper.	15			
5.	Place a cotton ball between any hinged instruments and keep all ratchets open during the sterilization process.	15			
6.	Wrap item(s), using the first square by folding the corner of the paper toward the center and turning a small corner back toward you.	15			
7.	Continue wrapping the items by folding one side toward the center, leaving a small corner toward you back on itself, and then do the same with the other side.	15			
8.	Fold the package up from the bottom and secure, folding the last corner back on itself.	15			
9.	Wrap the package in the second square of paper using the same technique; be sure there is no opening and seal with autoclave tape. Wrap item(s) snugly.	15			
10.	Label the contents and write the date and your initials on the tape.	15			
11.	If using a plastic pouch for sterilization, place item into the pouch, seal, and label.	15			
12.	Place wrapped instruments in the autoclave for sterilizing and return all unused supplies to the proper storage area when finished.	15			
13.	Wash hands.	15			
	Points Awarded / Points Possible	_____/ **190**			

Competency Checklist
Procedure 34–8: Perform Autoclave Sterilization

ABHES Curriculum

MA.A.1.9.a   Practice standard precautions and perform disinfection/sterilization techniques

CAAHEP Core Curriculum

III.P.5   Perform sterilization procedures
III.A.1   Recognize the implications for failure to comply with Centers for Disease Control (CDC) regulations in health care settings

---

Task:	To sterilize instruments or supplies that will penetrate a patient's skin or be in contact with otherwise sterile areas of a patient's body.
Supplies & Conditions:	Items properly sanitized and wrapped or sealed in pouches, disposable gloves, protective mitts, and sterile transfer forceps.
Standards:	A maximum of three attempts may be used to complete the task. The time limit for each attempt is 15 minutes, with a minimum score of 70 percent. **Scoring:** Determine student's score by dividing points awarded by total points possible and multiplying results by 100.

EVALUATION

Evaluator Signature: _____   Date: _____

Evaluator Comments:

497

Name: _____ Date: _____ Score: _____

Procedure 34–8 Steps

Start Time: _____ End Time: _____ Total Time: _____

	Steps	Possible Points	First Attempt	Second Attempt	Third Attempt
1.	Check the water level in the reservoir and add distilled water to the fill line if required.	15			
2.	Any quality control procedures required must be performed with the load to be sterilized and documented. ***Recognize the implications for failure to comply with Centers for Disease Control (CDC) regulations in health care settings.***	15			
3.	Wash your hands and apply gloves.	15			
4.	Load the wrapped or pouched items in the autoclave, allowing adequate space around the packs to ensure that steam will reach all the areas.	15			
5.	Remove gloves and wash hands.	15			
6.	Select the appropriate sterilization cycle, depending on the contents loaded, and press the start button.	15			
7.	After the cycle has ended, the autoclave will vent on its own. Open the autoclave door to allow the packs to dry before removing them from the autoclave. The door should be ajar only slightly, $\frac{1}{4}$ to $\frac{1}{2}$ inch.	15			
8.	When the drying cycle is completed, wear protective mitts to unload the items, making sure not to unload any packs that are damp.	15			
9.	Check the items to be sure that the stripes on the autoclave tape or indicators on the plastic pouches turned the appropriate color.	15			
10.	If any individual items have been placed in the autoclave unwrapped, sterile transfer forceps must be used to remove the item and placed in appropriate storage area.	15			
11.	Remove the mitts and wash your hands.	15			
	Points Awarded / Points Possible	_____/ **165**			

Competency Checklist
Procedure 35–1: Perform Patient Screening

ABHES Curriculum

MA.A.1.4.a	Follow documentation guidelines
MA.A.1.8.f	Display professionalism through written and verbal communications
MA.A.1.9.b	Formulate chief complaint

CAAHEP Core Curriculum

I.P.3	Perform patient screening using established protocols
I.A.1	Incorporate critical thinking skills when performing patient assessment
I.A.2	Incorporate critical thinking skills when performing patient care
V.P.1	Use feedback techniques to obtain patient information including: (a) reflection, (b) restatement, and (c) clarification
V.P.3	Use medical terminology correctly and pronounced accurately to communicate information to providers and patients
V.P.11	Report relevant information concisely and accurately
V.A.1	Demonstrate: (a) empathy, (b) active listening, and (c) nonverbal communication
V.A.2	Demonstrate the principles of self-boundaries
X.A.1	Demonstrate sensitivity to patient rights

Task: To conduct an in-person screening to identify and accurately record the patient's chief complaint (CC) and related symptoms in the patient's medical record.

Supplies & Conditions: Patient's chart or computer with appropriate software, pen, and any supplies or equipment needed to set up the room according to the reason for the patient being seen.

Standards: A maximum of three attempts may be used to complete the task. The time limit for each attempt is 10 minutes, with a minimum score of 70 percent. **Scoring:** Determine student's score by dividing points awarded by total points possible and multiplying results by 100.

EVALUATION

Evaluator Signature: _____ Date: _____

Evaluator Comments:

Name: _____ Date: _____ Score: _____

Procedure 35–1 Steps

Start Time: _____ End Time: _____ Total Time: _____

	Steps	Possible Points	First Attempt	Second Attempt	Third Attempt
1.	*Demonstrate sensitivity to patient rights.*	10			
2.	Review any completed office forms, including the HIPAA authorization agreement.	10			
3.	Call the patient by name from the reception room.	15			
4.	*Demonstrate the principles of self-boundaries.*	15			
5.	Restate the patient's name and introduce yourself.	15			
6.	Explain what you will be doing and request participation. *Incorporate critical thinking skills when performing patient assessment and care.*	15			
7.	Ask what brings the person to the office today. *Demonstrate empathy, active listening, and nonverbal communication.*	15			
8.	Use questioning to focus on the CC, its characteristics, and any related symptoms.	15			
9.	Identify and record any secondary concerns.	15			
10.	Ask the patient whether he or she is taking any medications.	15			
11.	Ask the patient whether he or she has any allergies.	15			
12.	Reconfirm the CC, symptoms, and any other concerns with the patient.	15			
13.	Record the CC statement and related information on the chart or EMR.	15			
14.	Set up the room according to the patient's complaint, demonstrating time management and anticipation skills.	15			
15.	Dismiss yourself in a professional manner and indicate to the patient the approximate wait time.	15			
16.	Notify the provider that the patient is ready to be seen.	15			
	Points Awarded / Points Possible	____/ **230**			

Competency Checklist
Procedure 35–2: Obtain and Record a Patient Health History

ABHES Curriculum

MA.A.1.4.a	Follow documentation guidelines
MA.A.1.8.f	Display professionalism through written and verbal communications
MA.A.1.9.b	Obtain patient history and formulate chief complaint

CAAHEP Core Curriculum

I.P.3.b	Perform patient screening using established protocols
I.A.1	Incorporate critical thinking skills when performing patient assessment
I.A.2	Incorporate critical thinking skills when performing patient care
V.P.1	Use feedback techniques to obtain patient information including: (a) reflection, (b) restatement, and (c) clarification
V.P.3	Use medical terminology correctly and pronounced accurately to communicate information to providers and patients
V.P.11	Report relevant information concisely and accurately
V.A.1	Demonstrate: (a) empathy, (b) active listening, and (c) nonverbal communication
V.A.2	Demonstrate the principles of self-boundaries
X.A.1	Demonstrate sensitivity to patient rights

Task: To obtain and record a comprehensive health history of a patient, including family, occupational, and social factors, to facilitate the diagnosis and health care plan for the patient.

Supplies & Conditions: Health history form and pen or computer with appropriate software.

Standards: A maximum of three attempts may be used to complete the task. The time limit for each attempt is 25 minutes, with a minimum score of 70 percent. **Scoring:** Determine student's score by dividing points awarded by total points possible and multiplying results by 100.

Forms: Procedure 35–2 Form (optional; may use EHR software program for charting, if available). Procedure forms can be downloaded from the Student Companion website.

EVALUATION

Evaluator Signature: _____   Date: _____

Evaluator Comments:

Name: _____   Date: _____   Score: _____

Procedure 35–2 Steps

Start Time: _____   End Time: _____   Total Time: _____

	Steps	Possible Points	First Attempt	Second Attempt	Third Attempt
1.	If using a paper system, obtain the medical history form and pen. If using an EHR, access history area.	10			
2.	*Demonstrate sensitivity to patient rights.*	10			
3.	*Demonstrate the principles of self-boundaries.*	15			
4.	Explain the purpose of the health history and inform the patient that all the information obtained is confidential. *Incorporate critical thinking skills when performing patient assessment and care.*	15			
5.	If the patient completed the form prior to the visit, review the information with the patient, clarifying information and ensuring no omissions. Use reflection, restatement, and clarification techniques. *Demonstrate empathy, active listening and nonverbal communication.*	15			
6.	If you are completing the form with the patient, be sure to ask all necessary questions and record or enter answers neatly and accurately. Use reflection, restatement, and clarification techniques. If using EHR software, bring up the patient's medical history section on the screen and enter the information appropriately.	15			
7.	When finished with the form or entering the data, summarize and clarify the information with the patient.	15			
8.	Thank the patient and explain the next step in the examination. Ensure that the patient is comfortable and explain whether there will be a wait.	15			
9.	Chart a summary of the findings on the patient's chart or EMR. Highlight significant information as instructed.	15			
10.	Assemble all necessary forms into the patient's chart or templates within EHR software and have them ready for the provider to use during the examination.	15			
	Points Awarded / Points Possible	____/ **140**			

Competency Checklist
Procedure 36–1: Measure Height and Weight Using a Balance Beam Scale

ABHES Curriculum

MA.A.1.4.a	Follow documentation guidelines
MA.A.1.9.b	Obtain vital signs

CAAHEP Core Curriculum

I.P.1.e	Measure and record height
I.P.1.f	Measure and record weight
I.P.3	Perform patient screening using established protocols
I.A.1	Incorporate critical thinking skills when performing patient assessment
I.A.2	Incorporate critical thinking skills when performing patient care
V.A.4	Explain to a patient the rationale for performance of a procedure

---

Task: To obtain an accurate measurement of a patient's height and weight.

Supplies & Conditions: Balance beam scale with extension measuring bar, paper towel, patient's chart/EHR, pen.

Standards: A maximum of three attempts may be used to complete the task. The time limit for each attempt is 5 minutes, with a minimum score of 70 percent. **Scoring:** Determine student's score by dividing points awarded by total points possible and multiplying results by 100.

EVALUATION

Evaluator Signature: _____   Date: _____

Evaluator Comments:

Name: _____ Date: _____ Score: _____

Procedure 36–1 Steps

Start Time: _____ End Time: _____ Total Time: _____

	Steps	Possible Points	First Attempt	Second Attempt	Third Attempt
1.	Wash hands.	15			
2.	Identify the patient and introduce yourself.	15			
3.	**Explain the rationale for performance of the procedure,** and instruct the patient to remove shoes and any heavy clothing.	15			
4.	Place a paper towel on the scale platform.	5			
5.	Assist patient to the center of the scale. **Incorporate critical thinking skills when performing patient assessment and care.**	15			
6.	Move the lower weight bar (measured in 50-pound increments) to the estimated number and slowly slide the upper bar until the balance beam point is centered.	15			
7.	Read the weight by adding the upper bar measurement to the lower bar measurement. Round to the nearest ¼ pound.	15			
8.	Raise the measuring bar beyond the patient's height and lift the extension.	15			
9.	Lower measuring bar until firmly resting on top of patient's head.	15			
10.	Assist patient off the scale and allow the patient to sit and put on shoes.	15			
11.	Read line where measurement falls. Round to the nearest ¼ inch.	15			
12.	Lower measuring bar to its original position and return the weights to zero.	15			
13.	Document in the patient's chart.	15			
	Points Awarded / Points Possible	____/ **185**			

Competency Checklist
Procedure 36–2: Measure and Record Oral Temperature with an Electronic Thermometer

ABHES Curriculum

MA.A.1.4.a	Follow documentation guidelines
MA.A.1.9.b	Obtain vital signs

CAAHEP Core Curriculum

I.P.1.b	Measure and record temperature
I.P.3	Perform patient screening using established protocols
I.A.1	Incorporate critical thinking skills when performing patient assessment
I.A.2	Incorporate critical thinking skills when performing patient care
V.A.4	Explain to a patient the rationale for performance of a procedure

---

Task: To determine a patient's oral temperature with an electronic thermometer.

Supplies & Conditions: Electronic thermometer unit, oral probe, probe cover, waste container, patient chart/EHR, pen.

Standards: A maximum of three attempts may be used to complete the task. The time limit for each attempt is 5 minutes, with a minimum score of 70 percent. **Scoring:** Determine student's score by dividing points awarded by total points possible and multiplying results by 100.

EVALUATION

Evaluator Signature: _____ Date: _____

Evaluator Comments:

505

Name: _____ Date: _____ Score: _____

Procedure 36–2 Steps

Start Time: _____ End Time: _____ Total Time: _____

	Steps	Possible Points	First Attempt	Second Attempt	Third Attempt
1.	Wash hands; assemble equipment.	15			
2.	Identify the patient and introduce yourself.	15			
3.	*Explain the rationale for performance of the procedure.*	15			
4.	Ensure that the patient has not smoked or consumed anything hot or cold in past 15 minutes.	5			
5.	Correctly prepare the thermometer. *Incorporate critical thinking skills when performing patient assessment and care.*	15			
6.	Insert the covered probe into the patient's mouth. Instruct the patient to keep his or her lips pursed around the probe and not to bite down. Maintain the covered probe in position until the unit signals, approximately 10 to 15 seconds.	15			
7.	Remove the probe from the patient. Do not touch the probe cover.	15			
8.	Read and note the temperature.	15			
9.	Press the eject button to discard the used probe cover into the waste container.	15			
10.	Return the probe to the stored position in the unit and store the unit in the charging stand.	15			
11.	Wash hands.	15			
12.	Document in the patient's chart.	15			
	Points Awarded / Points Possible	_____/ **170**			

Competency Checklist
Procedure 36–3: Measure and Record Rectal Temperature with an Electronic Thermometer

ABHES Curriculum

MA.A.1.4.a   Follow documentation guidelines
MA.A.1.9.b   Obtain vital signs

CAAHEP Core Curriculum

I.P.1.b   Measure and record temperature
I.P.3   Perform patient screening using established protocols
I.A.1   Incorporate critical thinking skills when performing patient assessment
I.A.2   Incorporate critical thinking skills when performing patient care
I.A.3   Show awareness of a patient's concerns related to the procedure being performed.
V.A.4   Explain to a patient the rationale for performance of a procedure

---

Task: To determine a patient's rectal temperature with an electronic thermometer.

Supplies & Conditions: Mannequin (if simulated), electronic thermometer, rectal probe, probe cover, drape (if adult), gloves, lubricant, tissues, waste container, patient chart/EHR, pen.

Standards: A maximum of three attempts may be used to complete the task. The time limit for each attempt is 5 minutes, with a minimum score of 70 percent. **Scoring:** Determine student's score by dividing points awarded by total points possible and multiplying results by 100.

EVALUATION

Evaluator Signature: _____   Date: _____

Evaluator Comments:

Name: _____ Date: _____ Score: _____

Procedure 36–3 Steps

Start Time: _____ End Time: _____ Total Time: _____

	Steps	Possible Points	First Attempt	Second Attempt	Third Attempt
1.	Wash hands, assemble equipment, and put on gloves.	15			
2.	Identify the patient and introduce yourself.	15			
3.	**Explain the rationale for performance of the procedure,** and instruct the patient to remove appropriate clothing, assisting as needed.	15			
4.	Assist the adult patient onto the examining table, position the patient on his or her side (lateral or Sims position), and cover with a drape, **showing awareness of the patient's concerns related to the procedure being performed.**	15			
5.	Place a small amount of lubricant onto a tissue and place it within reach.	5			
6.	Correctly prepare the thermometer. **Incorporate critical thinking skills when performing patient assessment and care.**	15			
7.	Apply lubricant to the end of the probe cover.	10			
8.	Arrange the drape to expose the buttocks, raise the upper buttock to expose the anus, and carefully insert the lubricated thermometer probe into the anal canal approximately 1 inch for adults and ½ inch for infants and children. Hold the thermometer in place until the unit signals.	15			
9.	Withdraw the thermometer. Eject the probe cover into the waste container.	15			
10.	Read the temperature, noting the temperature.	15			
11.	Replace the probe in the unit and return the thermometer to the charging stand.	15			
12.	Remove any excess lubricant from the anal area with a tissue.	10			
13.	• If the patient is an adult, assist him or her from the examining table and instruct him or her to dress. • If the patient is an infant or child, ask the parent or accompanying adult to dress him or her.	10			
14.	Remove and discard gloves in the waste container.	15			
15.	Wash hands.	15			
16.	Document the temperature in the patient's chart, placing an (R) after the finding.	15			
	Points Awarded / Points Possible	_____ / **215**			

Competency Checklist
Procedure 36–4: Measure Axillary Temperature

ABHES Curriculum

MA.A.1.4.a   Follow documentation guidelines
MA.A.1.9.b   Obtain vital signs

CAAHEP Core Curriculum

I.P.1.b   Measure and record temperature
I.P.3   Perform patient screening using established protocols
I.A.1   Incorporate critical thinking skills when performing patient assessment
I.A.2   Incorporate critical thinking skills when performing patient care
V.A.4   Explain to a patient the rationale for performance of a procedure

---

Task: To determine a patient's axillary temperature with an electronic thermometer.

Supplies & Conditions: Electronic thermometer, probe, probe cover, tissues, waste container, patient chart/EHR, pen.

Standards: A maximum of three attempts may be used to complete the task. The time limit for each attempt is 5 minutes, with a minimum score of 70 percent. **Scoring:** Determine student's score by dividing points awarded by total points possible and multiplying results by 100.

EVALUATION

Evaluator Signature: _____ Date: _____

Evaluator Comments:

Name: _____ Date: _____ Score: _____

Procedure 36–4 Steps

Start Time: _____ End Time: _____ Total Time: _____

	Steps	Possible Points	First Attempt	Second Attempt	Third Attempt
1.	Wash hands; assemble equipment.	15			
2.	Identify the patient and introduce yourself.	15			
3.	***Explain the rationale for performance of the procedure.***	15			
4.	Assist the patient, as necessary, to expose the axilla. Pat the axillary space with a tissue to remove perspiration.	10			
5.	Correctly prepare the thermometer. ***Incorporate critical thinking skills when performing patient assessment and care.***	15			
6.	Insert the covered probe deep in the axillary space.	15			
7.	Hold the arm tightly against the body. Maintain the covered probe in position until the thermometer unit signals, approximately 10 to 15 seconds.	15			
8.	Remove the probe from the patient. Do not touch the probe cover, and discard the used probe cover into the waste container.	15			
9.	Read and note the temperature.	15			
10.	Disinfect thermometer and return the probe to the stored position in the unit. Store the unit in the charging stand.	5			
11.	Help the patient replace his or her clothing.	15			
12.	Wash hands.	15			
13.	Document the temperature in the patient's chart, placing an (Ax) after the finding.	15			
	Points Awarded / Points Possible	_____/ **180**			

Competency Checklist
Procedure 36–5: Measure Core Body Temperature with a Tympanic (Aural) Thermometer

ABHES Curriculum

MA.A.1.4.a	Follow documentation guidelines
MA.A.1.9.b	Obtain vital signs

CAAHEP Core Curriculum

I.P.1.b	Measure and record temperature
I.P.3	Perform patient screening using established protocols
I.A.1	Incorporate critical thinking skills when performing patient assessment
I.A.2	Incorporate critical thinking skills when performing patient care
V.A.4	Explain to a patient the rationale for performance of a procedure

---

Task: To determine a patient's core body temperature using an infrared tympanic thermometer.

Supplies & Conditions: Tympanic thermometer unit, probe cover, waste container, patient chart/EHR, pen.

Standards: A maximum of three attempts may be used to complete the task. The time limit for each attempt is 5 minutes, with a minimum score of 70 percent. **Scoring:** Determine student's score by dividing points awarded by total points possible and multiplying results by 100.

EVALUATION

Evaluator Signature: _____   Date: _____

Evaluator Comments:

Name: _____ Date: _____ Score: _____

Procedure 36–5 Steps

Start Time: _____ End Time: _____ Total Time: _____

	Steps	Possible Points	First Attempt	Second Attempt	Third Attempt
1.	Wash hands; assemble equipment.	15			
2.	Identify the patient and introduce yourself.	15			
3.	*Explain the rationale for performance of the procedure.*	15			
4.	Correctly prepare the thermometer. *Incorporate critical thinking skills when performing patient assessment and care.*	15			
5.	Insert the covered probe into the ear canal, sealing the opening.	15			
6.	Press the scan button to activate the thermometer. Wait until the temperature reading is displayed on the screen.	15			
7.	Withdraw the thermometer. Observe the display window, noting the temperature.	15			
8.	Press the release button on the thermometer to eject the probe cover into a waste container and return the thermometer to the base.	15			
9.	Document the temperature in the patient's chart, using (T) or (Tym) to indicate tympanic temperature.	15			
	Points Awarded / Points Possible	_____/ **135**			

Competency Checklist
Procedure 36–6: Measure Temperature with a Temporal Artery Thermometer

ABHES Curriculum

MA.A.1.4.a	Follow documentation guidelines
MA.A.1.9.b	Obtain vital signs

CAAHEP Core Curriculum

I.P.1.b	Measure and record temperature
I.P.3	Perform patient screening using established protocols
I.A.1	Incorporate critical thinking skills when performing patient assessment
I.A.2	Incorporate critical thinking skills when performing patient care
V.A.4	Explain to a patient the rationale for performance of a procedure

---

Task:	To measure a patient's temperature with a temporal artery thermometer.
Supplies & Conditions:	Temporal artery thermometer, alcohol wipe or cover, patient chart/EHR, pen.
Standards:	A maximum of three attempts may be used to complete the task. The time limit for each attempt is 5 minutes, with a minimum score of 70 percent. **Scoring:** Determine student's score by dividing points awarded by total points possible and multiplying results by 100.

EVALUATION

Evaluator Signature: _____ Date: _____

Evaluator Comments:

Name: _____   Date: _____   Score: _____

Procedure 36–6 Steps

Start Time: _____   End Time: _____   Total Time: _____

	Steps	Possible Points	First Attempt	Second Attempt	Third Attempt
1.	Wash hands; assemble equipment. Clean the probe with alcohol or attach a cover.	15			
2.	Identify the patient and introduce yourself.	15			
3.	*Explain the rationale for performance of the procedure.*	15			
4.	Observe the forehead for perspiration and exposure to the environment. Adjust as necessary (e.g., remove hat, hold back hair).	15			
5.	Position the probe at the midline of the forehead. *Incorporate critical thinking skills when performing patient assessment and care.*	15			
6.	Keeping the probe flush on the skin, press and hold the scan button while slowly sliding the thermometer across the forehead until reaching the hairline.	15			
7.	When scanning is completed, release the button and lift the probe from the forehead or neck. Read the temperature on the display and return the thermometer to storage.	15			
8.	Document the temperature in the patient's chart, using (TA) to indicate temporal artery temperature.	15			
	Points Awarded / Points Possible	_____ / **120**			

514

Competency Checklist
Procedure 36–7: Measure the Apical Pulse

ABHES Curriculum

MA.A.1.4.a	Follow documentation guidelines
MA.A.1.9.b	Obtain vital signs

CAAHEP Core Curriculum

I.P.1.c	Measure and record pulse
I.P.3	Perform patient screening using established protocols
I.A.1	Incorporate critical thinking skills when performing patient assessment
I.A.2	Incorporate critical thinking skills when performing patient care
I.A.3	Show awareness of a patient's concerns related to the procedure being performed
V.A.4	Explain to a patient the rationale for performance of a procedure

---

Task:	To determine the rate, rhythm, and quality of a patient's apical pulse.
Supplies & Conditions:	Watch with second hand, stethoscope, alcohol wipe, patient chart/ EHR, pen.
Standards:	A maximum of three attempts may be used to complete the task. The time limit for each attempt is 5 minutes, with a minimum score of 70 percent. **Scoring:** Determine student's score by dividing points awarded by total points possible and multiplying results by 100.

EVALUATION

Evaluator Signature: _____ Date: _____

Evaluator Comments:

515

Name: _____ Date: _____ Score: _____

Procedure 36–7 Steps

Start Time: _____ End Time: _____ Total Time: _____

	Steps	Possible Points	First Attempt	Second Attempt	Third Attempt
1.	Wash hands; assemble equipment. Clean the stethoscope.	15			
2.	Identify the patient and introduce yourself.	15			
3.	*Explain the rationale for performance of the procedure.*	15			
4.	Uncover the left side of the chest. *Show awareness of the patient's concerns related to the procedure being performed. Incorporate critical thinking skills when performing patient assessment and care.*	10			
5.	Place the stethoscope earpieces in your ears.	15			
6.	Locate the apex.	15			
7.	Place the chest piece of the stethoscope at the apex.	15			
8.	Count the beats for a full minute. Note the rate.	15			
9.	Determine the quality of the heart sounds and remove the earpieces from your ears.	15			
10.	Assist or instruct the patient to dress.	15			
11.	Clean the earpieces and chest piece of the stethoscope.	15			
12.	Document the rate and quality of the heart sounds in the patient's chart.	15			
13.	Wash hands.	15			
	Points Awarded / Points Possible	_____ / **190**			

Name: _____ Date: _____ Score: _____

Competency Checklist
Procedure 36–8: Measure the Radial Pulse and Respirations

ABHES Curriculum

MA.A.1.4.a	Follow documentation guidelines
MA.A.1.9.b	Obtain vital signs

CAAHEP Core Curriculum

I.P.1.c	Measure and record pulse
I.P.1.d	Measure and record respirations
I.P.3	Perform patient screening using established protocols
I.A.1	Incorporate critical thinking skills when performing patient assessment
I.A.2	Incorporate critical thinking skills when performing patient care
V.A.4	Explain to a patient the rationale for performance of a procedure

---

Task: To determine the rate, rhythm, and quality of a patient's radial pulse and determine the rate, rhythm, sound, and depth of a patient's respirations.

Supplies & Conditions: Watch with second hand, patient chart/EHR, pen.

Standards: A maximum of three attempts may be used to complete the task. The time limit for each attempt is 5 minutes, with a minimum score of 70 percent. **Scoring:** Determine student's score by dividing points awarded by total points possible and multiplying results by 100.

EVALUATION

Evaluator Signature: _____ Date: _____

Evaluator Comments:

Name: _____ Date: _____ Score: _____

Procedure 36–8 Steps

Start Time: _____ **End Time:** _____ **Total Time:** _____

	Steps	Possible Points	First Attempt	Second Attempt	Third Attempt
1.	Wash hands; assemble equipment.	15			
2.	Identify the patient and introduce yourself.	15			
3.	***Explain the rationale for performance of the procedure.***	15			
4.	Determine the patient's recent activity.	10			
5.	Position the patient with the wrist supported on a table or lap.	15			
6.	Locate the radial artery on the thumb side of the wrist and observe the quality of the pulse before beginning to count. Determine whether it is regular, strong, weak, or thready. ***Incorporate critical thinking skills when performing patient assessment and care.***	15			
7.	Count a *regular* pulse for 30 seconds and multiply the results by two.	15			
8.	Assess respiration quality.	15			
9.	Count respirations for 30 seconds and multiply the results by two.	15			
10.	Document the patient's pulse and respiration (including quality characteristics) in the chart.	15			
11.	Wash hands.	15			
	Points Awarded / Points Possible	_____/ **160**			

Competency Checklist
Procedure 36–9: Measure Blood Pressure

ABHES Curriculum

MA.A.1.4.a	Follow documentation guidelines
MA.A.1.9.b	Obtain vital signs

CAAHEP Core Curriculum

I.P.1.a	Measure and record blood pressure
I.P.3	Perform patient screening using established protocols
I.A.1	Incorporate critical thinking skills when performing patient assessment
I.A.2	Incorporate critical thinking skills when performing patient care
V.A.4	Explain to a patient the rationale for performance of a procedure

---

Task:	To determine a patient's palpatory and auscultatory blood pressure measurements.
Supplies & Conditions:	Stethoscope, aneroid manometer, alcohol wipe, patient chart/EHR, pen.
Standards:	A maximum of three attempts may be used to complete the task. The time limit for each attempt is 5 minutes, with a minimum score of 70 percent. **Scoring:** Determine student's score by dividing points awarded by total points possible and multiplying results by 100.

EVALUATION

Evaluator Signature: _____ Date: _____

Evaluator Comments:

519

Name: _____ Date: _____ Score: _____

Procedure 36–9 Steps

Start Time: _____ End Time: _____ Total Time: _____

	Steps	Possible Points	First Attempt	Second Attempt	Third Attempt
1.	Wash hands; assemble equipment. Clean the earpieces and head of the stethoscope with antiseptic.	15			
2.	Identify the patient and introduce yourself.	15			
3.	*Explain the rationale for performance of the procedure.*	15			
4.	Place the patient in a relaxed and comfortable sitting or lying position. Expose the patient's upper arm well above the elbow, extending the arm with the palm up. *Incorporate critical thinking skills when performing patient assessment and care.*	10			
5.	With the valve of the inflation bulb open, squeeze all air from the bladder and place it over the brachial artery. Be sure the aneroid dial is in direct view.	15			
6.	With *one hand*, close the valve on the bulb, turning clockwise.	15			
7.	Position your other hand to palpate the radial pulse.	15			
8.	While observing the manometer, rapidly inflate the cuff to 30 mm above the level where radial pulse disappears.	15			
9.	Open the valve, slowly releasing the air until the radial pulse is detected. Observe the dial reading.	15			
10.	Deflate the cuff rapidly and completely.	15			
11.	Position the earpieces of the stethoscope in your ears.	10			
12.	Palpate the brachial artery at the medial antecubital space with your fingertips.	15			
13.	Place the head of the stethoscope directly over the palpated pulse.	15			
14.	Close the valve on the bulb and rapidly inflate the cuff to 30 mm above the palpated systolic pressure.	15			
15.	Open the valve, slowly deflating the cuff. Note the reading at which you hear the systolic pressure.	15			
16.	Allow the pressure to lower steadily until you note a change in sound to a softer, more muffled sound. Note this as diastolic pressure (if so instructed).	15			
17.	Continue to release pressure until all sound disappears. Note this point as diastolic pressure (if so instructed).	15			
18.	Remove the stethoscope from your ears and release the remaining air from the cuff.	15			
19.	Remove the cuff from the patient's arm. Assist the patient with clothing if necessary.	15			
20.	Reevaluate, if indicated, after a minimum of 15 seconds.	15			
21.	Clean the stethoscope. Fold the cuff properly and place it with the manometer and stethoscope in storage.	10			
22.	Wash hands and document the systolic and whichever diastolic reading the provider prefers in the patient's chart.	15			
	Points Awarded / Points Possible	____/ **315**			

Name: _____ Date: _____ Score: _____

Competency Checklist
Procedure 37–1: Prepare and Maintain Examination and Treatment Areas

ABHES Curriculum

MA.A.1.9.a   Practice standard precautions and perform disinfection/sterilization techniques

CAAHEP Core Curriculum

III.C.3.a   Define the following as practiced within an ambulatory care setting: medical asepsis

---

Task:	To provide an examination room that is comfortable, clean, and has the usual equipment and supplies necessary for an examination.
Supplies & Conditions:	Disposable gloves, disinfectant, disposable cloth, exam table, pillow, table paper, patient gowns, drapes, hand-washing liquid, paper towels, gauze squares, examination light, biohazard and regular waste container, and appropriate supplies and equipment (stethoscope, otoscope, ophthalmoscope, percussion hammer, pinwheel, hemoccult supplies, lubricant, pelvic exam supplies, tissues, tape measure).
Standards:	A maximum of three attempts may be used to complete the task. The time limit for each attempt is 15 minutes, with a minimum score of 70 percent. **Scoring:** Determine student's score by dividing points awarded by total points possible and multiplying results by 100.

EVALUATION

Evaluator Signature: _____   Date: _____

Evaluator Comments:

Name: _____ Date: _____ Score: _____

Procedure 37–1 Steps

Start Time: _____ End Time: _____ Total Time: _____

	Steps	Possible Points	First Attempt	Second Attempt	Third Attempt
1.	Assess the room condition, temperature, furniture, and equipment.	15			
2.	Wash hands and put on disposable gloves.	15			
3.	Place used supplies and disposable examination equipment in the waste or biohazard container. Check the waste container for space; replace it if the bag is full.	15			
4.	Tear the table paper near the top and roll it up with the pillow cover.	10			
5.	Wipe permanent examination equipment with disposable cloth or gauze squares and disinfectant.	15			
6.	Wipe the examination room tabletops with disposable cloth and disinfectant if contaminated from discarded examination supplies. Prepare the exam table for the next patient: a. Pull down clean table paper, fold the ragged edge, and place it under the table seat. b. Place a clean cover on the pillow. c. Check the table paper supply, gowns, and drapes.	15			
7.	Wipe any other equipment contaminated by the provider, such as a stool or exam lamp.	15			
8.	Disinfect the examination table and dispose of the cloth in the appropriate container.	15			
9.	Remove gloves and dispose in the appropriate container; wash hands.	15			
10.	Check the hand-washing dispenser and stock the supply.	10			
11.	Check the paper towel dispenser and supply more if needed.	10			
12.	Check the supplies in the cabinet and the examination table drawers, and replace as needed.	10			
13.	Make a final visual check of the room.	15			
	Points Awarded / Points Possible	_____ / **175**			

Name: _____ Date: _____ Score: _____

Competency Checklist
Procedure 37–2: Transfer a Patient from a Wheelchair to the Examination Table

ABHES Curriculum

MA.A.1.9.j   Make adaptations with patients with special needs

CAAHEP Core Curriculum

I.A.1   Incorporate critical thinking skills when performing patient assessment
I.A.2   Incorporate critical thinking skills when performing patient care
V.A.4   Explain to a patient the rationale for performance of a procedure
XII.P.3   Use proper body mechanics

Task: To safely move a patient from a wheelchair to an examination table.

Supplies & Conditions: Examination table, wheelchair and gait belt.

Standards: A maximum of three attempts may be used to complete the task. The time limit for each attempt is 10 minutes, with a minimum score of 70 percent. **Scoring:** Determine student's score by dividing points awarded by total points possible and multiplying results by 100.

EVALUATION

Evaluator Signature: _____   Date: _____

Evaluator Comments:

Name: _____ Date: _____ Score: _____

Procedure 37–2 Steps

Start Time: _____ End Time: _____ Total Time: _____

	Steps	Possible Points	First Attempt	Second Attempt	Third Attempt
1.	Unlock the wheels of the chair and wheel the patient to the examination room. *Incorporate critical thinking skills in performing patient assessment and care.*	15			
2.	Position the chair as near as possible to the place you want the patient to sit on the table. Lock the wheels on the chair.	15			
3.	Lower the table to chair level.	15			
4.	*Explain to the patient the rationale for performance of the procedure.* Apply the gait belt and fold the footrests back.	15			
5.	Stand directly in front of the patient with your feet slightly apart.	15			
6.	Use proper body mechanics; bend your knees and have the patient place his or her hands on your shoulders while you place your hands under the gait belt and assist the patient to a standing position.	15			
7.	Maintaining the position of your hands, pivot or sidestep to a position beside the table.	15			
8.	Place one foot slightly behind you for support and help the patient to a sitting position on the table.	15			
9.	If it is necessary to use a stool, determine the assistance required and enlist the needed help *before* taking the patient from the wheelchair.	15			
10.	While supporting the patient, stabilize the stool by placing your feet on the outside next to the legs and assist the patient to step onto the stool.	15			
11.	Assist the patient to sit on the table.	15			
12.	If the patient needs assistance to lie down, place one hand around the patient's back. Help the patient raise his or her legs to the table by placing your free arm under his or her legs and lifting them as the patient turns.	15			
13.	Place a pillow under the patient's head. Drape the patient appropriately.	15			
14.	Unlock the chair wheels and move the chair out of the way.	15			
	Points Awarded / Points Possible	_____ / **210**			

Competency Checklist
Procedure 37–3: Transfer a Patient from an Examination Table to a Wheelchair

ABHES Curriculum

MA.A.1.9.j   Make adaptations with patients with special needs

CAAHEP Core Curriculum

I.A.1	Incorporate critical thinking skills when performing patient assessment
I.A.2	Incorporate critical thinking skills when performing patient care
V.A.4	Explain to a patient the rationale for performance of a procedure
XII.P.3	Use proper body mechanics

Task:	To safely move a patient from the examination table to a wheelchair.
Supplies & Conditions:	Examination table, wheelchair, and gait belt.
Standards:	A maximum of three attempts may be used to complete the task. The time limit for each attempt is 10 minutes, with a minimum score of 70 percent. **Scoring:** Determine student's score by dividing points awarded by total points possible and multiplying results by 100.

EVALUATION

Evaluator Signature: _____   Date: _____

Evaluator Comments:

Name: _____ Date: _____ Score: _____

Procedure 37–3 Steps

Start Time: _____ **End Time:** _____ **Total Time:** _____

	Steps	Possible Points	First Attempt	Second Attempt	Third Attempt
1.	Reposition the chair and lock the wheels. ***Incorporate critical thinking skills in performing patient assessment and care.***	15			
2.	Assist the patient to a sitting position on the table.	15			
3.	***Explain to the patient the rationale for performance of the procedure,*** outlining what you will do and enlisting the patient's help. Assist the patient to dress if needed.	15			
4.	Apply a gait belt to the patient.	15			
5.	Use proper body mechanics; move so you are directly in front of the patient. Grasp the patient on the sides by the waist, parallel to below the armpits, by placing your hands under the gait belt. Plant your feet a shoulder's width apart and bend your knees. Ask the patient to put his or her hands on your shoulders. Assist the patient to step onto the floor (or have a stepstool in place if the table cannot be lowered to chair height).	15			
6.	Support the patient into a standing position on the stool or floor. (If using a stool, help the patient step down from the stool.) Sidestep or pivot the patient to a position in front of the chair.	15			
7.	Have the patient reach back to the arms of the chair as you help lower him or her into the chair. Ensure that the patient is comfortably seated.	15			
8.	Remove the gait belt from the patient and adjust the footrests.	15			
9.	Unlock the wheels and return the patient to the reception room.	15			
	Points Awarded / Points Possible	_____/ **135**			

Competency Checklist
Procedure 37–4: Positioning the Patient for an Exam

ABHES Curriculum

MA.A.1.9.c   Assist provider with general/physical exam

CAAHEP Core Curriculum

I.A.1   Incorporate critical thinking skills when performing patient assessment
I.A.2   Incorporate critical thinking skills when performing patient care
I.P.9   Assist provider with a patient exam
V.A.4   Explain to a patient the rationale for performance of a procedure

---

Task: To assist the patient into a variety of positions used in general physical and other examinations.

Supplies & Conditions: Adjustable exam table, table paper, gown, drape, pillow, disposable pillow cover.

Standards: A maximum of three attempts may be used to complete the task. The time limit for each attempt is 25 minutes, with a minimum score of 70 percent. **Scoring:** Determine student's score by dividing points awarded by total points possible and multiplying results by 100.

EVALUATION

Evaluator Signature: _____   Date: _____

Evaluator Comments:

Name: _____   Date: _____   Score: _____

Procedure 37–4 Steps

Start Time: _____   End Time: _____   Total Time: _____

	Steps	Possible Points	First Attempt	Second Attempt	Third Attempt
1.	Check the examination room for cleanliness. *Incorporate critical thinking skills in performing patient assessment and care.*	15			
2.	Identify the patient and introduce yourself.	15			
3.	*Explain to the patient the rationale for performance of the procedure.*	15			
4.	Give clear instructions to the patient regarding the amount of clothing to be removed and where it is to be placed, and instruct the patient in the use of the gown.	15			
5.	Assist the patient with gown if help is needed.	15			
6.	Assist the patient onto the examination table if help is needed.	15			
7.	Explain to the patient the necessary exam and the position required.	15			
8.	Assist the patient into the required position: • Anatomical	15			
	• Sitting	15			
	• Horizontal recumbent (supine)	15			
	• Dorsal recumbent	15			
	• Prone	15			
	• Sims'	15			
	• Knee-chest	15			
	• Trendelenburg	15			
	• Fowler's	15			
	• Semi-Fowler's	15			
	• Lithotomy	15			
9.	Drape the sheet evenly over the patient, but leave loose on all sides.	15			
10.	Assist the patient from the table when the examination is complete.	15			
	Points Awarded / Points Possible	_____/ **300**			

Competency Checklist
Procedure 38–1 Prepare a Patient for and Assist with a Routine Physical Examination

ABHES Curriculum

MA.A.1.9.c	Assist provider with general/physical examination
MA.A.1.9.h	Teach self-examination, disease management and health promotion

CAAHEP Core Curriculum

I.A.1	Incorporate critical thinking skills when performing patient assessment
I.A.2	Incorporate critical thinking skills when performing patient care
I.P.8	Instruct and prepare a patient for a procedure or a treatment
I.P.9	Assist provider with a patient exam
V.P.3	Use medical terminology correctly and pronounced accurately to communicate information to providers and patients
V.A.4	Explain to a patient the rationale for performance of a procedure

---

Task:	To have the patient, the room, and the examination equipment prepared for the provider to complete a physical examination as you assist with the process as needed.
Supplies and Conditions:	Gown, drape, stethoscope, ophthalmoscope, otoscope, tongue depressors, sterile gauze squares, tuning fork, nasal speculum, tape measure, percussion hammer, vaginal speculum, guaiac test kit, disposable gloves, lubricant, tissues, towel, Mayo tray, examination stool, exam lamp, regular and biohazardous waste container, patient chart or EMR, and a pen.
Standards:	A maximum of three attempts may be used to complete the task. The time limit for each attempt is 25 minutes, with a minimum score of 70 percent. **Scoring:** Determine student's score by dividing points awarded by total points possible and multiplying results by 100.

EVALUATION

Evaluator Signature: _____ Date: _____

Evaluator Comments:

Name: _____ Date: _____ Score: _____

Procedure 38–1 Steps

Start Time: _____ End Time: _____ Total Time: _____

	Steps	Possible Points	First Attempt	Second Attempt	Third Attempt
1.	Prepare the examination room as in Procedure 37–1.	15			
2.	Review the patient's chart for completed history and the physical examination form.	5			
3.	Wash hands.	15			
4.	Prepare the examination equipment on the Mayo tray in order of use and cover with a towel. ***Incorporate critical thinking skills when performing patient assessment and care.***	15			
5.	Pull out the step from the table. Place a gown and drape on the table.	5			
6.	Identify the patient, introduce yourself, check the chart, and ***explain to the patient the rationale for performance of the procedure***; use medical terminology correctly and pronounced accurately to communicate information to providers and the patient.	15			
7.	Measure and record vital signs, height, and weight.	15			
8.	Instruct the patient to go to the bathroom to empty the bladder.	5			
9.	Instruct the patient to remove clothing and place it on a chair, to put on the gown with the opening (according to the provider's preference), to sit at the end of the table, and to cover the legs with the drape.	5			
10.	Ensure that the patient is ready and notify the provider.	5			
11.	Assist the provider as needed with the examination. Position and drape the patient, adjust lights, and hand equipment as appropriate for each body system.	15			
12.	When the exam is completed, allow the patient to relax a moment and then help to sitting position.	5			
13.	Provide tissues to remove excess lubricant and instruct the patient to dress.	5			
14.	Take specimens from the room to the laboratory for testing.	15			
15.	Return to the room, provide patient instructions, and see the patient out.	15			
16.	Properly clean the room and prepare it for the next patient.	15			
17.	Give the room a visual check for completeness.	5			
	Points Awarded / Points Possible	____/ **175**			

Competency Checklist
Procedure 39-1 Irrigate the Ear

ABHES Curriculum

MA.A.1.4.a	Follow documentation guidelines
MA.A.1.9.a	Practice standard precautions and perform disinfection/sterilization techniques
MA.A.1.9.e	Perform specialty procedures

CAAHEP Core Curriculum

I.P.8	Instruct and prepare a patient for a procedure or a treatment
I.A.1	Incorporate critical thinking skills when performing patient assessment
I.A.2	Incorporate critical thinking skills when performing patient care
I.A.3	Show awareness of a patient's concerns related to the procedure being performed
V.A.4	Explain to a patient the rationale for performance of a procedure
X.P.3	Document patient care accurately in the medical record

Task: To irrigate the ear canal to remove foreign objects, impacted cerumen, or drainage.

Supplies and Conditions: Gloves, small basin, ordered lukewarm irrigation solution, water absorbent pad or towel, ear basin, elephant ear system, gauze squares, otoscope, ear speculum, tissues, patient chart/ EHR, and a pen.

Standards: A maximum of three attempts may be used to complete the task. The time limit for each attempt is 20 minutes, with a minimum score of 70 percent. **Scoring:** Determine student's score by dividing points awarded by total points possible and multiplying results by 100.

EVALUATION

Evaluator Signature: _____   Date: _____

Evaluator Comments:

531

Name: _____ Date: _____ Score: _____

Procedure 39-1 Steps

Start Time: _____ End Time: _____ Total Time: _____

	Steps	Possible Points	First Attempt	Second Attempt	Third Attempt
1.	Wash hands. Prepare the solution as ordered and assemble the necessary items for the procedure. *Incorporate critical thinking skills when performing patient assessment and care*.	15			
2.	Identify the patient, introduce yourself, and *explain the rationale for performance of the procedure. Show awareness of the patient's concerns related to the procedure being performed.*	15			
3.	Assist the patient onto the examination table or to a chair.	10			
4.	Put on gloves.	15			
5.	View the affected ear with an otoscope to see where cerumen or the foreign object is located so that the flow of solution can be directed properly.	15			
6.	Ask the patient to turn his or her head to the affected side and toward the back. Place a water absorbent pad or towel over the patient's shoulder to protect his or her clothing.	10			
7.	Use a gauze square to wipe away any particles from the outer ear before proceeding.	15			
8.	Fill the water bottle on the elephant ear system with body temperature water or other solution ordered by the provider. Twist on the disposable tip.	15			
9.	Position the ear basin under the ear for the patient to hold to catch the solution.	15			
10.	Use two hands to direct the flow of the solution. With one hand, place the tip end into the ear canal; with the other use the trigger handle to spray solution into the ear canal.	15			
11.	Use gauze squares to wipe the excess solution from the outside of the patient's ear.	10			
12.	Inspect the ear canal with an otoscope to determine whether the desired results have been obtained. Repeat irrigation if necessary.	15			
13.	Give the patient several gauze squares or tissues and have the patient tilt his or her head to the side to allow drainage of excess solution from the canal.	10			
14.	Discard the disposable tip into the waste receptacle and wash equipment. Return it to the proper storage area.	15			
15.	Remove gloves and wash hands.	15			
16.	Provide patient education and document the procedure in the patient's chart.	15			
	Points Awarded / Points Possible	_____ / **220**			

532

Competency Checklist
Procedure 39-2 Perform Audiometry Screening

ABHES Curriculum

MA.A.1.4.a	Follow documentation guidelines
MA.A.1.9.a	Practice standard precautions and perform disinfection/sterilization techniques
MA.A.1.9.e	Perform specialty procedures

CAAHEP Core Curriculum

I.P.8	Instruct and prepare a patient for a procedure or a treatment
I.A.1	Incorporate critical thinking skills when performing patient assessment
I.A.2	Incorporate critical thinking skills when performing patient care
I.A.3	Show awareness of a patient's concerns related to the procedure being performed
V.A.4	Explain to a patient the rationale for performance of a procedure
X.P.3	Document patient care accurately in the medical record

Task:	To screen patients for hearing loss.
Supplies and Conditions:	Audiometer with headphones, quiet room, audiogram chart, patient chart/EHR, and a pen.
Standards:	A maximum of three attempts may be used to complete the task. The time limit for each attempt is 15 minutes, with a minimum score of 70 percent. **Scoring:** Determine student's score by dividing points awarded by total points possible and multiplying results by 100.

EVALUATION

Evaluator Signature: _____ Date: _____

Evaluator Comments:

Name: _____ Date: _____ Score: _____

Procedure 39–2 Steps

Start Time: _____ End Time: _____ Total Time: _____

	Steps	Possible Points	First Attempt	Second Attempt	Third Attempt
1.	Wash hands. Assemble equipment and supplies. Prepare room. ***Incorporate critical thinking skills when performing patient assessment and care.***	15			
2.	Identify the patient, introduce yourself, ***and explain the rationale for performance of the procedure. Show awareness of the patient's concerns related to the procedure being performed.***	15			
3.	Assist the patient into sitting position in a chair.	10			
4.	Have patient put headphones on. Place the red on the right ear and the blue on the left.	15			
5.	Complete the test following the manufacturer's guidelines. The patient is asked to raise the hand coinciding to the ear the sound is heard in.	15			
6.	Continue testing until both ears are evaluated at all frequencies.	15			
7.	Plot the findings on the audiogram chart according to the manufacturer's guidelines.	15			
8.	Give the results to the provider for interpretation.	15			
9.	Clean equipment following manufacturer's guidelines.	10			
10.	Wash hands.	15			
11.	Document procedure in the patient's chart or EHR.	15			
	Points Awarded / Points Possible	_____ / **155**			

Competency Checklist
Procedure 39–3 Irrigate the Eye

ABHES Curriculum

MA.A.1.4.a	Follow documentation guidelines
MA.A.1.9.a	Practice standard precautions and perform disinfection/sterilization techniques
MA.A.1.9.e	Perform specialty procedures

CAAHEP Core Curriculum

I.P.8	Instruct and prepare a patient for a procedure or a treatment
I.A.1	Incorporate critical thinking skills when performing patient assessment
I.A.2	Incorporate critical thinking skills when performing patient care
I.A.3	Show awareness of a patient's concerns related to the procedure being performed
V.A.4	Explain to a patient the rationale for performance of a procedure
X.P.3	Document patient care accurately in the medical record

Task: To irrigate the patient's eye(s) to soothe tissues, relieve inflammation, and remove foreign objects and discharge.

Supplies and Conditions: Gloves, small basin of lukewarm irrigation solution, towel, emesis basin, irrigation syringe or bottle of solution, gauze squares, patient chart/ EHR, and a pen.

Standards: A maximum of three attempts may be used to complete the task. The time limit for each attempt is 10 minutes, with a minimum score of 70 percent. **Scoring:** Determine student's score by dividing points awarded by total points possible and multiplying results by 100.

EVALUATION

Evaluator Signature: _____ Date: _____

Evaluator Comments:

Name: _____ Date: _____ Score: _____

Procedure 39–3 Steps

Start Time: _____ End Time: _____ Total Time: _____

	Steps	Possible Points	First Attempt	Second Attempt	Third Attempt
1.	Wash hands. Assemble the items needed for the procedure; prepare lukewarm solution. ***Incorporate critical thinking skills when performing patient assessment and care.***	15			
2.	Identify the patient, introduce yourself, and ***explain the rationale for performance of the procedure. Show awareness of the patient's concerns related to the procedure being performed.***	15			
3.	Ask the patient which position would be more comfortable, sitting or lying down. Drape the patient with a towel to protect clothing.	10			
4.	Put on gloves.	15			
5.	Ask patient to tilt his or her head back and to the side. Place the emesis basin against the head. Instruct patient to hold the basin to catch the solution during irrigation.	15			
6.	Gently wipe eye with gauze square from the inner to outer canthus to remove any particles before proceeding with irrigation.	15			
7.	Fill syringe with ordered solution.	15			
8.	Hold the affected eye open with the thumb and index finger, and slowly release the solution over the eye gently and steadily.	15			
9.	When irrigation is completed, use gauze squares or tissues to blot the area dry.	10			
10.	Record the procedure in the patient's chart.	15			
11.	Wash the items and return them to the proper storage area.	15			
12.	Remove gloves and wash hands.	15			
	Points Awarded / Points Possible	_____ / 170			

Competency Checklist
Procedure 39–4 Screen Visual Acuity with a Snellen Chart

ABHES Curriculum

MA.A.1.4.a	Follow documentation guidelines
MA.A.1.9.a	Practice standard precautions and perform disinfection/sterilization techniques
MA.A.1.9.e	Perform specialty procedures

CAAHEP Core Curriculum

I.P.8	Instruct and prepare a patient for a procedure or a treatment
I.A.1	Incorporate critical thinking skills when performing patient assessment
I.A.2	Incorporate critical thinking skills when performing patient care
I.A.3	Show awareness of a patient's concerns related to the procedure being performed
V.A.4	Explain to a patient the rationale for performance of a procedure
X.P.3	Document patient care accurately in the medical record

Task: To measure the distant visual acuity of a patient.

Supplies and Conditions: Snellen chart, pointer, ocular eye occluder, patient chart/ EHR, and a pen.

Standards: A maximum of three attempts may be used to complete the task. The time limit for each attempt is 10 minutes, with a minimum score of 70 percent. **Scoring:** Determine student's score by dividing points awarded by total points possible and multiplying results by 100.

EVALUATION

Evaluator Signature: _____ Date: _____

Evaluator Comments:

Name: _____ Date: _____ Score: _____

Procedure 39–4 Steps

Start Time: _____ End Time: _____ Total Time: _____

	Steps	Possible Points	First Attempt	Second Attempt	Third Attempt
1.	Identify the patient, introduce yourself, and *explain the rationale for performance of the procedure. Show awareness of the patient's concerns related to the procedure being performed.*	15			
2.	Ask the patient to read the chart with both eyes (OU) first, standing 20 feet from the chart. *Incorporate critical thinking skills when performing patient assessment and care.*	15			
3.	To test acuity of the right eye, have the patient cover the left eye with an occluder.	15			
4.	Record the smallest line the patient can read without making a mistake.	15			
5.	Have the patient cover his or her right eye and test acuity of the left, following the same procedure.	15			
6.	Record the number of the smallest line the patient can read.	15			
	Points Awarded / Points Possible	___/ **90**			

Competency Checklist
Procedure 39–5 Screen Visual Acuity with the Jaeger System

ABHES Curriculum

MA.A.1.4.a	Follow documentation guidelines
MA.A.1.9.a	Practice standard precautions and perform disinfection/sterilization techniques
MA.A.1.9.e	Perform specialty procedures

CAAHEP Core Curriculum

I.P.8	Instruct and prepare a patient for a procedure or a treatment
I.A.1	Incorporate critical thinking skills when performing patient assessment
I.A.2	Incorporate critical thinking skills when performing patient care
I.A.3	Show awareness of a patient's concerns related to the procedure being performed
V.A.4	Explain to a patient the rationale for performance of a procedure
X.P.3	Document patient care accurately in the medical record

Task: To determine near distance visual acuity of a patient by using the Jaeger system.

Supplies and Conditions: Jaeger near vision acuity chart, patient chart/EHR, and a pen.

Standards: A maximum of three attempts may be used to complete the task. The time limit for each attempt is 10 minutes, with a minimum score of 70 percent. **Scoring:** Determine student's score by dividing points awarded by total points possible and multiplying results by 100.

EVALUATION

Evaluator Signature: _____ Date: _____

Evaluator Comments:

Procedure 39–5 Steps

Start Time: _____ End Time: _____ Total Time: _____

	Steps	Possible Points	First Attempt	Second Attempt	Third Attempt
1.	Identify the patient, introduce yourself, and *explain the rationale for performance of the procedure. Show awareness of the patient's concerns related to the procedure being performed. Incorporate critical thinking skills when performing patient assessment and care.*	15			
2.	Have the patient sit up straight but comfortably in a well-lighted area.	15			
3.	Hand the Jaeger chart to the patient to hold, between 14 inches and 16 inches from the eyes.	15			
4.	Instruct the patient to read (out loud to you) the various paragraphs of the card with both eyes open, first without wearing corrective lenses and then with.	15			
5.	Record the results and problems, if any, on the patient's chart to assist the provider in determining the visual acuity of the patient.	15			
6.	Thank the patient for cooperation and answer any questions.	10			
7.	Return the Jaeger chart to proper storage.	10			
	Points Awarded / Points Possible	____/ 95			

Competency Checklist
Procedure 39–6 Determine Color Vision Acuity by the Ishihara Method

ABHES Curriculum

MA.A.1.4.a	Follow documentation guidelines
MA.A.1.9.a	Practice standard precautions and perform disinfection/sterilization techniques
MA.A.1.9.e	Perform specialty procedures

CAAHEP Core Curriculum

I.P.8	Instruct and prepare a patient for a procedure or a treatment
I.A.1	Incorporate critical thinking skills when performing patient assessment
I.A.2	Incorporate critical thinking skills when performing patient care
I.A.3	Show awareness of a patient's concerns related to the procedure being performed
V.A.4	Explain to a patient the rationale for performance of a procedure
X.P.3	Document patient care accurately in the medical record

Task: To determine color vision acuity of a patient by using the Ishihara method.

Supplies and Conditions: Ishihara book, proper lighting, occluder, patient chart/EHR, and a pen.

Standards: A maximum of three attempts may be used to complete the task. The time limit for each attempt is 10 minutes, with a minimum score of 70 percent. **Scoring:** Determine student's score by dividing points awarded by total points possible and multiplying results by 100.

EVALUATION

Evaluator Signature: _____ Date: _____

Evaluator Comments:

Procedure 39–6 Steps

Start Time: _____ End Time: _____ Total Time: _____

	Steps	Possible Points	First Attempt	Second Attempt	Third Attempt
1.	Obtain the chart from the back of the book. ***Incorporate critical thinking skills when performing patient assessment and care.***	15			
2.	Identify the patient, introduce yourself, and ***explain the rationale for performance of the procedure. Show awareness of the patient's concerns related to the procedure being performed.***	w15			
3.	Ask the patient to hold the book 34 inches from his or her face and read the plates with both eyes.	15			
4.	Have the patient cover the left eye to test the right eye and then cover the right to test the left.	15			
5.	Compare answers given with those on the chart. Record those frames the patient misses and write down what the patient reports so that the degree of color deficiency may be determined by the provider.	15			
6.	Document results in the patient's chart.	15			
	Points Awarded / Points Possible	____/ **90**			

Competency Checklist
Procedure 39–7 Perform Spirometry Testing

ABHES Curriculum

MA.A.1.4.a	Follow documentation guidelines
MA.A.1.9.a	Practice standard precautions and perform disinfection/sterilization techniques
MA.A.1.9.e	Perform specialty procedures

CAAHEP Core Curriculum

I.P.2.d	Perform pulmonary function testing
I.P.8	Instruct and prepare a patient for a procedure or a treatment
I.A.1	Incorporate critical thinking skills when performing patient assessment
I.A.2	Incorporate critical thinking skills when performing patient care
I.A.3	Show awareness of a patient's concerns related to the procedure being performed
V.A.4	Explain to a patient the rationale for performance of a procedure
X.P.3	Document patient care accurately in the medical record

Task:	Evaluate patients suspected of having pulmonary insufficiency.
Supplies and Conditions:	Spirometer and disposable mouthpieces, patient chart/EHR, and a pen.
Standards:	A maximum of three attempts may be used to complete the task. The time limit for each attempt is 20 minutes, with a minimum score of 70 percent. **Scoring:** Determine student's score by dividing points awarded by total points possible and multiplying results by 100.

EVALUATION

Evaluator Signature: _____ Date: _____

Evaluator Comments:

543

Procedure 39–7 Steps

Start Time: _____ **End Time:** _____ **Total Time:** _____

	Steps	Possible Points	First Attempt	Second Attempt	Third Attempt
1.	Obtain the spirometer machine; assemble the necessary equipment and supplies; wash hands. *Incorporate critical thinking skills when performing patient assessment and care.*	15			
2.	Identify the patient, introduce yourself, and *explain the rationale for performance of the procedure. Show awareness of the patient's concerns related to the procedure being performed.*	15			
3.	Be sure the patient is in a comfortable position and any restrictive clothing (such as a tie or collar) is loosened before initiating the procedure.	15			
4.	Instruct the patient to sit or stand as straight as possible and not bend at the waist while blowing into the disposable mouthpiece.	15			
5.	Instruct the patient to make a tight seal around the mouthpiece with the lips.	15			
6.	After telling the patient to take deep breaths in (inhalation), coach the patient to breathe all the air out of the lungs until unable to exhale any longer, usually about 15 seconds.	15			
7.	Allow the patient to have a practice run before performing the actual test.	15			
8.	Support the patient during the test and have the patient keep blowing into the mouthpiece until told to stop.	15			
9.	Document the procedure in the patient's chart and place the results in the chart for the provider's review.	15			
	Points Awarded / Points Possible	____ / **135**			

Competency Checklist
Procedure 39–8 Perform Peak Flow Testing

ABHES Curriculum

MA.A.1.4.a	Follow documentation guidelines
MA.A.1.9.a	Practice standard precautions and perform disinfection/sterilization techniques
MA.A.1.9.e	Perform specialty procedures

CAAHEP Core Curriculum

I.P.8	Instruct and prepare a patient for a procedure or a treatment
I.A.1	Incorporate critical thinking skills when performing patient assessment
I.A.2	Incorporate critical thinking skills when performing patient care
I.A.3	Show awareness of a patient's concerns related to the procedure being performed
V.A.4	Explain to a patient the rationale for performance of a procedure
X.P.3	Document patient care accurately in the medical record

Task:	Correctly instruct the patient to measure his or her peak expiratory flow rate.
Supplies and Conditions:	Peak flow meter, mouthpiece, medical order, waste container, patient chart/EHR, and a pen.
Standards:	A maximum of three attempts may be used to complete the task. The time limit for each attempt is 20 minutes, with a minimum score of 70 percent. **Scoring:** Determine student's score by dividing points awarded by total points possible and multiplying results by 100.

EVALUATION

Evaluator Signature: _____ Date: _____

Evaluator Comments:

545

Name: _____ Date: _____ Score: _____

Procedure 39–8 Steps

Start Time: _____ End Time: _____ Total Time: _____

	Steps	Possible Points	First Attempt	Second Attempt	Third Attempt
1.	Assemble equipment and supplies; wash hands. *Incorporate critical thinking skills when performing patient assessment and care.*	15			
2.	Identify the patient, introduce yourself, and *explain the rationale for performance of the procedure. Show awareness of the patient's concerns related to the procedure being performed.*	15			
3.	Be sure the patient is in a comfortable position and any restrictive clothing (such as a tie or collar) is loosened before initiating the procedure.	15			
4.	Set the indicator to the bottom (lowest number) of the scale.	15			
5.	Instruct the patient to take in a deep breath, place the meter to mouth, close lips around the mouthpiece, and blow as hard as he or she can.	15			
6.	Write down the number the patient achieved.	15			
7.	Repeat steps 5 and 6 two more times.	15			
8.	Instruct the patient to do a peak flow 2–3 times a day.	15			
9.	Explain to the patient how to establish his or her "personal best"; explain the "Three Zone" system and how to record results in his or her peak flow diary.	15			
10.	Dispose of mouthpiece in the waste container.	15			
11.	Document.	15			
	Points Awarded / Points Possible	____/ **165**			

Competency Checklist
Procedure 39–9 Measure and Record Pulse Oximetry Testing

ABHES Curriculum

MA.A.1.4.a	Follow documentation guidelines
MA.A.1.9.a	Practice standard precautions and perform disinfection/sterilization techniques
MA.A.1.9.d	Assist provider with specialty examination
MA.A.1.9.e	Perform specialty procedures

CAAHEP Core Curriculum

I.P.1.i	Measure and record pulse oximetry
I.P.8	Instruct and prepare a patient for a procedure or a treatment
I.A.1	Incorporate critical thinking skills when performing patient assessment
I.A.2	Incorporate critical thinking skills when performing patient care
I.A.3	Show awareness of a patient's concerns related to the procedure being performed
V.A.4	Explain to a patient the rationale for performance of a procedure
X.P.3	Document patient care accurately in the medical record

Task:	To measure and record a patient's oxygen level in the blood.
Supplies and Conditions:	Pulse oximeter, alcohol wipes, nail polish remover if needed, patient chart/EHR, and a pen.
Standards	A maximum of three attempts may be used to complete the task. The time limit for each attempt is 5 minutes, with a minimum score of 70 percent. **Scoring:** Determine student's score by dividing points awarded by total points possible and multiplying results by 100.

EVALUATION

Evaluator Signature: _____ Date: _____

Evaluator Comments:

Name: _____ Date: _____ Score: _____

Procedure 39–9 Steps

Start Time: _____ End Time: _____ Total Time: _____

	Steps	Possible Points	First Attempt	Second Attempt	Third Attempt
1.	Wash hands and assemble equipment. *Incorporate critical thinking skills when performing patient assessment and care.*	15			
2.	Identify the patient, introduce yourself, and *explain the rationale for performance of the procedure. Show awareness of the patient's concerns related to the procedure being performed.*	15			
3.	Select a site for the sensor.	15			
4.	Clean the site with alcohol. Remove nail polish if needed. Wash with soap and water.	15			
5.	Apply sensor; read results.	15			
6.	Note the results (including pulse) according to the manufacturer's instructions. (Take reading after 10 seconds.)	15			
7.	Notify provider immediately of abnormal results. Abnormal results are less than 95 percent.	15			
8.	Document procedure, site of application (sensor applied to left index finger), and results.	15			
	Points Awarded / Points Possible	____/ **120**			

548

Competency Checklist
Procedure 39–10 Assist with a Flexible Sigmoidoscopy

ABHES Curriculum

MA.A.1.4.a	Follow documentation guidelines
MA.A.1.9.a	Practice standard precautions and perform disinfection/sterilization techniques
MA.A.1.9.d	Assist provider with specialty examination
MA.A.1.9.e	Perform specialty procedures

CAAHEP Core Curriculum

I.P.8	Instruct and prepare a patient for a procedure or a treatment
I.P.9	Assist provider with a patient exam
I.A.1	Incorporate critical thinking skills when performing patient assessment
I.A.2	Incorporate critical thinking skills when performing patient care
I.A.3	Show awareness of a patient's concerns related to the procedure being performed
V.A.4	Explain to a patient the rationale for performance of a procedure
X.P.3	Document patient care accurately in the medical record

Task:	To assist in examination of the sigmoid colon.
Supplies and Conditions:	Gloves; water-soluble lubricant; gauze squares; flexible sigmoidoscope; long cotton-tipped swabs; drape sheet (fenestrated optional); suction machine (container with room temperature water); tissues; if ordered by provider: biopsy forceps, specimen container for transport to lab, lab request form, patient chart/EHR, and a pen.
Standards:	A maximum of three attempts may be used to complete the task. The time limit for each attempt is 20 minutes, with a minimum score of 70 percent. **Scoring:** Determine student's score by dividing points awarded by total points possible and multiplying results by 100.

EVALUATION

Evaluator Signature: _____ Date: _____

Evaluator Comments:

Name: _____ Date: _____ Score: _____

Procedure 39–10 Steps

Start Time: _____ End Time: _____ Total Time: _____

	Steps	Possible Points	First Attempt	Second Attempt	Third Attempt
1.	Identify patient, introduce yourself, and *explain the rationale for performance of the procedure. Show awareness of the patient's concerns related to the procedure being performed. Incorporate critical thinking skills when performing patient assessment and care.*	15			
2.	Assemble all needed items on a Mayo tray near the end of the examination table.	15			
3.	Plug in cord of light source to make sure it works properly; then turn it off.	5			
4.	Instruct the patient to disrobe from the waist down and let you know when he or she is ready. Assist the patient to sit at the end of the table and cover him or her with the drape sheet for privacy.	15			
5.	Wash hands and put on gloves.	15			
6.	Just before the provider is ready to begin the exam, assist the patient into a knee-chest or Sims' position, whichever the provider prefers.	15			
7.	Assist the provider by applying about two tablespoons of lubricant on gauze square for the tip of the gloved fingers.	15			
8.	As the provider finishes the digital exam, plug the sigmoidoscope into the light source. Secure the air-inflation tubing and have it ready to hand to the provider; activate the switches for air inflation and light.	15			
9.	As the provider inserts the sigmoidoscope, be ready to hand items as needed.	15			
10.	Be prepared to rinse the suction tip in water if it becomes clogged.	15			
11.	If biopsy is indicated, hand biopsy forceps to the provider and have a specimen container open so the provider can place tissue in it. Place the cap on the container securely.	15			
12.	Use tissues to clean lubricant and waste from the patient's anal area and discard it into the waste container.	15			
13.	Place a small pad or dressing over the anal area in case of light bleeding.	15			
14.	Assist the patient to resting prone position (or return table to starting position).	15			
15.	Assist the patient to a sitting position, allowing time for balance to return before helping him or her down from the table. Instruct the patient to dress.	15			

16.	Wear gloves to clean the exam table and instruments. The scope and suction tip should be cleaned with detergent and water and placed in a disinfectant to be sterilized.	15			
17.	Remove gloves and wash hands.	15			
18.	Attach a label and the completed requisition form to the specimen container. Place the specimen container in the area for laboratory pickup.	15			
19.	Restock the room and return the instruments to storage.	15			
20.	Document the procedure on the patient's chart.	15			
	Points Awarded / Points Possible	___/ **290**			

Competency Checklist
Procedure 40–1 Prepare the Patient for and Assist with a Gynecological Exam and Pap Test

ABHES Curriculum

MA.A.1.4.a	Follow documentation guidelines
MA.A.1.9.a	Practice standard precautions and perform disinfection/sterilization techniques
MA.A.1.9.c	Assist providers with general/physical examination
MA.A.1.9.d	Assist provider with specialty examination including OB-GYN

CAAHEP Core Curriculum

I.P.9	Assist provider with a patient exam
I.A.1	Incorporate critical thinking skills when performing patient assessment
I.A.2	Incorporate critical thinking skills when performing patient care
I.A.3	Show awareness of a patient's concerns related to the procedure being performed
V.A.1	Demonstrate (a) empathy, (b) active listening, and (c) nonverbal communication
V.A.2	Demonstrate the principles of self-boundaries
V.A.4	Explain to a patient the rationale for performance of a procedure
X.P.3	Document patient care accurately in the medical record

Task: To prepare the patient and assist the provider to complete a pelvic examination and obtain a Pap test to determine a patient's gynecological health.

Supplies and Conditions: Mayo tray, two cloth or paper towels, three pairs of disposable gloves, water-soluble lubricant, vaginal speculum, tissues, endocervical broom, ThinPrep bottle, label, laboratory requisition, patient's chart/EHR, and pen.

Standards: A maximum of three attempts may be used to complete the task. The time limit for each attempt is 25 minutes, with a minimum score of 70 percent. **Scoring:** Determine student's score by dividing points awarded by total points possible and multiplying results by 100.

EVALUATION

Evaluator Signature: _____ Date: _____

Evaluator Comments:

Name: _____ Date: _____ Score: _____

Procedure 40–1 Steps

Start Time: _____ End Time: _____ Total Time: _____

	Steps	Possible Points	First Attempt	Second Attempt	Third Attempt
1.	Wash hands.	15			
2.	Prepare the room and equipment. *Incorporate critical thinking skills when performing patient assessment and care.*	15			
3.	Call the patient from the reception room; introduce yourself and identify the patient.	5			
4.	Instruct the patient to go to the bathroom to empty the bladder.	15			
5.	*Explain the rationale for performance of the procedure. Show awareness of the patient's concerns related to the procedure being performed. Demonstrate empathy, active listening, and nonverbal communication.*	15			
6.	Obtain the necessary information to complete the cytology requisition form.	15			
7.	Attach a label to the ThinPrep bottle and place it on the Mayo tray.	15			
8.	Instruct the patient to remove all clothing and put on the examination gown with the opening in front. *Demonstrate the principles of self-boundaries.*	15			
9.	When the patient is gowned, enter the room and pull out the step from the end of the table. Ask the patient sit on the table. Cover the patient's legs with the drape. Push in the table step.	15			
10.	Notify the provider that the patient is ready.	5			
11.	Accompany the provider into the room and apply critical thinking skills to provide assistance as needed. Be sure to use proper body mechanics when positioning the patient.	5			
12.	Position the patient in a sitting position for basic assessment and initial breast examination. *Be sure to show awareness to any patient concerns regarding the procedure.*	5			
13.	Assist the patient to a supine position for a continued breast exam.	15			
14.	When the breast exam is completed, assist the patient to cover her chest with the gown and drape and prepare for the pelvic exam.	5			
15.	Assist the patient into a lithotomy position, helping her place her feet into the stirrups, and adjust as needed.	15			
16.	Place the drape over the patient from the chest to the feet. Push the drape down between her legs until it touches the table. Instruct the patient to slide her buttocks down to the end of the table.	15			

554

17.	The provider will take his or her position on the exam stool at the end of the table. Remove the cover from the Mayo tray if not previously done. Hand gloves to the provider.	15			
18.	Adjust the lamp so that the light facilitates inspection of the perineal and anal areas.	15			
19.	Put on gloves and run warm water over the speculum.	15			
20.	Hand the speculum, handle first, to the provider.	15			
21.	Hand the endocervical broom, handle first, to the provider.	15			
22.	Open the labeled specimen bottle and be ready to accept the endocervical broom.	15			
23.	The provider will stand to perform the bimanual pelvic and rectal exam. Apply lubricant to the gloved index and middle fingers of the examining hand.	15			
24.	When the provider has finished the exam, have the patient push back up the table, help her get her feet out of the stirrups, and push the stirrups in.	15			
25.	Assist the patient to sit up. Pull out the table step. When the patient's sense of balance has returned, assist her down from the table.	15			
26.	Hand tissues to the patient to remove any residual lubricant.	5			
27.	Instruct the patient to dress. Provide assistance as needed. Remove gloves and wash hands.	5			
28.	Advise the patient when results will be available and schedule a follow-up appointment if indicated.	5			
29.	Provide any patient teaching information pamphlets that are appropriate, and dismiss the patient. Record exam, Pap test, and any teaching in the chart.	15			
30.	Apply gloves; properly clean and disinfect the room and all instruments and restock supplies.	15			
31.	Place the labeled specimen bottle with the attached requisition in the lab pickup area.	15			
32.	Pull down fresh table paper on the exam table.	15			
33.	Remove gloves and wash hands.	15			
	Points Awarded / Points Possible	____/ **415**			

Competency Checklist
Procedure 41–1 Measure Length, Weight, and Head and Chest Circumference of an Infant or Child

ABHES Curriculum

MA.A.1.4.a	Follow documentation guidelines
MA.A.1.9.d	Assist provider with specialty examination

CAAHEP Core Curriculum

I.A.1	Incorporate critical thinking skills when performing patient assessment
I.A.2	Incorporate critical thinking skills when performing patient care
I.A.3	Show awareness of a patient's concerns related to the procedure being performed
I.P.1.g	Measure and record length (infant)
I.P.1.h	Measure and record head circumference (infant)
I.P.8	Instruct and prepare a patient for a procedure or a treatment
I.P.9	Assist provider with a patient exam
II.P.4	Document on a growth chart
V.A.4	Explain to a patient the rationale for performance of a procedure.
X.P.3	Document patient care accurately in the medical record

Task: To obtain an accurate measurement of an infant or child's length, weight, and head and chest circumference.

Supplies and Conditions: Exam table with table paper, portable measurement chart board, measuring tape, patient's chart with growth chart or EMR; parents' record booklet, pediatric scale, and pen.

Standards: A maximum of three attempts may be used to complete the task. The time limit for each attempt is 25 minutes, with a minimum score of 70 percent. **Scoring:** Determine student's score by dividing points awarded by total points possible and multiplying results by 100.

EVALUATION

Evaluator Signature: _____ Date: _____

Evaluator Comments:

557

Name: _____ Date: _____ Score: _____

Procedure 41–1 Steps

Start Time:_____   End Time:_____   Total Time:_____

Steps		Possible Points	First Attempt	Second Attempt	Third Attempt
MEASURING WEIGHT					
1.	Introduce yourself, identify the patient, *and explain the rationale for performance of the procedure* to the parent or caregiver, *showing awareness of the patient's concerns related to the procedure.* Wash hands.	15			
2.	Ask the parent to undress the infant or child, including diaper.	15			
3.	Place both weights to the left of the scale to check the balance. *Apply critical thinking skills when performing patient assessment and care.*	15			
4.	Place a water-absorbent pad on the scale; reset scale to zero if necessary.	15			
5.	Gently place the infant on his or her back on the scale; place your hand slightly above the child to ensure safety.	15			
6.	Place the bottom weight to the highest measurement that will not cause the balance bar to drop to the bottom edge.	15			
7.	Slowly move upper weight until the balance bar rests in the center of the indicator. Read the infant's weight while he or she is lying still.	15			
8.	Return both weights to their resting position to the extreme left.	15			
9.	Gently remove infant and assist parent to apply diaper.	15			
10.	Discard the used absorbent pad.	15			
MEASURING LENGTH					
1.	*Explain the rationale for performance of the procedure* to the parent or caregiver, *showing awareness of the patient's concerns related to the procedure.*	15			
2.	Gently place infant on his or her back on the portable measurement chart board with the top of the infant's head flush to the top of the board. Keep the legs straight and slide the footboard up so it is flush with the infant's heels. *Apply critical thinking skills when performing patient assessment and care.*	15			
3.	Gently remove the infant. Measure the distance between the headboard and the footboard. Read the length in inches to the nearest ¼, ½, or ¾ inch.	15			

MEASURING HEAD CIRCUMFERENCE					
1.	***Explain the rationale for performance of the procedure*** to the parent or caregiver, ***showing awareness of the patient's concerns related to the procedure.***	15			
2.	Place measuring tape snug around the forehead just above the eyebrows and the most prominent portion of the back of the head.	15			
3.	Read measurement to the nearest ¼, ½, or ¾ inch.	15			
MEASURING CHEST CIRCUMFERENCE					
1.	***Explain the rationale for performance of the procedure*** to the parent or caregiver, ***showing awareness of the patient's concerns related to the procedure.***	15			
2.	Use one thumb to hold the tape measure at the zero mark against the infant's chest at the midsternal area and around the nipples. ***Apply critical thinking skills when performing patient assessment and care.***	15			
3.	Read measurement to the nearest ¼, ½, or ¾ inch.	15			
4.	Document the measurements in the patient's medical record and growth chart.	15			
	Points Awarded / Points Possible	____/ **300**			

Competency Checklist
Procedure 41–2 Plot Data on a Growth Chart

ABHES Curriculum

MA.A.1.4.a	Follow documentation guidelines
MA.A.1.9.d	Assist provider with specialty examination

CAAHEP Core Curriculum

I.A.1	Incorporate critical thinking skills when performing patient assessment
I.A.2	Incorporate critical thinking skills when performing patient care
I.P.8	Instruct and prepare a patient for a procedure or a treatment
II.P.4	Document on a growth chart
X.P.3	Document patient care accurately in the medical record

Task: To record the growth and development of a patient accurately on a growth chart.

Supplies and Conditions: Patient's chart and growth chart; pen or EHR.

Standards: A maximum of three attempts may be used to complete the task. The time limit for each attempt is 20 minutes, with a minimum score of 70 percent. **Scoring:** Determine student's score by dividing points awarded by total points possible and multiplying results by 100.

EVALUATION

Evaluator Signature: _____ Date: _____

Evaluator Comments:

561

Name: _____ Date: _____ Score: _____

Procedure 41–2 Steps

Start Time: _____   End Time: _____   Total Time: _____

	Steps	Possible Points	First Attempt	Second Attempt	Third Attempt
1.	Obtain measurement data from the patient's chart and the appropriate growth chart depending on the infant or childs age. ***Apply critical thinking skills when performing patient assessment and care.***	15			
2.	Using the Length-for-age and Weight-for-age percentiles chart, locate the patient's age on the growth chart.	15			
3.	Locate the patient's height on the growth chart.	15			
4.	Locate the patient's weight on the growth chart.	15			
5.	Find where the age on the horizontal line and child's stature or length (height) on the vertical line intersect, and plot the measurement by making a dot on the chart.	15			
6.	Do the same for the child's weight. You can also determine the child's percentile by following the line on which the measurement is plotted to the side of the paper where the percentiles are indicated.	15			
7.	Using the Head circumference-for-age and Weight-for-length percentiles chart, locate the graph for the head circumference and plot it the same way. The weight-for-length percentile is also determined on this graph by plotting them both and finding their intersection.	15			
8.	Fill in the box chart on the growth chart with the date, patient's age, weight, height, and head circumference.	15			
9.	Some providers want you to connect the dots of the measurements over time with a thin line as shown in Figure 41-9.	15			
	Points Awarded / Points Possible	____/ 135			

Name: _____ Date: _____ Score: _____

Competency Checklist
Procedure 41–3 Screen Pediatric Visual Acuity with a Modified Snellen Chart

ABHES Curriculum

M.A.A.1.4.a   Follow documentation guidelines
M.A.A.1.9.d   Assist provider with specialty examination

CAAHEP Core Curriculum

I.P.8   Instruct and prepare a patient for a procedure or a treatment
I.P.9   Assist provider with a patient exam
V.A.4   Explain to a patient the rationale for performance of a procedure
X.P.3   Document patient care accurately in the medical record

---

Task: To measure distant visual acuity of a child.

Supplies and Conditions: Modified Snellen chart, pointer, eye occluder, patient's chart or EHR, and pen.

Standards: A maximum of three attempts may be used to complete the task. The time limit for each attempt is 20 minutes, with a minimum score of 70 percent. **Scoring:** Determine student's score by dividing points awarded by total points possible and multiplying results by 100.

EVALUATION

Evaluator Signature: _____   Date: _____

Evaluator Comments:

Name: _____ Date: _____ Score: _____

Procedure 41–3 Steps

Start Time: _____ End Time: _____ Total Time: _____

	Steps	Possible Points	First Attempt	Second Attempt	Third Attempt
1.	Identify the patient and introduce yourself.	15			
2.	**Explain to the patient the rationale for performance of the procedure,** using language that is appropriate for the patient.	15			
3.	Ask the patient to read the chart with both eyes at a distance of 20 feet from the chart.	15			
4.	Have the patient cover the left eye with the occluder to test the acuity of the right eye.	15			
5.	Record the smallest line the patient reads without making a mistake.	15			
6.	Have the patient cover the right eye with the occluder to test the acuity of the left eye.	15			
7.	Record the smallest line read.	15			
	Points Awarded / Points Possible	___/ **105**			

Competency Checklist
Procedure 42–1: Complete an Incident Exposure Report Related to an Error in Patient Care

ABHES Curriculum

MA.A.1.4.e   Perform risk management procedures

MA.A.1.4.f   Comply with federal, state, and local health laws and regulations as they relate to health care settings

CAAHEP Core Curriculum

X.P.7   Complete an incident report related to an error in patient care

---

Task: To provide documentation required by the risk management department in the event an error occurs in regard to patient care.

Supplies & Conditions: Unusual Occurrence Form (UOR) form, pen

Standards: A maximum of three attempts may be used to complete the task. The time limit for each attempt is 15 minutes, with a minimum score of 70 percent. **Scoring:** Determine student's score by dividing points awarded by total points possible and multiplying results by 100.

Forms: Procedure Form 42–1 (UOR form). Procedure forms can be downloaded from the Student Companion website.

EVALUATION

Evaluator Signature: _____   Date: _____

Evaluator Comments:

Name: _____ Date: _____ Score: _____

Procedure 42–1 Steps

Start Time: _____ **End Time:** _____ **Total Time:** _____

	Steps	Possible Points	First Attempt	Second Attempt	Third Attempt
1.	Report the incident immediately to a supervisor for documentation.	15			
2.	Assemble equipment.	15			
3.	Fill in the demographic information about the patient.	15			
4.	Fill in location of the event.	15			
5.	Complete the section regarding information about the patient factors prior to the event.	15			
6.	Fill in the categories of event section.	15			
7.	In the space provided, give a written description of the event.	15			
8.	Add any additional persons involved.	15			
9.	Complete the review section.	15			
10.	Complete the corrective action section.	15			
11.	Complete the procedures followed section.	15			
12.	Complete the family/patient attitude after the event section.	15			
13.	Add any additional information that may be warranted and obtain signatures, titles, and dates.	15			
14.	Forward form to the risk management department following the office protocol so proper action can occur.	15			
	Points Awarded / Points Possible	_____/ **210**			

Competency Checklist
Procedure 42–2 Comply with Safety Signs, Symbols, and Labels

ABHES Curriculum

MA.A.1.10.c   Dispose of biohazardous materials

CAAHEP Core Curriculum

XII.C.1   Identify: (a) safety signs, (b) symbols, and (c) labels
XII.P.1   Comply with: (a) safety signs, (b) symbols, and (c) labels

---

Task: Ensure that designated laboratory areas, chemicals and reagents, and equipment such as the refrigerator and biohazard waste receptacles are labeled appropriately.

Supplies & Conditions: OSHA Hazard Communication Standard Labels and appropriate safety signs.

Standards: A maximum of three attempts may be used to complete the task. The time limit for each attempt is 15 minutes, with a minimum score of 70 percent. **Scoring:** Determine student's score by dividing points awarded by total points possible and multiplying results by 100.

EVALUATION

Evaluator Signature: _____   Date: _____

Evaluator Comments:

Name: _____ Date: _____ Score: _____

Procedure 42–2 Steps

Start Time: _____ End Time: _____ Total Time: _____

	Steps	Possible Points	First Attempt	Second Attempt	Third Attempt
1.	Ensure the refrigerator used to store reagents, test kits, or any biological specimens is labeled appropriately.	5			
2.	Ensure the biohazard receptacles are labeled appropriately.	15			
3.	Ensure all chemicals and reagents are labeled appropriately.	15			
4.	Ensure all designated areas within the facility have the proper signage in place.	15			
	Points Awarded / Points Possible	_____/ **50**			

Competency Checklist
Procedure 42–3 Clean a Spill

ABHES Curriculum

MA.A.1.9.g	Recognize and respond to medical office emergencies
MA.A.1.10.c	Dispose of biohazardous materials

CAAHEP Core Curriculum

III.P.2	Select appropriate barrier/personal protective equipment (PPE)
III.P.10	Demonstrate proper disposal of biohazardous material: (a) sharps, and (b) regulated wastes
XII.P.2.c	Demonstrate proper use of sharps disposal containers
XII.P.4	Participate in a mock exposure event with documentation of specific steps

---

Task:	Following the steps listed in the procedure, clean a spill (when blood or other body fluids are involved), observing universal precautions.
Supplies & Conditions:	Gloves, eye protection, plastic apron with sleeves, hair and shoe covers, biohazard bags, disinfectant, and paper or cloth towels and/or spill kit; in a simulated office lab environment.
Standards:	A maximum of three attempts may be used to complete the task. The time limit for each attempt is 20 minutes, with a minimum score of 70 percent. **Scoring:** Determine student's score by dividing points awarded by total points possible and multiplying results by 100.

EVALUATION

Evaluator Signature: _____   Date: _____

Evaluator Comments:

569

Name: _____ Date: _____ Score: _____

Procedure 42–3 Steps

Start Time: _____ End Time: _____ Total Time: _____

	Steps	Possible Points	First Attempt	Second Attempt	Third Attempt
1.	Select and apply appropriate barrier or personal protective equipment.	5			
2.	Locate the office spill kit or other appropriate cleaning supplies and follow office protocol for cleaning spills. Follow instructions on the spill kit appropriate to the hazard.	15			
3.	Thoroughly clean area with an effective disinfectant or a 10 percent solution of household bleach.	15			
4.	If the spill involves bodily fluids, dispose of materials in biohazard waste container.	15			
5.	If glass fragments or sharps are involved, use a brush or broom and dustpan to clean up items and place in a puncture-proof biohazard sharps container. Never place your fingers or hand into the top of the sharps container (as an accidental exposure could occur).	15			
6.	Document the incident, findings, and actions taken, and then date and sign.	5			
	Points Awarded / Points Possible	____/ 70			

Competency Checklist
Procedure 42–4 Demonstrate Proper Use of Eyewash Equipment

ABHES Curriculum

MA.A.1.9.g   Recognize and respond to medical office emergencies

CAAHEP Core Curriculum

III.P.2   Select appropriate barrier/personal protective equipment (PPE)
XII.P.2.a   Demonstrate proper use of eyewash equipment
XII.P.4   Participate in a mock exposure event with documentation of specific steps

---

Task:	Following the steps listed in the procedure, identify and respond to accidental chemical exposure to the eyes; describe and demonstrate how to properly use the eyewash station.
Supplies & Conditions:	Eyewash station, quality control log.
Standards:	A maximum of three attempts may be used to complete the task. The time limit for each attempt is 10 minutes, with a minimum score of 70 percent. **Scoring:** Determine student's score by dividing points awarded by total points possible and multiplying results by 100.
Forms:	Procedure Form 42–4 (Eyewash quality control form). Procedure forms can be downloaded from the Student Companion website.

EVALUATION

Evaluator Signature: _____ Date: _____

Evaluator Comments:

Name: _____ Date: _____ Score: _____

Procedure 42–4 Steps

Start Time: _____ **End Time:** _____ **Total Time:** _____

	Steps	Possible Points	First Attempt	Second Attempt	Third Attempt
1.	Locate the eyewash station and make sure it is accessible and in proper working condition.	5			
2.	Check that the bowl is free of rust/trash and that water drains from the bowl.	15			
3.	Document in the quality control log.	15			
	Points Awarded / Points Possible	____/ **35**			

Competency Checklist
Procedure 42–5 Demonstrate Fire Preparedness

CAAHEP Core Curriculum

XII.P.2.b   Demonstrate proper use of fire extinguishers

Task: Following the steps listed in the procedure, identify and respond to fire hazards; describe and demonstrate how to operate a fire extinguisher correctly, using the PASS acronym.

Supplies & Conditions: Fire extinguisher.

Standards: A maximum of three attempts may be used to complete the task. The time limit for each attempt is 15 minutes, with a minimum score of 85 percent. **Scoring:** Determine student's score by dividing points awarded by total points possible and multiplying results by 100.

EVALUATION

Evaluator Signature: _____   Date: _____

Evaluator Comments:

Name: _____ Date: _____ Score: _____

Procedure 42–5 Steps

Start Time: _____ **End Time:** _____ **Total Time:** _____

	Steps	Possible Points	First Attempt	Second Attempt	Third Attempt
1.	Read the following scenarios and identify the fire hazards presented. Then describe how to respond to (correct) each hazard. A. Multiple pieces of equipment are plugged into extension cords (copy machine, fax machine, computer station with printer, coffeepot). _____ _____ _____ B. Keyboard cleaning fluid and spray are located next to the outlet strip on the counter. _____ _____ _____ C. During the course of the day, Sally the Medical Assistant student spilled a cup of coffee on the keyboard. _____ _____ _____	15			
2.	Describe how to operate a fire extinguisher, explaining what the PASS acronym means.	15			
3.	Correctly operate the fire extinguisher, using the PASS method.	15			
	Points Awarded / Points Possible	_____/ **45**			

Competency Checklist
Procedure 42–6 Use a Microscope

CAAHEP Core Curriculum

VI.P.8   Perform routine maintenance of administrative or clinical equipment

---

Task: Following the steps listed in the procedure, gain skill in use of the microscope.

Supplies & Conditions: Microscope, electrical outlet for light source of microscope, specimen on disposable glass slide with frosted end, cover glass (used usually for wet specimens only), lens cleaning tissues, latex or vinyl gloves.

Standards: Provided with all necessary equipment and supplies, follow the steps in the procedure with the instructor observing each step. A maximum of three attempts may be used to complete the task. Students must complete all procedure steps in 30 minutes, with a minimum score of 70 percent. **Scoring:** Determine student's score by dividing points awarded by total points possible and multiplying results by 100.

EVALUATION

Evaluator Signature: _____   Date: _____

Evaluator Comments:

575

Name: _____ Date: _____ Score: _____

Procedure 42–6 Steps

Start Time: _____ End Time: _____ Total Time: _____

	Steps	Possible Points	First Attempt	Second Attempt	Third Attempt
1.	Wash hands and put on latex or vinyl gloves.	10			
2.	Assemble the necessary equipment.	5			
3.	Clean the ocular lens with lens cleaning tissues.	5			
4.	Plug the microscope light source into an electrical outlet and turn on the light switch at the front base of the microscope.	5			
5.	Place the specimen slide on the stage with the frosted end up between the clips and secure it over the opening of the stage.	5			
6.	Watch carefully as you raise the substage so that it does not come in direct contact with the slide.	5			
7.	Turn the revolving nosepiece to low-power objective (10×) and begin to focus the coarse-adjustment dial until a wide shaft can be seen.	5			
8.	When the outline of the specimen is in view, turn the fine-adjustment dial until the specimen can be seen in detail.	5			
9.	Adjust the substage diaphragm level or adjust the mirror to obtain proper lighting.	5			
10.	If sharper detail is needed, carefully turn the revolving nosepiece to the intermediate-power objective and adjust the fine-focus dial.	5			
11.	When using the oil-immersion lens objective or hpf, oil should be used very sparingly.	5			
12.	When the specimen has been identified, turn off the light and return all items to the proper storage area. The microscope stage should be cleaned and recorded in the maintenance log.	10			
13.	Remove gloves and wash hands.	10			
	Points Awarded / Points Possible	____/ 80			

Name: _____ Date: _____ Score: _____

Competency Checklist
Procedure 43–1 Instruct a Patient on the Collection of a Clean-Catch, Midstream Urine Specimen

ABHES Curriculum

MA.A.1.10.e(1)   Instruct patients in the collection of a clean-catch, midstream urine specimen

MA.A.1.10.d   Collect, label, and process specimens

CAAHEP Core Curriculum

I.A.3   Show awareness of a patient's concerns related to the procedure being performed

V.A.4   Explain to a patient the rationale for performance of a procedure

---

Task: To instruct patients in the collection of a clean-catch, midstream urine specimen.

Supplies & Conditions: Sterile container, antiseptic wipes, disposable gloves, pen, and label for container.

Standards: Provided with all necessary equipment and supplies, follow the steps in the procedure with the instructor observing each step. A maximum of three attempts may be used to complete the task. Students must complete all procedure steps in 25 minutes (not including preparation of the brochure), with a minimum score of 70 percent. **Scoring:** Determine student's score by dividing points awarded by total points possible and multiplying results by 100.

EVALUATION

Evaluator Signature: _____ Date: _____

Evaluator Comments:

Name: _____ Date: _____ Score: _____

Procedure 43–1 Steps

Start Time: _____ End Time: _____ Total Time: _____

	Steps	Possible Points	First Attempt	Second Attempt	Third Attempt
1.	Obtain or locate instructions for instructing male and female patients in the proper collection of urine specimens.	30			
2.	Assemble supplies to provide to the patient.	10			
3.	Identify the patient and instruct him or her for the collection as outlined in the instructions, *including the rationale for performing the procedure. Show awareness to the patient's concerns related to the procedure being performed.*	15			
4.	Provide the patient with the labeled sterile cup and antiseptic wipes. Direct the patient to the restroom and ask him or her to collect the specimen.	5			
5.	Obtain the specimen from the patient upon exit from the restroom using your facilities protocols.	5			
	Points Awarded / Points Possible	_____/ **65**			

Competency Checklist
Procedure 43–2 Perform Screening for Pregnancy

ABHES Curriculum

MA.A.1.10.a	Practice quality control
MA.A.1.10.b(6)(a)	Perform selected CLIA-waived tests that assist with diagnosis and treatment: Kit testing: Pregnancy
MA.A.1.10.b(6)(c)	Perform selected CLIA-waived tests that assist with diagnosis and treatment: Kit testing: Dip Sticks
M.A.A.1.10.d	Collect, label, and process specimens

CAAHEP Core Curriculum

I.P.10	Perform a quality control measure
I.P.11.d	Obtain specimens and perform: CLIA-waived immunology test
II.P.3	Maintain lab test results using flow sheets

Task:	Following the steps listed in the procedure, perform a pregnancy screening on a urine sample to determine the presence (or absence) of human chorionic gonadotropin (hCG).
Supplies & Conditions:	Disposable gloves, other personal protective equipment (PPE) per laboratory policies, urine specimen, quality control materials, reagents, black or blue pen/EHR, and biohazard waste container.
Standards:	Provided with all necessary equipment and supplies, follow the steps in the procedure with the instructor observing each step. A maximum of three attempts may be used to complete the task. Students must complete all procedure steps in 25 minutes, with a minimum score of 70 percent. **Scoring:** Determine student's score by dividing points awarded by total points possible and multiplying results by 100.
Forms Needed:	Procedure 43–2 Forms (quality control log, laboratory report form). Procedure forms can be downloaded from the Student Companion website.

EVALUATION

Evaluator Signature: _____ Date: _____

Evaluator Comments:

Name: _____ Date: _____ Score: _____

Procedure 43–2 Steps

Start Time: _____ End Time: _____ Total Time: _____

	Steps	Possible Points	First Attempt	Second Attempt	Third Attempt
1.	Assemble the necessary equipment and supplies.	10			
2.	Wash hands and don disposable gloves and other PPE as required.	5			
3.	Perform quality control testing on two reagent cards, one negative and one positive.	15			
4.	Record the results of the quality control analyses in the quality control log; do not report patient results if quality control results are not in the acceptable range.	15			
5.	Prepare the reagent for patient testing and process the test according to the manufacturer's directions.	15			
6.	If the test is negative you must perform a specific gravity test with a urine dipstick or refractometer to determine concentration of the urine.	15			
7.	Dispose of contaminated waste in the biohazard waste container.	5			
8.	Remove gloves and wash hands.	5			
9.	Record the results of the test on the patient's health record and on the laboratory log sheet.	15			
	Points Awarded / Points Possible	_____ / **100**			

Competency Checklist
Procedure 43–3 Test Urine with Reagent Strips

ABHES Curriculum

MA.A.1.10.b(1)	Perform selected CLIA-waived tests that assist with diagnosis and treatment: Urinalysis
M.A.A.1.10.b(6)(c)	Perform selected CLIA-waived tests that assist with diagnosis and treatment: Kit testing: Dip Sticks
M.A.A.1.10.d	Collect, label, and process specimens

CAAHEP Core Curriculum

I.P.11.c	Obtain specimens and perform: CLIA-waived urinalysis
II.P.3	Maintain lab test results using flow sheets

Task:	Following the steps listed in the procedure, demonstrate the steps required to test urine with reagent strips to detect pH, protein, glucose, ketones, blood, bilirubin, urobilinogen, leukocytes, and specific gravity in urine.
Supplies & Conditions:	Multistix 10 SG reagent strips, fresh urine specimen, disposable gloves, watch with second hand or timer, patient's chart/EHR, pen, and adequate lighting to read color chart on reagent bottle (for accurate test results).
Standards:	Provided with all necessary equipment and supplies, follow the steps in the procedure with the instructor observing each step. A maximum of three attempts may be used to complete the task. Students must complete all procedure steps in 15 minutes, with a minimum score of 70 percent. **Scoring:** Determine student's score by dividing points awarded by total points possible and multiplying results by 100.
Forms:	Procedure 43-3 Form (Urinalysis laboratory log sheet). Procedure forms can be downloaded from the Student Companion website.

EVALUATION

Evaluator Signature: _____   Date: _____

Evaluator Comments:

Name: _____   Date: _____   Score: _____

Procedure 43–3 Steps

Start Time: _____   End Time: _____   Total Time: _____

	Steps	Possible Points	First Attempt	Second Attempt	Third Attempt
1.	Assemble the necessary equipment and supplies.	10			
2.	Wash hands and don disposable gloves and other PPE as required.	5			
3.	Stir the urine by rotating the UA container in a circular motion to distribute solutes evenly throughout the specimen.	5			
4.	Remove the cap from the bottle and take out one reagent strip without touching the test paper end. Place the cap securely back on bottle.	5			
5.	Dip the test paper end of the reagent strip into the urine specimen. With the reagent side of the strip down, pull it across the inside of the specimen container opening to remove excess urine. Blot side of strip on an absorbent pad.	5			
6.	Begin timing tests immediately.	15			
7.	Place the bottle on its side and hold it at the bottom with your left hand. Place the reagent strip next to the color chart on the bottle.	5			
8.	Read the test results from the bottom to the top in order of shorter to longer timings.	5			
9.	Discard the used reagent strip, gloves, and other disposables in the proper receptacle. Wash hands. Return reagent strips to the proper storage area.	5			
10.	Record the results as indicated for each section on the patient's chart and in the laboratory log book.	15			
	Points Awarded / Points Possible	_____/ 75			

Competency Checklist
Procedure 43–4 Obtain Urine Sediment for Microscopic Examination

ABHES Curriculum

M.A.A.1.10.d   Collect, label, and process specimens

Task:	Following the steps listed in the procedure, obtain urine sediment to prepare a specimen for microscopic examination.
Supplies & Conditions:	In a simulated medical office situation, students will be provided the equipment and supplies necessary to perform the procedure: fresh urine specimen, disposable latex or vinyl gloves, two centrifuge tubes, centrifuge, frosted-end glass slides with cover glass, tapered pipette, patient's chart/EHR, pen, pencil, tongue depressor, microscope with light source, urine sediment chart, timer, and sharps container.
Standards:	Provided with all necessary equipment and supplies, follow the steps in the procedure with the instructor observing each step. A maximum of three attempts may be used to complete the task. Students must complete all procedure steps in 20 minutes, with a minimum score of 70 percent. **Scoring:** Determine student's score by dividing points awarded by total points possible and multiplying results by 100.

EVALUATION

Evaluator Signature: _____ Date: _____

Evaluator Comments:

Name: _____ Date: _____ Score: _____

Procedure 43–4 Steps

Start Time: _____ End Time: _____ Total Time: _____

	Steps	Possible Points	First Attempt	Second Attempt	Third Attempt
1.	Wash hands, put on gloves, and assemble all the needed items on a cleared counter surface near the centrifuge.	10			
2.	Stir the urine specimen by rotating the container and pour equal amounts (approximately 10 mL) into each of two test tubes or use plain water in one of the test tubes.	5			
3.	To balance the centrifuge, place the centrifuge tubes on opposite sides. Urine should be spun at 1,500 revolutions per minute for three to five minutes.	5			
4.	When the centrifuge has completely stopped, lift out the tube containing the urine specimen and carefully pour off the urine (supernatant).	5			
5.	There will still be a few drops of urine in the bottom of the test tube with the sediment. Gently tap the bottom of the tube on the counter or against your palm to mix the urine and sediment together.	5			
6.	Obtain a drop or two of urine sediment with a disposable pipette and place it on a clean frosted-end glass slide.	5			
7.	Place a cover slip over the specimen, allow it to settle, and place it on the microscope stage.	5			
	Points Awarded / Points Possible	_____/ **40**			

Competency Checklist
Procedure 43–5 Screen and Follow Up Test Results

CAAHEP Core Curriculum

II.P.2	Differentiate between normal and abnormal test results
II.A.1	Reassure a patient of the accuracy of the test results

---

Task:	Following the steps listed in the procedure, screen and follow up lab results for normal and abnormal values to relay information to the health care provider.
Supplies & Conditions:	Scenarios of simulated lab reports for examination and analysis and reference materials supplied by the instructor (e.g., Internet, laboratory reference manuals, textbook, and so on).
Standards:	Provided with all necessary equipment and supplies, follow the steps in the procedure with the instructor observing each step. A maximum of three attempts may be used to complete the task. Students must complete all procedure steps in 15 minutes, with a minimum score of 70 percent. **Scoring:** Determine student's score by dividing points awarded by total points possible and multiplying results by 100.
Forms:	Procedure 43–5 Form (laboratory report form). Procedure forms can be downloaded from the Student Companion website.

EVALUATION

Evaluator Signature: _____ Date: _____

Evaluator Comments:

585

Name: _____ Date: _____ Score: _____

Procedure 43–5 Steps

Start Time: _____ End Time: _____ Total Time: _____

	Steps	Possible Points	First Attempt	Second Attempt	Third Attempt
1.	Screen the test results to determine whether they are normal or abnormal.	15			
2.	Screen the test results to determine whether laboratory reports are missing any key elements.	15			
3.	Identify the appropriate action for the abnormal values with the health care provider.	15			
4.	Identify the appropriate action for the normal values with the health care provider.	15			
5.	After reviewing the results, the provider may order you to call the patient with the results and any actions that may be warranted.	15			
6.	Call the patient to advise the results per the provider's orders and *reassure the patient of the accuracy of the test results*.	15			
7.	Accurately chart action taken in the patient's medical record.	15			
	Points Awarded / Points Possible	_____ / **105**			

Competency Checklist
Procedure 43–6 Instruct a Patient to Collect a Stool Specimen

ABHES Curriculum

M.A.A.1.10.d   Collect, label, and process specimens

MA.A.1.10.e(2)   Instruct patients in the collection of a fecal specimen

CAAHEP Core Curriculum

I.P.11.e   Obtain specimens and perform: CLIA-waived microbiology test

I.A.3   Show awareness of a patient's concerns related to the procedure being performed

V.A.4   Explain to a patient the rationale for performance of a procedure

---

Task:	Following the steps listed in the procedure, instruct patients to collect an adequate stool specimen for laboratory analysis.
Supplies & Conditions:	In a simulated medical office situation, students will be provided the equipment and supplies necessary to perform the procedure: specimen container with lid, lab request form, pen, patient's chart/EHR, label, printed instructions (optional), and tongue depressors.
Standards:	Provided with all necessary equipment and supplies, follow the steps in the procedure with the instructor observing each step. A maximum of three attempts may be used to complete the task. Students must complete all procedure steps in 30 minutes, with a minimum score of 70 percent. **Scoring:** Determine student's score by dividing points awarded by total points possible and multiplying results by 100.

EVALUATION

Evaluator Signature: _____   Date: _____

Evaluator Comments:

Name: _____ Date: _____ Score: _____

Procedure 43–6 Steps

Start Time: _____ End Time: _____ Total Time: _____

	Steps	Possible Points	First Attempt	Second Attempt	Third Attempt
1.	Assemble the items next to the patient.	5			
2.	Write identifying information on the request form and specimen container labels.	15			
3.	Identify the patient and explain the provider's orders, *including the rationale for performing the procedure. Show awareness of the patient's concerns related to the procedure* by answering any questions the patient might have. Give printed instructions or write out if necessary.	15			
4.	Instruct the patient to obtain the amount of stool required. The stool culture and ova and parasite containers must be filled to the designated line on the container. For other stool testing, three or four tablespoons are needed. Explain that nothing else should be placed in the cup besides stool (no tissue paper, urine, etc.).	5			
5.	Instruct the patient to place the specimen in the containers specified, secure the covers tightly, and write the date and time the specimen was obtained on the labels of the containers. Record that the patient was given instructions.	5			
6.	Advise patient to return the specimens to the lab or medical office when complete. Place the specimens with the request form in the designated area to be sent to the reference lab for testing.	5			
7.	Record that the specimen was returned to the lab and sent to the reference lab for processing.	15			
	Points Awarded / Points Possible	____/ 65			

Competency Checklist
Procedure 43–7 Perform an Occult Blood Test

ABHES Curriculum

M.A.A.1.10.d   Collect, label, and process specimens
M.A.A.1.10.e(2)   Instruct patients in the collection of a fecal specimen

CAAHEP Core Curriculum

I.P.10   Perform a quality control measure

Task:	Following the steps listed in the procedure, determine the presence of occult blood in the stool.
Supplies & Conditions:	Hemoccult slides prepared by patient, developer, timer, patient's chart/EHR, pen, biohazard bag, and latex or vinyl gloves.
Standards:	Provided with all necessary equipment and supplies, follow the steps in the procedure with the instructor observing each step. A maximum of three attempts may be used to complete the task. Students must complete all procedure steps in 30 minutes, with a minimum score of 70 percent. **Scoring:** Determine student's score by dividing points awarded by total points possible and multiplying results by 100.

EVALUATION

Evaluator Signature: _____ Date: _____

Evaluator Comments:

Name: _____ Date: _____ Score: _____

Procedure 43–7 Steps

Start Time: _____ End Time: _____ Total Time: _____

	Steps	Possible Points	First Attempt	Second Attempt	Third Attempt
1.	Wash hands and assemble items needed for testing on counter. Put on gloves.	10			
2.	Open the test side of the hemoccult paper slide.	5			
3.	Remove the cap from the bottle of developer.	5			
4.	Place two drops of developer on each section of the reagent paper slide: A, B.	5			
5.	Immediately begin timing for 1 minute. At 30 seconds, watch closely for any change of color that might be developing. Read at 60 seconds.	5			
6.	Compare the test with the control color and read the results.	5			
7.	Place one drop of developer between the positive and negative control. Read within 10 seconds.	5			
8.	Discard the test in a biohazard waste bag. Remove gloves and wash hands.	15			
9.	Record test results on the patient's chart and laboratory log sheet as either positive or negative and sign.	15			
	Points Awarded / Points Possible	_____/ **70**			

Competency Checklist
Procedure 43–8 Instruct a Patient to Collect a Sputum Specimen

ABHES Curriculum

M.A.A.1.10.d   Collect, label, and process specimens
M.A.A.1.10.e(3) Instruct patients in the collection of sputum specimens

CAAHEP Core Curriculum

I.A.3   Show awareness of a patient's concerns related to the procedure being performed
V.A.4   Explain to a patient the rationale for performance of a procedure

---

Task: Following the steps listed in the procedure, instruct a patient in the collection of an adequate sputum specimen for laboratory analysis.

Supplies & Conditions: Sputum specimen container and lid, label, pen, patient's chart/EHR, label, request form, and printed instruction sheet (optional).

Standards: Provided with all necessary equipment and supplies, follow the steps in the procedure with the instructor observing each step. A maximum of three attempts may be used to complete the task. Students must complete all procedure steps in 30 minutes, with a minimum score of 70 percent. **Scoring:** Determine student's score by dividing points awarded by total points possible and multiplying results by 100.

EVALUATION

Evaluator Signature: _____   Date: _____

Evaluator Comments:

Name: _____ Date: _____ Score: _____

Procedure 43–8 Steps

Start Time: _____ End Time: _____ Total Time: _____

	Steps	Possible Points	First Attempt	Second Attempt	Third Attempt
1.	Assemble the items next to the patient.	10			
2.	Write the patient's name on a specimen cup label and complete the lab request form.	15			
3.	Identify the patient and explain the provider's orders. Explain the procedure, *including the rationale for performing the procedure. Show awareness of the patient's concerns related to the procedure* by answering any questions the patient might have. Give printed instructions or write them out if you feel the patient has a difficult time understanding you.	15			
4.	Instruct the patient to remove the lid from the sterile specimen container and to expel secretions from a first morning coughing episode into the center of the cup, being careful not to touch the inside of the cup. The container should not be more than half full.	5			
5.	Instruct the patient not to allow saliva, tears, sweat, mucus from the nose or mouth, or any other substance to enter the cup.	5			
6.	When secretions have been obtained and the cup sealed with its cover, the patient should write the time and date that it was obtained on the label and the lab request form and bring them to the lab or medical office as soon as possible.	5			
7.	Place the completed lab request form and the specimen container in the transfer bag. Send it to the lab.	5			
8.	Record that instruction was given to the patient in sputum collecting.	15			
	Points Awarded / Points Possible	_____/ **75**			

Competency Checklist
Procedure 43–9 Perform a Wound Collection for Microbiologic Testing

ABHES Curriculum

MA.A.1.10.d(3) Perform wound collection procedures

CAAHEP Core Curriculum

I.A.3   Show awareness of a patient's concerns related to the procedure being performed
I.P.11.e   Obtain specimens and perform: CLIA-waived microbiology test
V.A.4   Explain to a patient the rationale for performance of a procedure

---

Task: Following the steps listed in the procedure, obtain a wound culture from a patient, using sterile technique.

Supplies & Conditions: Sterile culturette, gloves, other personal protective equipment as required by the collection procedure, pen, and simulated patient chart/EHR.

Standards: Provided with all necessary equipment and supplies, follow the steps in the procedure with the instructor observing each step. A maximum of three attempts may be used to complete the task. Students must complete all procedure steps in 20 minutes, with a minimum score of 70 percent. **Scoring:** Determine student's score by dividing points awarded by total points possible and multiplying results by 100.

EVALUATION

Evaluator Signature: _____ Date: _____

Evaluator Comments:

Name: _____ Date: _____ Score: _____

Procedure 43–9 Steps

Start Time: _____ End Time: _____ Total Time: _____

	Steps	Possible Points	First Attempt	Second Attempt	Third Attempt
1.	Assemble necessary supplies for collection of the specimen and ascertain that the culturette is not expired.	10			
2.	Identify the patient and explain the procedure, *including the rationale for performing the procedure. Show awareness of the patient's concerns related to the procedure* by answering any questions the patient might have and assisting the patient into a comfortable position before you proceed.	15			
3.	Verify the health care provider's order.	5			
4.	Remove the sterile swab from the sleeve.	15			
5.	Collect an adequate specimen without touching any other area except for the exudate and gently rolling the swab in the affected area.	5			
6.	Reinsert the sterile swab in the sleeve and break the ampule.	5			
7.	Record the patient information on the culturette (not the wrapper); if required, complete a lab requisition form for an outside laboratory.	5			
8.	Correctly document the procedure in the patient's medical record.	15			
	Points Awarded / Points Possible	_____/ **75**			

Competency Checklist
Procedure 43–10 Obtain a Throat Culture

ABHES Curriculum

MA.A.1.10.d(4) Obtain throat specimens for microbiologic testing

CAAHEP Core Curriculum

I.A.3	Show awareness of a patient's concerns related to the procedure being performed
I.P.11.e	Obtain specimens and perform: CLIA-waived microbiology test
V.A.4	Explain to a patient the rationale for performance of a procedure

---

Task:	Following the steps listed in the procedure, perform the procedure for obtaining a throat culture by isolating a disease-causing organism to determine effective treatment of the patient.
Supplies & Conditions:	Sterile swabs, sterile tongue depressor, disposable gloves, pen, patient's chart, penlight (optional), and label.
Standards:	Provided with all necessary equipment and supplies, follow the steps in the procedure with the instructor observing each step. A maximum of three attempts may be used to complete the task. Students must complete all procedure steps in 30 minutes, with a minimum score of 70 percent. **Scoring:** Determine student's score by dividing points awarded by total points possible and multiplying results by 100.

EVALUATION

Evaluator Signature: _____ Date: _____

Evaluator Comments:

595

Name: _____ Date: _____ Score: _____

Procedure 43–10 Steps

Start Time: _____ End Time: _____ Total Time: _____

	Steps	Possible Points	First Attempt	Second Attempt	Third Attempt
1.	Assemble the needed items near the identified patient. Label the culturette swab and complete a request form. Wash hands and put on gloves.	10			
2.	Identify the patient and explain the procedure, *including the rationale for performing the procedure. Show awareness of the patient's concerns related to the procedure* by answering any questions the patient might have and assisting the patient into a comfortable position before you proceed.	15			
3.	Open a sterile swab and ask the patient to open the mouth as wide as possible.	5			
4.	Depress the tongue with a sterile tongue depressor held in one hand. Hold the sterile swab in the other. Ask the patient to say "ah" to assist depression of the tongue. Quickly insert the swab into the back of the throat and roll over the peritonsillar areas, touching areas with obvious exudate.	15			
5.	Remove the swab and depressor from the patient's mouth. Attend to the patient's needs and offer tissues.	5			
6.	Place the swab in the culturette container for transportation to the lab. Place in the transport bag with the request form. Place in the proper storage area for transport to the reference lab.	5			
7.	Discard all disposable items in the proper receptacle. Remove gloves and wash hands.	5			
8.	Record the procedure on the patient's chart and initial.	15			
	Points Awarded / Points Possible	_____/ **75**			

Competency Checklist
Procedure 43–11 Perform a Rapid Strep Screening Test for Group A Strep

ABHES Curriculum

MA.A.1.10.a	Practice quality control
MA.A.1.10.b(6)(b)	Perform selected CLIA-waived tests that assist with diagnosis and treatment: Kit testing: Quick strep
MA.A.1.10.d(4)	Obtain throat specimens for microbiologic testing

CAAHEP Core Curriculum

I.P.10	Perform a quality control measure
I.P.11.e	Obtain specimens and perform: CLIA-waived microbiology test
I.A.3	Show awareness of a patient's concerns related to the procedure being performed
V.A.4	Explain to a patient the rationale for performance of a procedure

---

Task:	Following the steps listed in the procedure, screen a patient specimen for the presence of group A strep by testing a throat swab for group A strep with a rapid diagnostic test and interpreting the results.
Supplies & Conditions:	Gloves, sterile throat swab, tongue blade, commercial test kit for group A strep with positive and negative controls, patient's chart/EHR, laboratory report form, biohazard container.
Standards:	Provided with all necessary equipment and supplies, follow the steps in the procedure with the instructor observing each step. A maximum of three attempts may be used to complete the task. Students must complete all procedure steps in 30 minutes, with a minimum score of 70 percent. **Scoring:** Determine student's score by dividing points awarded by total points possible and multiplying results by 100.
Forms Needed:	Procedure 43–11 Forms (quality control log and laboratory log sheet). Procedure forms can be downloaded from the Student Companion website.

EVALUATION

Evaluator Signature: _____ Date: _____

Evaluator Comments:

Name: _____ Date: _____ Score: _____

Procedure 43–11 Steps

Start Time: _____ End Time: _____ Total Time: _____

	Steps	Possible Points	First Attempt	Second Attempt	Third Attempt
1.	Assemble supplies.	10			
2.	Identify the patient and explain the procedure, *including the rationale for performing the procedure. Show awareness of the patient's concerns related to the procedure* by answering any questions the patient might have and assisting the patient into a comfortable position before you proceed.	15			
3.	Wash your hands and don gloves.	5			
4.	Using the tongue blade to keep the tongue out of the way, insert the sterile swab into the back of the oral cavity to collect the specimen from the peritonsillar area.	15			
5.	Label the reagent chamber for the test with the patient's name.	5			
6.	Following the manufacturer's instructions exactly, perform the test on the patient's specimen.	15			
7.	Perform the positive and negative controls, recording the results in the laboratory log record, knowing what action must be taken if the results of the quality control are not within the manufacturer's prescribed range.	15			
8.	Dispose of waste in a biohazard waste container.	5			
9.	Properly complete the lab report form and accurately enter the results on the patient's chart.	15			
	Points Awarded / Points Possible	_____/ **100**			

Competency Checklist
Procedure 44–1 Puncture Skin with a Sterile Lancet

ABHES Curriculum

MA.A.1.9.a   Practice standard precautions
MA.A.1.10.d(2) Perform capillary puncture

CAAHEP Core Curriculum

I.P.2.c   Perform capillary puncture
I.A.3   Show awareness of a patient's concerns related to the procedure being performed
III.P.2   Select appropriate barrier/personal protective equipment (PPE)
V.A.4   Explain to a patient the rationale for performance of a procedure

---

Task: Following the steps listed in the procedure, puncture skin with a sterile lancet to obtain a few drops of capillary blood for screening tests.

Supplies & Conditions: Latex or vinyl gloves, sterile lancet, alcohol, cotton balls, sharps container, flat, stable surface.

Standards: Provided with all necessary equipment and supplies, follow the steps in the procedure with the instructor observing each step. A maximum of three attempts may be used to complete the task. Students must complete all procedure steps in 15 minutes, with a minimum score of 70 percent. **Scoring:** Determine student's score by dividing points awarded by total points possible and multiplying results by 100.

EVALUATION

Evaluator Signature: _____ Date: _____

Evaluator Comments:

Name: _____   Date: _____   Score: _____

Procedure 44–1 Steps

Start Time: _____   End Time: _____   Total Time: _____

	Steps	Possible Points	First Attempt	Second Attempt	Third Attempt
1.	Identify the patient.	15			
2.	***Explain the rationale for performing the procedure to the patient. Show awareness of the patient's concerns related to the procedure being performed.***	15			
3.	Inspect the patient's fingers (or other puncture site) and select the most desirable site.	5			
4.	Wash hands, put on gloves, and assemble the needed items on the flat surface.	5			
5.	Wipe the desired site with an alcohol-prep pad and let dry.	5			
6.	Take the sterile lancet out of the package without contaminating the point.	5			
7.	Hold the patient's finger (or other site) securely between your thumb and great finger. In your other hand, hold the lancet, pointed downward, with your thumb and index or great finger. Puncture the site quickly with a firm, steady, down-and-up motion to approximately a 2-mm depth.	15			
8.	Discard the first drop of blood by blotting it away with a dry gauze square (unless the test being performed indicates not to).	10			
9.	Keep applying gentle pressure on either side of the puncture site until the necessary amount of blood has been obtained.	5			
10.	Wipe the site with a gauze pad and ask the patient to hold it gently for a minute or two.	5			
11.	Remove gloves, wash hands, and discard used items in the proper receptacle.	10			
12.	Record the procedure in the patient's chart.	15			
	Points Awarded / Points Possible	_____/ **110**			

Competency Checklist
Procedure 44–2 Obtain Venous Blood with a Sterile Needle and Syringe

ABHES Curriculum

MA.A.1.9.a   Practice standard precautions and perform disinfection/sterilization techniques
MA.A.1.10.d(1)   Perform venipuncture

CAAHEP Core Curriculum

I.P.2.b   Perform venipuncture
I.A.3   Show awareness of a patient's concerns related to the procedure being performed
III.P.2   Select appropriate barrier/personal protective equipment (PPE)
V.A.4   Explain to a patient the rationale for performance of a procedure

---

Task: Following the steps listed in the procedure, obtain venous blood specimens with a sterile needle and syringe.

Supplies & Conditions: Sterile safety needle (19–23 G, 1 to $1\frac{1}{2}$ inches in length), 10–20 mL syringe for specimen tubes, laboratory specimen packaging materials, pen, patient's chart/EHR, alcohol-prep pads, latex or vinyl gloves, tourniquet, lab request form (labeled appropriately with the vacuum blood specimen tubes that were ordered), gauze squares, adhesive bandage, spirits of ammonia, emesis basin, biohazard waste container (should be within reach), and sharps container.

Standards: Provided with all necessary equipment and supplies, follow the steps in the procedure with the instructor observing each step. A maximum of three attempts may be used to complete the task. Students must complete all procedure steps in 15 minutes, with a minimum score of 70 percent. **Scoring:** Determine student's score by dividing points awarded by total points possible and multiplying results by 100.

EVALUATION

Evaluator Signature: _____   Date: _____

Evaluator Comments:

Name: _____ Date: _____ Score: _____

Procedure 44–2 Steps

Start Time: _____ End Time: _____ Total Time: _____

	Steps	Possible Points	First Attempt	Second Attempt	Third Attempt
1.	Identify the patient by using two identifiers.	15			
2.	Assemble all needed items on a flat, stable surface next to the patient. Wash hands. Put on gloves.	15			
3.	Secure a needle onto a syringe by holding the needle guard in one hand and turning the syringe barrel clockwise. Push in the plunger of the syringe all the way to release any air from the barrel.	10			
4.	Explain the procedure to the patient, *including the rationale for performing the procedure. Show awareness of the patient's concerns related to the procedure being performed.* After consulting the patient, select a vein that can be palpated.	15			
5.	Apply a tourniquet to the patient's upper arm, about three inches above the bend in the elbow.	5			
6.	Clean the site lightly with an alcohol-prep pad and let it air-dry.	10			
7.	Ask the patient to clench the fist only if the vein does not stand out.	5			
8.	Take off the needle guard, and, with the bevel of the needle up, insert the needle tip into the vein with a quick and steady motion, following the path of the vein at approximately a 15–30° angle.	15			
9.	Hold the barrel of the syringe in one hand and, with the other hand, pull the plunger back slowly and steadily until the barrel is filled with the amount of blood needed to fill the specimen tubes. As you observe the blood flow into the syringe, ask the patient to open the fist slowly; release the tourniquet.	15			
10.	Pull the needle out in the same path as it was inserted and place a gauze square over the site as the needle is withdrawn. Have the patient apply gentle pressure and slightly elevate the arm. Activate the needle safety device and discard the needle into a sharps container.	15			
11.	Attach a blood transfer device to the syringe and allow the blood to transfer using the tube's vacuum. Do not depress the plunger of the syringe. Fill the tubes with blood from the syringe according to the correct order of draw. Blood smears should be made at this time if needed.	10			
12.	Invert the tubes 8–10 times and stand red-stoppered tubes vertically to clot so that serum can be drawn after centrifugation.	5			

13.	Deposit the entire syringe and blood transfer device intact in the sharps biohazard waste container. Label all required specimen tubes and complete a lab request form. The completed lab request form is usually placed in one side of the lab-provided biobag and the specimens in the other, protected (sealed and leak-proof), side to be sent to a reference lab for analysis.	15			
14.	Once it is determined that the patient doesn't have an allergy to adhesives, apply a bandage over the puncture site.	5			
15.	Discard disposables in the proper receptacles. Remove gloves, wash hands, and return items to the proper storage area.	5			
16.	Record the procedure in the log book and on the patient's chart and initial.	15			
	Points Awarded / Points Possible	_____/ **175**			

Competency Checklist
Procedure 44–3 Obtain Venous Blood with a Vacuum Tube

ABHES Curriculum

MA.A.1.9.a   Practice standard precautions and perform disinfection/sterilization techniques
MA.A.1.10.d(1) Perform venipuncture

CAAHEP Core Curriculum

I.P.2.b   Perform venipuncture
I.A.3   Show awareness of a patient's concerns related to the procedure being performed
III.P.2   Select appropriate barrier/personal protective equipment (PPE)
V.A.4   Explain to a patient the rationale for performance of a procedure

---

Task: Following the steps listed in the procedure, obtain venous blood with a vacuum tube.

Supplies & Conditions: Disposable vacuum-tube holder with safety needle (19–23 G, 1 to $1\frac{1}{2}$ inch in length), labeled specimen tubes (vacuum), alcohol-prep pads, latex or vinyl gloves, sharps container, gauze squares, tourniquet, lab request forms, pen, patient's chart/EHR, bandages, biohazard waste container, and laboratory specimen packaging material.

Standards: Provided with all necessary equipment and supplies, follow the steps in the procedure with the instructor observing each step. A maximum of three attempts may be used to complete the task. Students must complete all procedure steps in 15 minutes, with a minimum score of 70 percent. **Scoring:** Determine student's score by dividing points awarded by total points possible and multiplying results by 100.

EVALUATION

Evaluator Signature: _____   Date: _____

Evaluator Comments:

Name: _____ Date: _____ Score: _____

Procedure 44–3 Steps

Start Time: _____   End Time: _____   Total Time: _____

	Steps	Possible Points	First Attempt	Second Attempt	Third Attempt
1.	Identify the patient by using two identifiers.	15			
2.	Assemble all needed items on a flat, stable surface next to the patient. For needle assembly, secure a safety needle onto the Vacutainer holder by screwing the grooved end of the needle into the grooved tip of the adapter, holding the needle guard, and turning the adapter in a clockwise motion. Set aside. Wash hands. Put on gloves.	15			
3.	*Explain the rationale of the procedure being performed to the patient. Show awareness of the patient's concerns related to the procedure.* After consulting the patient, select a vein that can be palpated.	10			
4.	Apply a tourniquet to the patient's upper arm, about three inches above the bend in the elbow.	15			
5.	Clean the site with an alcohol-prep pad and let it air-dry.	5			
6.	Ask the patient to clench the fist only if the vein does not stand out.	10			
7.	Take off the needle guard and, with the bevel of the needle up, insert the tip of the needle into the vein with a quick and steady motion, following the path of the vein at approximately a 15-30° degree angle.	5			
8.	Hold the Vacutainer holder with one hand and, with the other hand, place your index and great fingers on either side of the protruding edges of the adapter. Push the vacuum tube completely into the adapter with your thumb, allowing the needle to puncture the stopper. Blood will flow into the tube by vacuum force if the other end of the needle is in the vein properly. As you observe blood flow into the tube, ask the patient to open the fist slowly and then release the tourniquet. When the tube is filled, pull it out of the adapter by holding it between your thumb and great finger and pushing against the adapter with your index finger.	15			
9.	Fill the required number of tubes for the tests ordered by the provider according to the correct order of draw. Blood smears should be made at this time if needed.	15			
10.	Pull the needle out in the path by which it was inserted and place a gauze square over the site as the needle is withdrawn. Have the patient apply gentle pressure and slightly elevate the arm. Activate the needle safety device and discard entire Vacutainer holder and needle into a sharps container.	15			
11.	Invert the tubes 8–10 times and stand red-stoppered tubes vertically to clot so that serum can be drawn after centrifugation.	10			

606

12.	Label all required specimen tubes and complete a lab request form.	5			
13.	Once it is determined that the patient does not have an allergy to adhesives, apply a bandage over the puncture site.	15			
14.	Discard disposables in the proper receptacle. Remove gloves, wash hands, and return items to the proper storage area.	5			
15.	Record the procedure in the log book and on the patient's chart and initial.	5			
16.	Place labeled specimen tubes with the lab request form securely in the appropriate specimen container for safe transport to the lab. The completed lab request form is usually placed in one side of the lab-provided biobag and the specimens in the other, protected (sealed and leak-proof), side to be sent to a reference lab for analysis.	15			
	Points Awarded / Points Possible	____/ **175**			

Competency Checklist
Procedure 44–4 Obtain Venous Blood with the Butterfly Needle Method

ABHES Curriculum

MA.A.1.9.a   Practice standard precautions and perform disinfection/sterilization techniques
MA.A.1.10.d(1) Perform venipuncture

CAAHEP Core Curriculum

I.P.2.b   Perform venipuncture
I.A.3   Show awareness of a patient's concerns related to the procedure being performed
III.P.2   Select appropriate barrier/personal protective equipment (PPE)
V.A.4   Explain to a patient the rationale for performance of a procedure

Task:	Following the steps listed in the procedure, obtain venous blood specimens from infants and children, elderly, or patients with veins that are difficult to draw (veins not easily seen or felt). Suggested sites to obtain blood are the antecubital or the back of the hand.
Supplies & Conditions:	Disposable vacuum-tube holder with sterile safety butterfly needle (22 G), syringe or appropriate vacuum tubes, pen, patient's chart/EHR, lab request form, spirits of ammonia, emesis basin, tourniquet, latex or vinyl gloves, alcohol-prep pads, gauze squares, bandage, Mayo tray table, and biohazard sharps container.
Standards:	Provided with all necessary equipment and supplies, follow the steps in the procedure with the instructor observing each step. A maximum of three attempts may be used to complete the task. Students must complete all procedure steps in 15 minutes, with a minimum score of 70 percent. **Scoring:** Determine student's score by dividing points awarded by total points possible and multiplying results by 100.

EVALUATION

Evaluator Signature: _____ Date: _____

Evaluator Comments:

Procedure 44–4 Steps

Start Time: _____   End Time: _____   Total Time: _____

	Steps	Possible Points	First Attempt	Second Attempt	Third Attempt
1.	Identify the patient by using two identifiers.	15			
2.	Assemble all needed items on a flat, stable surface next to the patient. For needle assembly, secure a needle onto the Vacutainer holder by screwing the grooved end of the needle into the grooved tip of the Vacutainer holder and turning the holder in a clockwise motion. If using a syringe, secure the needle directly to the syringe using the same method. Push any air out of syringe before using it to draw a blood specimen. Set aside. Wash hands. Put on gloves.	15			
3.	*Explain the rationale for performing the procedure. Show awareness of the patient's concerns related to the procedure.* After consulting the patient, select a vein that can be palpated.	10			
4.	Apply the tourniquet to the patient's arm, about three inches above the needle insertion site.	5			
5.	Clean the site lightly with an alcohol-prep pad and let it air-dry.	5			
6.	Ask the patient to make a fist and hold it until you say to release it.	10			
7.	Remove the needle guard and quickly insert the butterfly needle into the vein at a 5–10 degree angle if drawing from the hand and 15–30 degrees if using the antecubital by holding the wings together or holding the body of the needle (watch for a flash of blood).	15			
8.	Pull back on the plunger of the syringe slowly until an adequate amount of blood is obtained, and then ask the patient to release the fist. If using the Vacutainer method, press the appropriate tube onto the needle inside the Vacutainer holder until the blood starts to flow; switch tubes as needed.	15			
9.	Release the tourniquet and withdraw the needle quickly.	10			
10.	Apply gentle pressure over the site with gauze and ask the patient to hold the arm slightly up for a few minutes.	15			
11.	Retract the needle or activate the safety lock on the needle and then place the used needle, Vacutainer holder if used, and all other contaminated supplies in a biohazard sharps container.	10			
12.	If a syringe was used, attach a blood transfer device to the syringe and allow the blood to transfer using the tube's vacuum. Do not depress the plunger of the syringe. Fill the tubes with blood from the syringe according to the correct order of draw. Blood smears should be made at this time if needed.	15			

13.	Invert the tubes 8–10 times and stand red-stoppered tubes vertically to clot so that serum can be drawn after centrifugation.	5			
14.	Deposit the entire syringe and blood transfer device intact in the sharps biohazard waste container. Label all required specimen tubes and complete a lab request form. The completed lab request form is usually placed in one side of the lab-provided biobag and the specimens in the other, protected (sealed and leak-proof), side to be sent to a reference lab for analysis.	15			
15.	Once it is determined that the patient does not have an allergy to adhesives, apply a bandage to the site.	5			
16.	Place specimens in the appropriate lab transport container.	5			
17.	Remove gloves and discard them in a biohazard container or bag. Wash hands and return items to the proper storage area.	5			
18.	Record the procedure in the log book and on the patient's chart and initial.	15			
	Points Awarded / Points Possible	____/ 190			

Competency Checklist
Procedure 45–1 Determine Hemoglobin Using a Hemoglobinometer

ABHES Curriculum

MA.A.1.10.a   Practice quality control
MA.A.1.10.b(2) Perform selected CLIA-waived tests that assist with diagnosis and treatment: Hematology testing

CAAHEP Core Curriculum

I.P.10   Perform a quality control measure
I.P.11(a)   Obtain specimens and perform: CLIA-waived hematology test
I.A.3   Show awareness of patient's concerns related to the procedure being performed
V.A.4   Explain to a patient the rationale for performance of a procedure
II.P.3   Maintain lab test results using flow sheets.

Task: Following the steps listed in the procedure, perform a hemoglobin determination.

Supplies & Conditions: Hemoglobinometer, reagent card, sterile disposable lancet, gauze, alcohol-prep pads, gloves, other personal protective equipment (PPE) per laboratory policies, patient's chart/EHR, and pen.

Standards: Provided with all necessary equipment and supplies, follow the steps in the procedure with the instructor observing each step. A maximum of three attempts may be used to complete the task. Students must complete all procedure steps in 15 minutes, with a minimum score of 70 percent. **Scoring:** Determine student's score by dividing points awarded by total points possible and multiplying results by 100.

EVALUATION

Evaluator Signature: _____   Date: _____

Evaluator Comments:

613

Name: _____ Date: _____ Score: _____

Procedure 45–1 Steps

Start Time: _____ End Time: _____ Total Time: _____

	Steps	Possible Points	First Attempt	Second Attempt	Third Attempt
1.	Assemble all supplies and the hemoglobinometer; place them on a secure work surface.	10			
2.	Identify the patient. Explain the procedure to the patient, *including the rationale for performing the procedure. Show awareness of the patient's concerns related to the procedure.*	15			
3.	Wash hands; apply gloves and other PPE as required.	5			
4.	Perform a capillary puncture.	15			
5.	Place a large, beaded drop of blood on the reagent card while making sure the instrument is on. Wipe the patient's finger with a dry gauze pad and have the patient apply pressure to the site of the puncture.	15			
6.	After the instrument displays the results, chart this in the patient's medical record.	15			
7.	Dispose of the lancet in the biohazard sharps containers. Dispose of the remaining soiled articles in the biohazard trash container.	15			
8.	Take care of the patient's needs once it is determined that the patient does not have an allergy to adhesives, and put a bandage over puncture site.	5			
9.	Disinfect work area.	15			
10.	Remove gloves, dispose, and wash hands.	10			
11.	Record the results in the patient's chart, as well as the quality control sample results and test results, in the laboratory log book.	15			
	Points Awarded / Points Possible	____/ **135**			

Competency Checklist
Procedure 45–2 Determine Hematocrit (Hct) Using a Microhematocrit Centrifuge

ABHES Curriculum

MA.A.1.10.b(2) Perform selected CLIA-waived tests that assist with diagnosis and treatment: Hematology testing.

CAAHEP Core Curriculum

I.P.11.a	Obtain specimens and perform: CLIA-waived hematology test
I.A.3	Show awareness of patient's concerns related to the procedure being performed
V.A.4	Explain to a patient the rationale for performance of a procedure
II.P.3	Maintain lab test results using flow sheets.

Task: Following the steps listed in the procedure, determine hematocrit (Hct) readings using the microhematocrit centrifuge.

Supplies & Conditions: Sterile disposable lancet, self-sealed plastic microhematocrit tubes, microhematocrit centrifuge, latex or vinyl gloves, other personal protective equipment (PPE) per laboratory policies, gauze, alcohol-prep pads, patient's chart/EHR, pen (if hemoglobin is done by this procedure, conversion chart will also be needed to determine Hb), and Table 45–1.

Standards: Provided with all necessary equipment and supplies, follow the steps in the procedure with the instructor observing each step. A maximum of three attempts may be used to complete the task. Students must complete all procedure steps in 15 minutes, with a minimum score of 70 percent. **Scoring:** Determine student's score by dividing points awarded by total points possible and multiplying results by 100.

EVALUATION

Evaluator Signature: _____ Date: _____

Evaluator Comments:

Procedure 45–2 Steps

Start Time: _____ End Time: _____ Total Time: _____

	Steps	Possible Points	First Attempt	Second Attempt	Third Attempt
1.	Assemble the needed items. Check to see that the centrifuge is plugged into the electrical outlet.	10			
2.	Identify the patient. Explain the procedure to the patient, *including the rationale for performing the procedure. Show awareness of the patient's concerns related to the procedure.*	15			
3.	Wash hands; apply gloves and other PPE as required.	5			
4.	Perform a capillary puncture. Wipe away the first drop of blood with a gauze square.	15			
5.	Hold the microhematocrit tube as you would hold a pencil or pen, horizontally with the opening next to the drop of blood that appears at the puncture site and fill. Obtain as many tubes as ordered.	15			
6.	Wipe the outside end of the glass tube with a gauze square while still holding it horizontally.	10			
7.	Have the patient hold a dry gauze square on the puncture site. Make sure bleeding has stopped; offer the patient a bandage.	5			
8.	Secure the sealed end of the tube against the rubber padding in the centrifuge (sealed end of tube is always toward you). Balance the centrifuge with another tube opposite it.	5			
9.	Close the inside cover carefully over the tubes and lock it into place by turning the dial clockwise. Then close and lock the outside cover. Listen for it to click into place.	5			
10.	Turn the timer switch to three to five minutes. It will automatically turn off. Wait until the centrifuge has completely stopped spinning and unlock both covers.	5			
11.	Accurately read the results.	15			
12.	Disinfect work area.	15			
13.	Discard used items in the proper waste receptacles, remove gloves, and wash hands.	15			
14.	Record the reading in the patient's chart and on the laboratory log sheet.	15			
15.	Return items to the proper storage areas.	5			
	Points Awarded / Points Possible	_____/ **155**			

Competency Checklist
Procedure 45–3 Perform an Erythrocyte Sedimentation Rate (ESR)

ABHES Curriculum

MA.A.1.10.b(2) Perform selected CLIA-waived tests that assist with diagnosis and treatment: Hematology testing

CAAHEP Core Curriculum

I.P.11.a   Obtain specimens and perform: CLIA-waived hematology test
II.P.3   Maintain lab test results using flow sheets.

Task:	Following the steps listed in the procedure, measure the rate of fall of red blood cells within a prescribed time.
Supplies & Conditions:	Goggles or face shield, gloves, other personal protective equipment (PPE) per laboratory policies, prefilled vial, calibrated sed rate pipette, EDTA tube with patient's blood, sed rate stand, flat work surface, timer, patient's chart/EHR, laboratory report form, and blue or black pen.
Standards:	Provided with all necessary equipment and supplies, follow the steps in the procedure with the instructor observing each step. A maximum of three attempts may be used to complete the task. Students must complete all procedure steps in 70 minutes, with a minimum score of 70 percent. **Scoring:** Determine student's score by dividing points awarded by total points possible and multiplying results by 100.

EVALUATION

Evaluator Signature: _____   Date: _____

Evaluator Comments:

Procedure 45–3 Steps

Start Time: _____   **End Time:** _____   **Total Time:** _____

	Steps	Possible Points	First Attempt	Second Attempt	Third Attempt
1.	Assemble all supplies on a flat work surface.	10			
2.	Wash hands and apply gloves and other PPE as required before uncapping the mixed EDTA sample.	5			
3.	Remove the stopper on the prefilled sedivial; using a disposable pipette, fill to the indicated line with blood. Replace the stopper on the sedivial and invert several times to mix.	10			
4.	Place vial in sediplast rack on a level surface. Insert the pipette through the pierceable stopper, pushing down in a twisting motion until the pipette touches the bottom of the prefilled vial.	10			
5.	Set the timer.	5			
6.	After the appropriate time, read the numeric results of the test, using the designation of mm/hr after the numeric reading.	15			
7.	Dispose of the testing materials in a biohazard waste container.	5			
8.	Disinfect work area.	15			
9.	Remove gloves, dispose, and wash hands.	10			
10.	Record the reading in the patient's chart and on the laboratory log sheet.	15			
	Points Awarded / Points Possible	_____/ **100**			

Competency Checklist
Procedure 45–4 Screen Blood Sugar (Glucose) Level

ABHES Curriculum

MA.A.1.10.a   Practice quality control
MA.A.1.10.b(3) Perform selected CLIA-waived tests that assist with diagnosis and treatment: Chemistry testing

CAAHEP Core Curriculum

I.P.10   Perform a quality control measure
I.P.11.b   Obtain specimens and perform: CLIA-waived chemistry test
I.A.3   Show awareness of a patient's concerns related to the procedure being performed
V.A.4   Explain to a patient the rationale for performance of a procedure
II.P.3   Maintain lab test results using flow sheets.

Task: Following the steps listed in the procedure, determine the sugar (glucose) level in the blood.

Supplies & Conditions: Sterile disposable lancet, reagent strips, glucometer, latex or vinyl gloves, other personal protective equipment (PPE) per laboratory policies, alcohol-prep pads, and gauze squares.

Standards: Provided with all necessary equipment and supplies, follow the steps in the procedure with the instructor observing each step. A maximum of three attempts may be used to complete the task. Students must complete all procedure steps in 30 minutes, with a minimum score of 70 percent. **Scoring:** Determine student's score by dividing points awarded by total points possible and multiplying results by 100.

EVALUATION

Evaluator Signature: _____   Date: _____

Evaluator Comments:

Name: _____ Date: _____ Score: _____

Procedure 45–4 Steps

Start Time: _____ End Time: _____ Total Time: _____

	Steps	Possible Points	First Attempt	Second Attempt	Third Attempt
1.	Assemble all needed items on a flat, steady surface. Perform quality controls according to the manufacturer's guidelines.	10			
2.	Identify the patient. Explain the procedure to the patient, *including the rationale for performing the procedure. Show awareness of the patient's concerns related to the procedure.*	15			
3.	Wash hands; apply gloves and other PPE as required.	5			
4.	Perform a capillary puncture.	15			
5.	Complete the test per the manufacturer's directions for the instrument.	5			
6.	Give the patient a dry gauze square to hold over the puncture site after wiping it with an alcohol-prep pad. Offer a bandage.	15			
7.	Wait for the instrument to display the results. The number displayed is the blood glucose level.	15			
8.	Disinfect work area.	15			
9.	Discard all used items in the proper receptacle, remove gloves, and wash hands.	15			
10.	Document result in the patient's chart and laboratory log book. Record the controls in the control log as well as the lot number and the expiration date of the reagent test strips.	15			
	Points Awarded / Points Possible	_____/ **125**			

Competency Checklist
Procedure 45–5 Perform Hemoglobin A1C (Glycosylated Hemoglobin) Screening

ABHES Curriculum

MA.A.1.10.b(2) Perform selected CLIA-waived tests that assist with diagnosis and treatment: Hematology testing

CAAHEP Core Curriculum

I.P.11.a	Obtain specimens and perform: CLIA-waived hematology test
I.A.3	Show awareness of a patient's concerns related to the procedure being performed
V.A.4	Explain to a patient the rationale for performance of a procedure
II.P.3	Maintain lab test results using flow sheets.

Task:	Following the steps listed in the procedure, evaluate diabetic patients' overall compliance with diet regimen for management of blood glucose levels.
Supplies & Conditions:	Sterile disposable lancet, disposable gloves, other personal protective equipment (PPE) per laboratory policies, alcohol-prep pads, gauze, testing instrument, reagents, black or blue pen, biohazard waste container, and sharps container.
Standards:	Provided with all necessary equipment and supplies, follow the steps in the procedure with the instructor observing each step. A maximum of three attempts may be used to complete the task. Students must complete all procedure steps in 25 minutes, with a minimum score of 70 percent. **Scoring:** Determine student's score by dividing points awarded by total points possible and multiplying results by 100.

EVALUATION

Evaluator Signature: _____ Date: _____

Evaluator Comments:

Name: _____ Date: _____ Score: _____

Procedure 45–5 Steps

Start Time: _____ End Time: _____ Total Time: _____

	Steps	Possible Points	First Attempt	Second Attempt	Third Attempt
1.	Assemble the necessary equipment and supplies.	10			
2.	Identify the patient. Explain the procedure to the patient, *including the rationale for performing the procedure. Show awareness of the patient's concerns related to the procedure.*	15			
3.	Wash hands; apply gloves and other PPE as required.	5			
4.	Perform the capillary puncture and collect the blood sample per the manufacturer's directions for the instrument. Perform the test.	15			
5.	Check the patient's finger for excessive bleeding and provide clean gauze, instructing the patient to apply pressure to the site. Offer a bandage.	5			
6.	Dispose of contaminated sharps in the sharps container and other contaminated materials in the biohazard waste container.	15			
7.	Disinfect work area.	15			
8.	Remove gloves and wash hands.	5			
9.	Document result in the patient's chart and laboratory log book.	15			
	Points Awarded / Points Possible	____/ **100**			

Competency Checklist
Procedure 45–6 Perform a Cholesterol Screening

ABHES Curriculum

MA.A.1.10.a Practice quality control
MA.A.1.10.b(3) Perform selected CLIA-waived tests that assist with diagnosis and treatment: Chemistry testing

CAAHEP Core Curriculum

I.P.10 Perform a quality control measure
I.P.11.b Obtain specimens and perform: CLIA-waived chemistry test
I.A.3 Show awareness of a patient's concerns related to the procedure being performed
V.A.4 Explain to a patient the rationale for performance of a procedure
II.P.3 Maintain lab test results using flow sheets.

Task:	Following the steps listed in the procedure, screen a cholesterol level for hypercholesterolemia.
Supplies & Conditions:	Sterile disposable lancet, disposable gloves, other personal protective equipment (PPE) per laboratory policies, alcohol-prep pads, gauze, testing instrument (if indicated—some tests are done without an instrument), reagents, black or blue pen, biohazard waste container, and sharps container.
Standards:	Provided with all necessary equipment and supplies, follow the steps in the procedure with the instructor observing each step. A maximum of three attempts may be used to complete the task. Students must complete all procedure steps in 25 minutes, with a minimum score of 70 percent. **Scoring:** Determine student's score by dividing points awarded by total points possible and multiplying results by 100.

EVALUATION

Evaluator Signature: _____ Date: _____

Evaluator Comments:

Name: _____   Date: _____   Score: _____

Procedure 45–6 Steps

Start Time: _____   End Time: _____   Total Time: _____

	Steps	Possible Points	First Attempt	Second Attempt	Third Attempt
1.	Assemble the necessary equipment and supplies.	10			
2.	Identify the patient. Explain the procedure to the patient, *including the rationale for performing the procedure. Show awareness of the patient's concerns related to the procedure.*	15			
3.	Wash hands; apply gloves and other PPE as required.	5			
4.	Perform the capillary puncture and collect the blood sample per the manufacturer's directions for the instrument or the reagent card.	15			
5.	Record the results of the test on the patient's chart and on the laboratory log sheet.	15			
6.	Check the patient's finger for excessive bleeding and provide clean gauze, instructing the patient to apply pressure to the site. Offer a bandage.	5			
7.	Disinfect work area.	15			
8.	Dispose of contaminated sharps in the sharps container and other contaminated materials in the biohazard waste container.	15			
9.	Remove gloves and wash hands.	5			
	Points Awarded / Points Possible	_____/ **100**			

Competency Checklist
Procedure 45–7 Perform a Screening for Infectious Mononucleosis

ABHES Curriculum

MA.A.1.10.a   Practice quality control
MA.A.1.10.b(4) Perform selected CLIA-waived tests that assist with diagnosis and treatment: Immunology testing

CAAHEP Core Curriculum

I.P.10   Perform a quality control measure
I.P.11.d   Obtain specimens and perform: CLIA-waived immunology test
I.A.3   Show awareness of a patient's concerns related to the procedure being performed
V.A.4   Explain to a patient the rationale for performance of a procedure
II.P.3   Maintain lab test results using flow sheets.

Task: Following the steps listed in the procedure, determine the presence (or absence) of antibodies to the Epstein-Barr virus (EBV).

Supplies & Conditions: Sterile disposable lancet, disposable gloves, other personal protective equipment (PPE) per laboratory policies, alcohol-prep pads, gauze squares, quality control materials, reagents, black or blue pen, biohazard waste container, and sharps container.

Standards: Provided with all necessary equipment and supplies, follow the steps in the procedure with the instructor observing each step. A maximum of three attempts may be used to complete the task. Students must complete all procedure steps in 15 minutes, with a minimum score of 70 percent. **Scoring:** Determine student's score by dividing points awarded by total points possible and multiplying results by 100.

EVALUATION

Evaluator Signature: _____   Date: _____

Evaluator Comments:

Name: _____ Date: _____ Score: _____

Procedure 45–7 Steps

Start Time: _____ End Time: _____ Total Time: _____

	Steps	Possible Points	First Attempt	Second Attempt	Third Attempt
1.	Assemble the necessary equipment and supplies.	10			
2.	Identify the patient. Explain the procedure to the patient, *including the rationale for performing the procedure. Show awareness of the patient's concerns related to the procedure.*	15			
3.	Wash hands; apply gloves and other PPE as required.	5			
4.	Perform the capillary puncture and collect the blood sample per the manufacturer's directions.	15			
5.	Perform quality control testing on two additional cards, one negative and one positive, while performing testing on the patient's sample.	15			
6.	Record the results of the quality control analyses in the quality control log; do not report patient results if quality control results are not in the acceptable range.	15			
7.	Record the results of the test on the patient's chart.	15			
8.	Check the patient's finger for excessive bleeding and provide clean gauze pad, instructing the patient to apply pressure to the site. Offer a bandage.	5			
9.	Dispose of contaminated sharps in the sharps container and other contaminated materials in the biohazard waste container.	15			
10.	Disinfect work area.	15			
11.	Remove gloves and wash hands.	5			
	Points Awarded / Points Possible	_____/ 130			

Competency Checklist
Procedure 46–1 Perform Electrocardiography

ABHES Curriculum

MA.A.1.4.a	Follow documentation guidelines
MA.A.1.9.d	Assist provider with specialty examination
MA.A.1.9.e	Perform specialty procedures

CAAHEP Core Curriculum

I.P.2.a	Perform electrocardiography
I.P.8	Instruct and prepare a patient for a procedure or a treatment
I.A.1	Incorporate critical thinking skills when performing patient assessment
I.A.2	Incorporate critical thinking skills when performing patient care
V.A.4	Explain to a patient the rationale for performance of a procedure
X.P.3	Document patient care accurately in the medical record

Task: Following the steps listed in the procedure, obtain a graphic representation of the electrical activity of the patient's heart.

Supplies & Conditions: Electrocardiograph; ECG paper; disposable, pre-gelled adhesive electrodes as appropriate for use with patient cable of ECG machine; patient cable and lead wires with clips to attach to electrodes; exam table; pillow; drape sheet or patient gown; gauze squares; alcohol prep-pads; patient's chart or EHR; pen; and disposable razor.

Standards: A maximum of three attempts may be used to complete the task. The time limit for each attempt is 20 minutes, with a minimum score of 70 percent. **Scoring:** Determine student's score by dividing points awarded by total points possible and multiplying results by 100.

EVALUATION

Evaluator Signature: _____ Date: _____

Evaluator Comments:

Name: _____ Date: _____ Score: _____

Procedure 46–1 Steps

Start Time: _____ End Time: _____ Total Time: _____

	Steps	Possible Points	First Attempt	Second Attempt	Third Attempt
1.	Prepare the ECG machine and other equipment.	15			
2.	Wash hands and assemble other equipment.	15			
3.	Introduce yourself, identify the patient, and **explain the rationale for performing the procedure**.	15			
4.	Ask the patient to disrobe from the waist up and remove clothing from the lower legs.	5			
5.	Assist the patient onto the treatment table and cover the patient with a drape sheet.	5			
6.	Place the arm electrodes on the fleshy outer area of the upper arm, with the connectors pointing down. Leg electrodes should be placed on the fleshy inner area of the lower leg near the calf, with connectors pointing up. **Incorporate critical thinking skills when performing patient assessment and care.**	15			
7.	Connect the lead wire tips to the appropriate electrodes by clipping to the tab on the electrodes.	15			
8.	Attach and explain the anatomical positioning of all six disposable adhesive chest electrodes, V_1 through V_6.	15			
9.	Cover patient with the drape.	5			
10.	Enter patient information.	15			
11.	Remind the patient not to move, and press the Auto button.	15			
12.	Tear the tracing off from the machine.	15			
13.	Alert the provider of any complaints or unusual findings. With provider approval, remove the lead wires from the limb electrodes. Remove the electrodes from the patient.	15			
14.	Assist the patient to a sitting position and then down from the table when ready.	5			
15.	Change the table paper and pillow cover and discard used disposables.	15			
16.	Wash hands.	15			
17.	Give the tracing to the provider for interpretation.	15			
18.	Record the appropriate entry on the patient's chart.	15			
	Points Awarded / Points Possible	_____/ **230**			

Competency Checklist
Procedure 46–2 Holter Monitoring

ABHES Curriculum

M.A.A.1.4.a	Follow documentation guidelines
M.A.A.1.9.d	Assist provider with specialty examination
M.A.A.1.9.e	Perform specialty procedures

CAAHEP Core Curriculum

I.P.2.a	Perform electrocardiography
I.P.8	Instruct and prepare a patient for a procedure or a treatment
V.A.4	Explain to a patient the rationale for performance of a procedure
X.P.3	Document patient care accurately in the medical record

Task: Following the steps listed in the procedure, demonstrate the procedure for proper hookup of a Holter monitor to detect chest pain and cardiac arrhythmias, to evaluate chest pain and cardiac status following pacemaker implantation or after an acute myocardial infarction, and to determine correlation of symptoms and activity.

Supplies & Conditions: Holter monitor, disposable razor, alcohol prep-pads, disposable adhesive electrodes, blank magnetic tape or flash memory card, diary for patient, belt or shoulder strap for recorder, patient's chart or EHR, and pen.

Standards: A maximum of three attempts may be used to complete the task. The time limit for each attempt is 20 minutes, with a minimum score of 85 percent. **Scoring:** Determine student's score by dividing points awarded by total points possible and multiplying results by 100.

EVALUATION

Evaluator Signature: _____ Date: _____

Evaluator Comments:

Name: _____ Date: _____ Score: _____

Procedure 46–2 Steps

Start Time: _____ End Time: _____ Total Time: _____

	Steps	Possible Points	First Attempt	Second Attempt	Third Attempt
1.	Wash hands and assemble the equipment and supplies.	15			
2.	Introduce yourself, identify the patient, and *explain the rationale for performing the procedure.*	15			
3.	Ask the patient to remove clothing from the waist up. Assist the patient to sit at the end of the examination table.	10			
4.	Use the razor to remove chest hair if necessary.	15			
5.	Rub each site vigorously with gauze square and apply the electrodes and lead wires carefully, making sure there is good skin contact.	15			
6.	Place the belt around the patient's waist or drape around the patient's shoulder, and advise the patient about proper care of the recorder and precautions.	15			
7.	Instruct the patient to go about his or her routine daily activities but to be sure to note in the diary any symptoms or problems experienced. (Include the time it occurred and how long it lasted.)	15			
8.	Give the patient the diary to take for completion and arrange a return appointment time.	15			
9.	Document in patient's chart. Record the date and time the monitor began on the patient's chart and in the patient's diary and initial.	15			
10.	When the patient comes in for the appointment the next day, assist in disrobing. Remove the electrodes and wires; clean the electrode sites and remove the memory card or cassette from the recorder.	15			
11.	Document that the patient returned with equipment, place the diary in the patient's chart for evaluation by the provider, and initial.	15			
	Points Awarded / Points Possible	_____/ **160**			

Competency Checklist
Procedure 48–1 Prepare a Sterile Field

ABHES Curriculum

MA.A.1.9.a   Practice standard precautions and perform disinfection/sterilization techniques

CAAHEP Core Curriculum

III.P.6   Prepare a sterile field

Task: Following the steps listed in the procedure, set up a sterile tray for a minor surgical procedure, according to the provider's preference.

Supplies & Conditions: Disposable sterile poly-lined drapes or sterile towels (two); Mayo instrument tray or stand positioned above the waist with stem to the right, at right angle to the counter; disposable sterile field drapes; peel-apart sterile package or autoclaved sterile package; sterile cup; container of sterile solution.

Standards: A maximum of three attempts may be used to complete the task. The time limit for each attempt is 15 minutes, with a minimum score of 70 percent. **Scoring:** Determine student's score by dividing points awarded by total points possible and multiplying results by 100.

EVALUATION

Evaluator Signature: _____   Date: _____

Evaluator Comments:

Name: _____ Date: _____ Score: _____

Procedure 48–1 Steps

Start Time: _____ End Time: _____ Total Time: _____

	Steps	Possible Points	First Attempt	Second Attempt	Third Attempt
1.	Adjust the height of the Mayo tray so that the stand is at waist level.	5			
2.	Clean the Mayo tray, starting from the center and working in a circular pattern.	10			
3.	Place a sterile drape package on a clean, dry surface and open the pack, exposing the sterile drape with the corners facing you.	5			
4.	Grasp the sterile drape by the corner and lift up enough to unfold, but do not touch anything.	10			
5.	Grasp the opposite corner, allow the drape to unfold completely, and place the drape over the Mayo tray. Do not reach over the drape.	15			
6.	Properly open a fanfolded or prepackaged sterile pack and allow the contents to drop onto the sterile field.	30			
7.	After all supplies have been dropped onto the sterile field, apply sterile gloves or use sterile transfer forceps to arrange the instruments on the field according to the provider's preference. Pour any solutions as appropriate.	30			
8.	Place a sterile drape over the field to protect it until the procedure begins.	15			
	Points Awarded / Points Possible	_____/ **120**			

Competency Checklist
Procedure 48–2 Hand Washing for Surgical Asepsis

ABHES Curriculum

MA.A.1.9.a   Practice standard precautions and perform disinfection/sterilization techniques

CAAHEP Core Curriculum

III.P.3   Perform handwashing

Task: Following the steps listed in the procedure, perform a surgical scrub.

Supplies & Conditions: Personal protective equipment (eye protection, mask), sterile gloves, surgical scrub agent, surgical sink, sterile dry towel.

Standards: A maximum of three attempts may be used to complete the task. The time limit for each attempt is 10 minutes, with a minimum score of 100 percent. **Scoring:** Determine student's score by dividing points awarded by total points possible and multiplying results by 100.

EVALUATION

Evaluator Signature: _____   Date: _____

Evaluator Comments:

Name: _____ Date: _____ Score: _____

Procedure 48–2 Steps

Start Time: _____ End Time: _____ Total Time: _____

	Steps	Possible Points	First Attempt	Second Attempt	Third Attempt
1.	Don all personal protective equipment needed (eye protection, mask).	15			
2.	Lay out sterile dry towel and gloves.	5			
3.	Remove all hand and wrist jewelry.	5			
4.	Open surgical scrub agent and place in sink area.	5			
5.	Turn on water by using the automatic sensor or foot and knee controls. Wet hands and forearms, keeping hands and fingers pointed upward (during the entire procedure).	15			
6.	Using the nail stick, clean under each nail. Drop the nail stick in the sink and rinse hands.	15			
7.	Wet hands and forearms up to the elbow, starting with the fingers and working down.	15			
8.	Scrub one side (hands and forearms up to the elbow), using the surgical scrub agent, starting from the fingers and working down. Rinse.	15			
9.	Scrub the opposite side, using the same steps as in Step 8. Drop the scrub brush in the sink. Rinse. The entire rinse should take between two and six minutes.	15			
10.	Turn off the water with the automatic sensor or foot and knee control.	15			
11.	Pick up the sterile dry towel, and, keeping it several inches from your body, start at the fingertips of one side and pat dry all the way up to the elbow. Repeat this procedure with the opposite side of the arm, using the opposite side of the towel. Apply sterile gloves.	15			
	Points Awarded / Points Possible	____/ 135			

Competency Checklist
Procedure 48–3 Sterile Gloving

ABHES Curriculum

MA.A.1.9.a   Practice standard precautions and perform disinfection/sterilization techniques

CAAHEP Core Curriculum

III.P.2   Select appropriate barrier/personal protective equipment (PPE)

Task: Following the steps listed in the procedure, demonstrate the correct method of applying sterile gloves.

Supplies & Conditions: Package of sterile gloves of proper size and biohazard waste bag. To comply with standard precautions, gloves and other protective barriers must be worn if there is any possibility of coming in contact with blood or any body fluids.

Standards: A maximum of three attempts may be used to complete the task. The time limit for each attempt is **5 minutes**, with a minimum score of 100 percent. **Scoring:** Determine student's score by dividing points awarded by total points possible and multiplying results by 100.

EVALUATION

Evaluator Signature: _____ Date: _____

Evaluator Comments:

Name: _____ Date: _____ Score: _____

Procedure 48-3 Steps

Start Time: _____ End Time: _____ Total Time: _____

	Steps	Possible Points	First Attempt	Second Attempt	Third Attempt
1.	Remove your wristwatch, rings, and other jewelry from your hands and wrists and perform hand washing for surgical asepsis, following the instructions in Procedure 48–2.	15			
2.	Tear the seal and open the package of sterile gloves as you would open a book. Place it on a clean counter surface with the cuff end toward your body.	5			
3.	Grasp the glove for your dominant hand by the fold of the cuff with the finger and thumb of your nondominant hand. Insert your dominant hand, carefully pulling the glove on with the other hand, keeping the cuff turned back.	15			
4.	Place gloved fingers under the cuff of the other glove and insert your nondominant hand. Put the glove on by pulling on the inside fold of the cuff. Avoid touching the thumb of your dominant hand to the outside cuff of the other glove where it has been contaminated.	15			
5.	Now both hands are gloved and sterile. Place your fingers under the cuffs to smooth the gloves over the wrists and smooth out the fingers for better fit. Check for tears and holes.	15			
6.	Keep your hands above waist level. Do not touch anything other than items in the sterile field.	5			
7.	Remove the gloves by pulling the glove off your dominant hand with your thumb and fingers at the palm. Pull the glove off inside-out.	15			
8.	Slip your ungloved hand into the inside top cuff of the gloved hand and slip the glove off inside-out.	15			
9.	Deposit the gloves in a biohazard waste bag if they came in contact with body fluids or other potentially infectious material.	5			
10.	Wash hands.	5			
	Points Awarded / Points Possible	_____/ 110			

Competency Checklist
Procedure 48–4 Prepare Skin for Minor Surgery

ABHES Curriculum

MA.A.1.9.e   Perform specialty procedures including but not limited to minor surgery, cardiac, respiratory, OB-GYN, neurological, gastroenterology procedures

CAAHEP Core Curriculum

I.A.3   Show awareness of a patient's concerns related to the procedure being performed

V.A.4   Explain to a patient the rationale for performance of a procedure

---

Task: Following the steps listed in the procedure, demonstrate each of the steps required in the skin prep procedure. *In the institutional setting, preparing the forearm might be sufficient; moreover, the shaving process can be demonstrated by using a razor with no blade.*

Supplies & Conditions: Small basin for soap solution, 4 × 4-inch gauze squares (sponges), disposable razor, scissors, antiseptic soap solution, emesis basin for disposables, gooseneck lamp, sterile drape sheet or towels (or fenestrated drape sheet), latex or vinyl gloves, and skin antiseptic. To comply with standard precautions, gloves and other protective barriers must be worn if there is any possibility of coming in contact with blood or any body fluids.

Standards: A maximum of three attempts may be used to complete the task. The time limit for each attempt is 15 minutes, with a minimum score of 70 percent. **Scoring:** Determine student's score by dividing points awarded by total points possible and multiplying results by 100.

EVALUATION

Evaluator Signature: _____ Date: _____

Evaluator Comments:

Name: _____ Date: _____ Score: _____

Procedure 48–4 Steps

Start Time: _____ End Time: _____ Total Time: _____

	Steps	Possible Points	First Attempt	Second Attempt	Third Attempt
1.	Assemble all items and wash and glove hands.	15			
2.	Introduce yourself and identify the patient.	15			
3.	**Explain to the patient the rationale for performance of the procedure**. Answer any questions the patient may have. **Show awareness of the patient's concerns related to the procedure being performed**. Ask the patient to remove necessary clothing, and explain where the patient should put any belongings. Assist the patient if necessary.	15			
4.	Assist the patient into the proper position on the treatment table and drape with a sheet or light bath blanket as directed by the provider.	15			
5.	If appropriate, apply an absorbent towel underneath area to be shaved to catch water. Adjust the gooseneck lamp to light the area.	15			
6.	Place gauze squares in the soapy solution and use one at a time to soap the area to be shaved. After use, discard each in an emesis basin.	15			
7.	When the skin prep site is covered by scalp hair, beard, or pubic hair, use scissors to clip hair in preparation for shaving. Shave hair by placing the razor against the skin at about a 30-degree angle.	15			
8.	Remove all soap and hair from the area by wetting a sterile gauze square with sterile water and wiping the area. Dry the area with sterile gauze squares. Remove absorbent towel if used.	15			
9.	Apply antiseptic solution to the surgery site with a gauze square held by transfer forceps or disposable skin prep kit. Begin application in the center of the site and move outward in a circular motion.	15			
10.	Cover the prepared area with a sterile drape sheet or towel until the provider is ready to begin.	15			
11.	Discard disposable items and return other items to the proper storage area. Remove gloves and wash hands.	15			
12.	Attend to the patient's comfort. Patients are usually apprehensive about even minor surgical procedures. Reassurance at this time is most important.	15			
	Points Awarded / Points Possible	_____ / **180**			

Competency Checklist
Procedure 49–1 Perform Wound Collection

ABHES Curriculum

MA.A.1.9.a   Practice standard precautions and perform disinfection/sterilization techniques
MA.A.1.10.d(3) Perform wound collection procedures

CAAHEP Core Curriculum

I.P.8   Instruct and prepare a patient for a procedure or a treatment
III.P.2   Select appropriate barrier/personal protective equipment (PPE)
V.A.4   Explain to a patient the rationale for performance of a procedure

---

Task: Following the steps listed in the procedure, collect a wound culture while maintaining sterile technique.

Supplies & Conditions: Appropriate personal protective equipment as required by procedure, sterile gloves, sterile instrumentation, culture swab with transport media.

Standards: A maximum of three attempts may be used to complete the task. The time limit for each attempt is 15 minutes, with a minimum score of 70 percent. **Scoring:** Determine student's score by dividing points awarded by total points possible and multiplying results by 100.

EVALUATION

Evaluator Signature: _____   Date: _____

Evaluator Comments:

Name: _____ Date: _____ Score: _____

Procedure 49–1 Steps

Start Time: _____ **End Time:** _____ **Total Time:** _____

	Steps	Possible Points	First Attempt	Second Attempt	Third Attempt
1.	Assemble all necessary supplies.	5			
2.	Introduce yourself and identify the patient.	15			
3.	Verify the provider's orders.	15			
4.	*Explain to the patient the rationale for performance of the procedure.*	15			
5.	Remove the sterile swab from the container.	5			
6.	Collect a sterile specimen. Roll the sterile swab in the exudate.	15			
7.	Insert the sterile swab back into the culture swab container and crush the media ampule.	15			
8.	Record the patient information on the container.	15			
9.	Document the procedure in the patient's chart.	15			
	Points Awarded / Points Possible	____/ **115**			

Competency Checklist
Procedure 49–2 Assist with Minor Surgery

ABHES Curriculum

MA.A.1.9.a	Practice standard precautions and perform disinfection/sterilization techniques
MA.A.1.9.e	Perform specialty procedures including but not limited to minor surgery, cardiac, respiratory, OB-GYN, neurological, gastroenterology
MA.A.1.9.h	Teach self-examination, disease management and health promotion

CAAHEP Core Curriculum

I.P.8	Instruct and prepare a patient for a procedure or a treatment.
I.A.3	Show awareness of a patient's concerns related to the procedure being performed.
III.P.2	Select appropriate barrier/personal protective equipment (PPE)
III.P.7	Perform within a sterile field
V.A.4	Explain to a patient the rationale for performance of a procedure

---

Task: Following the steps listed in the procedure, demonstrate assisting with minor surgery. *In the instructional setting, the instructor will pose as provider and simulate the procedure with a mannequin to check the steps of the procedure.*

Supplies & Conditions: **Basic sterile setup:** needle and syringe; needle holder; appropriate suture, disposable scalpel; thumb forceps; surgical scissors; hemostats; retractor; three or four pairs of vinyl gloves; gauze squares; cotton-tipped applicators; alcohol prep-pads fenestrated sheet or towels; towel clamps; bandages; bandage scissors; tape; ordered anesthetic; antiseptic (small glass container for antiseptic solution); plastic biohazardous sharps container and waste bag (and waste receptacle); patient's EMR; pen; histology request form for laboratory analysis if a biopsy is indicated; Mayo tray table; proper lighting and extra backup sterile setup. ***Note:*** *Some of the equipment might differ according to the procedure performed and provider preference.*

Standards: A maximum of three attempts may be used to complete the task. The time limit for each attempt is 30 minutes, with a minimum score of 70 percent. **Scoring:** Determine student's score by dividing points awarded by total points possible and multiplying results by 100.

EVALUATION
Evaluator Signature: _____ Date: _____
Evaluator Comments:

Name: _____ Date: _____ Score: _____

Procedure 49–2 Steps

Start Time: _____ End Time: _____ Total Time: _____

	Steps	Possible Points	First Attempt	Second Attempt	Third Attempt
1.	Wash hands.	5			
2.	Assemble the appropriate equipment and supplies.	15			
3.	Correctly set up a sterile tray, maintaining sterile technique, and cover it with a sterile drape per office policy.	15			
4.	Introduce yourself and identify the patient.	15			
5.	***Explain to the patient the rationale for performance of the procedure.*** Ensure that the patient has signed the informed consent form. Advise the patient to empty the bladder. If a biopsy is to be taken, complete a lab request form for histology analysis.	15			
6.	When the patient returns, take vital signs and record.	15			
7.	Instruct the patient to disrobe as necessary for the procedure and advise where to place any belongings. Assist the patient if needed. ***Show awareness of the patient's concerns related to the procedure being performed.***	5			
8.	Assist the patient to the treatment table and into the desired position for surgery. Perform a skin prep procedure. Give the patient support and understanding and answer any questions at this time. Drape the patient appropriately.	15			
9.	When the provider is ready to begin the procedure, remove the sterile towel from the prepared sterile setup. Assist the provider by handing sterile gloves (if indicated) and assist with drawing up anesthesia as needed.	15			
10.	If you are to assist with the surgical procedure, wash hands and put on sterile gloves. Hand instruments and other sterile items to the provider as needed; mop excessive blood with gauze sponges as needed.	15			
11.	Assist with collecting any specimen as needed by the provider.	15			
12.	Assist with suturing or stapling the incision as needed by the provider.	15			
13.	When the surgery is completed, assist in (or perform) cleaning and bandaging the surgery site, remove gloves, and wash hands.	15			
14.	Attend to the patient's comfort by helping the patient into a sitting position to regain balance and, when stable, from the table. Assist in dressing if necessary.	5			
15.	Give the patient postoperative instructions.	5			
16.	Document the procedure in the patient's chart.	15			
17.	Put on gloves and clean up the treatment area. Wash hands and restock treatment room.	15			
	Points Awarded / Points Possible	____ / **215**			

Competency Checklist
Procedure 49–3 Assist with Suturing a Laceration

ABHES Curriculum

MA.A.1.9.a	Practice standard precautions and perform disinfection/sterilization techniques
MA.A.1.9.e	Perform specialty procedures including but not limited to minor surgery, cardiac, respiratory, OB-GYN, neurological, gastroenterology
MA.A.1.9.h	Teach self-examination, disease management and health promotion

CAAHEP Core Curriculum

I.P.8	Instruct and prepare a patient for a procedure or a treatment
I.A.3	Show awareness of a patient's concerns related to the procedure being performed
III.P.2	Select appropriate barrier/personal protective equipment (PPE)
III.P.7	Perform within a sterile field
V.A.4	Explain to a patient the rationale for performance of a procedure

---

Task: Demonstrate each of the steps required in the procedure to assist with suturing a laceration while maintaining sterile technique. *In the instructional setting, the instructor will pose as provider and simulate the procedure with a mannequin to check the steps of the procedure.*

Supplies & Conditions: Alcohol prep-pads, cotton balls, PPE, biohazard bag, gauze squares, bandages and tape, bandage scissors, antiseptic, ordered anesthetic, appropriate tetanus vaccine (if needed), patient's EMR, pen. **Sterile items:** swabs, needle and syringe, vinyl gloves, fenestrated drape, ordered suture material, gauze squares, hemostats, needle holder, scissors, sharps container.

Standards: A maximum of three attempts may be used to complete the task. The time limit for each attempt is 30 minutes, with a minimum score of 70 percent. **Scoring:** Determine student's score by dividing points awarded by total points possible and multiplying results by 100.

EVALUATION

Evaluator Signature: _____   Date: _____

Evaluator Comments:

Name: _____ Date: _____ Score: _____

Procedure 49–3 Steps

Start Time: _____ End Time: _____ Total Time: _____

	Steps	Possible Points	First Attempt	Second Attempt	Third Attempt
1.	Wash hands and assemble all needed items, using sterile technique.	15			
2.	Introduce yourself and identify the patient.	15			
3.	**Explain to the patient the rationale for performance of the procedure.** Advise the patient to empty the bladder.	15			
4.	When the patient returns, take and record vital signs.	15			
5.	**Show awareness of the patient's concerns related to the procedure being performed.** Ask the patient to remove necessary clothing. Explain where the patient should place any belongings. Assist the patient if needed. Allow privacy if needed.	5			
6.	Assist the patient into the appropriate position for skin prep of the wound. Proceed with the steps for preparing skin for minor surgery and then drape the patient appropriately.	15			
7.	Put on PPE and sterile gloves. Arrange the instruments and other sterile items in the order the provider will use them. Remove gloves and wash hands.	15			
8.	When the provider is ready to begin the suturing procedure, remove the sterile towel from the prepared sterile setup. Assist the provider by handing sterile gloves (if indicated) and assist with drawing up anesthesia as needed.	15			
9.	If you assist with the suturing procedure, wash hands and put on sterile gloves. Hand instruments and other sterile items to the provider as needed; absorb excessive blood from the wound with sterile gauze as needed.	15			
10.	When the wound has been closed with sutures, assist with (or perform) cleaning and bandaging the site per the provider's orders. When bandaging is done, remove and properly dispose of gloves and wash hands.	15			
11.	Administer appropriate tetanus vaccine if ordered by provider.	15			
12.	Tend to the patient's needs and comfort. Assist with sitting up, getting dressed, and helping from the treatment table as needed.	5			
13.	Give the patient postoperative instructions.	5			
14.	Document the procedure in the patient's chart.	15			
15.	Put on gloves and clean up the treatment area. Wash hands and restock treatment room.	15			
	Points Awarded / Points Possible	____/ 195			

Competency Checklist
Procedure 49–4 Remove Sutures or Staples

ABHES Curriculum

MA.A.1.9.a	Practice standard precautions and perform disinfection/sterilization techniques
MA.A.1.9.e	Perform specialty procedures including but not limited to minor surgery, cardiac, respiratory, OB-GYN, neurological, gastroenterology
MA.A.1.9.h	Teach self-examination, disease management and health promotion

CAAHEP Core Curriculum

I.P.8	Instruct and prepare a patient for a procedure or a treatment
I.A.3	Show awareness of a patient's concerns related to the procedure being performed
III.P.2	Select appropriate barrier/personal protective equipment (PPE)
III.P.7	Perform within a sterile field
III.P.9	Perform dressing change
V.A.4	Explain to a patient the rationale for performance of a procedure

---

Task:	Demonstrate the steps required to remove sutures or staples (using a mannequin or model as the patient).
Supplies & Conditions:	**Sterile items:** thumb forceps, suture-removal scissors (or staple extractor), gauze squares, vinyl gloves, cotton-tipped applicators, butterfly or Steri-Strip closures; **Skin care documentation:** antiseptic solution, hydrogen peroxide, tincture of benzoin, basin with warm soapy water, bandages, tape, towels, biohazard waste bag, sharps container, bandage scissors, patient's chart, and pen
Standards:	A maximum of three attempts may be used to complete the task. The time limit for each attempt is 30 minutes, with a minimum score of 70 percent. **Scoring:** Determine student's score by dividing points awarded by total points possible and multiplying results by 100.

EVALUATION

Evaluator Signature: _____ Date: _____

Evaluator Comments:

Name: _____ Date: _____ Score: _____

Procedure 49–4 Steps

Start Time: _____ End Time: _____ Total Time: _____

	Steps	Possible Points	First Attempt	Second Attempt	Third Attempt
1.	Wash hands and assemble all needed items, using sterile technique.	15			
2.	Introduce yourself and identify the patient.	15			
3.	*Explain to the patient the rationale for performance of the procedure.* Answer any questions. Ask the patient about the healing condition of the incision or laceration, take vital signs, and record them in the patient's chart.	15			
4.	*Show awareness of the patient's concerns related to the procedure being performed.* Ask the patient to remove necessary clothing for inspection of the healing incision. Explain where the patient should place any belongings. Assist the patient if needed. Allow privacy if needed.	5			
5.	Assist the patient to the treatment table and into the required position and drape appropriately.	5			
6.	Put on gloves and remove the bandage. Clean the incision with antiseptic solution, using cotton-tipped applicators. Advise the provider that the incision site is ready.	15			
7.	After the provider orders suture or staple removal, open a sterile package containing the necessary instruments on the Mayo tray and proceed.	10			
For Suture Removal:					
8.	Grasp the knot of the suture material with thumb forceps and gently but firmly pull up, making just enough space to place the suture removal scissors to clip the suture as close to the skin as possible. Pull the suture with the forceps (back) toward the healing incision so that no stress is put on it. Continue until all are removed. Count the number of sutures removed and compare with the number in the patient's chart.	15			
For Skin Staples:					
9.	If skin staples are to be removed, place the sterile staple extractor under a staple (one at a time) and squeeze the handles of the extractor completely closed. Lift the staple away from the skin and dispose in a sharps container. Continue until all are removed.	15			
10.	Apply antiseptic solution to the site and allow it to air-dry. Apply Steri-Strips or a butterfly closure if necessary for support during the healing process and bandage.	15			
11.	Remove gloves and wash hands.	5			
12.	Give the patient postoperative instructions.	5			
13.	Document the procedure in the patient's chart.	15			
14.	Put on gloves and clean up the treatment area. Wash hands and restock treatment room.	15			
	Points Awarded / Points Possible	_____/ **165**			

646

Competency Checklist
Procedure 50–1 Use the PDR or Other Drug Reference to Find Medication Information

ABHES Curriculum

MA.A.1.6.d   Properly utilize Physician's Desk Reference (PDR), drug handbook and other drug references to identify a drug's classification, usual dosage, usual side effects, and contraindications

---

Task:	Following the steps listed in the procedure, locate specific information on medications in a PDR or other drug reference.
Supplies & Conditions:	PDR or other drug reference.
Standards:	A maximum of three attempts may be used to complete the task. The time limit for each attempt is 10 minutes, with a minimum score of 100 percent. **Scoring:** Determine student's score by dividing points awarded by total points possible and multiplying results by 100.
Forms:	Procedure 50–1 Scenario (optional). Procedure scenario is included in the Instructor's Manual. Instructor may provide other medications to be used.

EVALUATION

Evaluator Signature: _____   Date: _____

Evaluator Comments:

Name: _____ Date: _____ Score: _____

Procedure 50–1 Steps

Start Time: _____ End Time: _____ Total Time: _____

	Steps	Possible Points	First Attempt	Second Attempt	Third Attempt
1.	Obtain name of ordered medication. Determine whether generic or trade name.	15			
2.	Note appearance of brand-name medication.	15			
3.	Locate prescribing information. Confirm order matches drug name.	15			
4.	Verify accuracy of order and medication.	15			
	Points Awarded / Points Possible	____/ 60			

Competency Checklist
Procedure 51–1 Calculate Proper Dosages of Medication for Administration

ABHES Curriculum

MA.A.1.6.b   Demonstrate accurate occupational math and metric conversions for proper medication administration

CAAHEP Core Curriculum

II.P.1   Calculate proper dosages of medication for administration

---

Task:	Perform calculation problems to reinforce your knowledge and prepare you for calculating dosages correctly and safely for patient administration.
Supplies & Conditions:	Calculation problems or access to online medication dosage administration site.
Standards:	A maximum of three attempts may be used to complete the task. The time limit for each attempt is 10 minutes, with a minimum score of 100 percent. **Scoring:** Determine student's score by dividing points awarded by total points possible and multiplying results by 100.

EVALUATION

Evaluator Signature: _____   Date: _____

Evaluator Comments:

Name: _____ Date: _____ Score: _____

Procedure 51–1 Steps

Start Time: _____ **End Time:** _____ **Total Time:** _____

	Steps	Possible Points	First Attempt	Second Attempt	Third Attempt
1.	Obtain a variety of calculation problems from your instructor or use an online medical dosage website.	15			
2.	Complete the problems and verify your answers with your instructor.	15			
	Points Awarded / Points Possible	_____/ **30**			

Competency Checklist
Procedure 52–1 Prepare a Prescription

ABHES Curriculum

MA.A.1.4.a	Follow documentation guidelines
MA.A.1.4.f (2)	Describe what procedures can and cannot be delegated to the medical assistant and by whom within various employment settings
MA.A.1.6.c	Prescriptions: (1) Identify parts of prescriptions, (2) Identify appropriate abbreviations that are accepted in prescription writing, (3) Comply with legal aspects of creating prescriptions, including federal and state laws
MA.A.1.6.e	Comply with federal, state, and local health laws and regulations

CAAHEP Core Curriculum

X.P.3	Document patient care accurately in the medical record

Task:	Prepare a prescription according to the provider's direction.
Supplies & Conditions:	Patient's chart/EHR, prescription pad, or electronic prescription.
Standards:	A maximum of three attempts may be used to complete the task. The time limit for each attempt is 10 minutes, with a minimum score of 100 percent. **Scoring:** Determine student's score by dividing points awarded by total points possible and multiplying results by 100.
Forms:	Procedure 52–1 Scenario with Procedure 52–1 Form. Procedure forms can be downloaded from the Student Companion website; Procedure scenarios are included in the Instructor's Manual.

EVALUATION

Evaluator Signature: _____ Date: _____

Evaluator Comments:

651

Name: _____ Date: _____ Score: _____

Procedure 52–1 Steps

Start Time: _____ **End Time:** _____ **Total Time:** _____

	Steps	Possible Points	First Attempt	Second Attempt	Third Attempt
1.	Obtain the order from the chart.	15			
2.	Compare patient identifiers.	15			
3.	Fill in prescription fields on the blank prescription pad or in the EHR.	15			
4.	Compare the completed prescription to the order.	15			
5.	Obtain prescriber's signature.	15			
6.	Compare the completed prescription to the order—again.	15			
7.	Present the completed prescription to the patient if paper copy. If using the EHR system, the provider will send it electronically to the pharmacy upon completion, or print for signature if warranted.	15			
8.	Document correctly in the patient's chart.	15			
	Points Awarded / Points Possible	____/ **120**			

Competency Checklist
Procedure 52–2 Record a Medication Entry in the Patient's Chart

ABHES Curriculum

MA.A.1.4.a   Follow documentation guidelines

CAAHEP Core Curriculum

I.P.4   Verify the rules of medication administration: (a) right patient, (b) right medication, (c) right dose, (d) right route, (e) right time, and (f) right documentation

X.P.3   Document patient care accurately in the medical record

---

Task: Record a medication entry in the patient's chart.

Supplies & Conditions: Patient medical record/EHR, black or blue pen.

Standards: A maximum of three attempts may be used to complete the task. The time limit for each attempt is 10 minutes, with a minimum score of 100 percent. **Scoring:** Determine student's score by dividing points awarded by total points possible and multiplying results by 100.

Forms: Procedure 52–2 Scenario. Procedure scenarios are included in the Instructor's Manual.

EVALUATION

Evaluator Signature: _____   Date: _____

Evaluator Comments:

Procedure 52–2 Steps

Start Time: _____   **End Time:** _____   **Total Time:** _____

	Steps	Possible Points	First Attempt	Second Attempt	Third Attempt
1.	Obtain the completed medication order and the medication record if separate documents.	15			
2.	Prepare and administer medication, following the Seven Rights.	15			
3.	Record the information in the medication record.	15			
4.	Sign off the order on the medication order sheet or chart.	15			
	Points Awarded / Points Possible	_____/ 60			

Competency Checklist
Procedure 52–3 Prepare and Administer Oral Medication

ABHES Curriculum

MA.A.1.4.a	Follow documentation guidelines
MA.A.1.9.f	Prepare and administer oral and parenteral medications and monitor intravenous (IV) infusions

CAAHEP Core Curriculum

I.P.4	Verify the rules of medication administration: (a) right patient, (b) right medication, (c) right dose, (d) right route, (e) right time, and (f) right documentation
I.P.6	Administer oral medications
I.A.1	Incorporate critical thinking skills when performing patient assessment
I.A.2	Incorporate critical thinking skills when performing patient care
I.A.3	Show awareness of a patient's concerns related to the procedure being performed
II.P.1	Calculate proper dosages of medication for administration
V.A.4	Explain to a patient the rationale for performance of a procedure
X.P.3	Document patient care accurately in the medical record

Task:	Measure and administer the ordered dose of oral medication.
Supplies & Conditions:	Medication order, medicine cup (disposable), disposable paper cup filled with water, medicine tray.
Standards:	A maximum of three attempts may be used to complete the task. The time limit for each attempt is 15 minutes, with a minimum score of 100 percent. **Scoring:** Determine student's score by dividing points awarded by total points possible and multiplying results by 100.

EVALUATION

Evaluator Signature: _____ Date: _____

Evaluator Comments:

Name: _____ Date: _____ Score: _____

Procedure 52–3 Steps

Start Time: _____ End Time: _____ Total Time: _____

	Steps	Possible Points	First Attempt	Second Attempt	Third Attempt
1.	Obtain the medication from the storage area. Read the label carefully, comparing it with the order. Follow the Seven Rights.	15			
2.	Calculate the dosage, if necessary, and wash hands.	15			
3.	Prepare the medication: a. Take the bottle cap off and place it inside-up on counter. b. If in pill or capsule form, pour the desired amount into the cap. Then pour the medication into a medicine cup. c. If in liquid form, pour it directly into a measuring device to the calibrated line of the ordered amount. Syrup or liquid medications may also be given in disposable plastic measuring spoons or droppers.	15			
4.	Place the medication container on a tray and the ordered dose in a medicine cup. Place a cup of water on the tray for the patient to drink with the medicine, if allowed. Read the label a second time and compare with the order.	15			
5.	Take the medication tray to the patient and confirm the patient's identity. Read the label a third time and compare it to the order prior to administering.	15			
6.	*Explain to a patient the rationale for performance of the procedure, showing awareness of the patient's concerns related to the procedure being performed.*	15			
7.	*Incorporate critical thinking skills when performing patient care.* Give the patient the medication and offer the cup of water, if allowed.	15			
8.	Discard any disposables and return the medication container and tray to the proper storage area. Read the label a fourth time.	15			
9.	Record the information in the medication record. Sign off the order on the medication order sheet or chart.	15			
	Points Awarded / Points Possible	_____/ **135**			

Competency Checklist
Procedure 52–4 Administer Eyedrops

ABHES Curriculum

MA.A.1.4.a	Follow documentation guidelines
MA.A.1.9.f	Prepare and administer oral and parenteral medications and monitor intravenous (IV) infusions

CAAHEP Core Curriculum

I.P.7	Administer parenteral (excluding IV) medications
I.A.1	Incorporate critical thinking skills when performing patient assessment
I.A.2	Incorporate critical thinking skills when performing patient care
I.A.3	Show awareness of a patient's concerns related to the procedure being performed
V.A.4	Explain to a patient the rationale for performance of a procedure
X.P.3	Document patient care accurately in the medical record

Task:	Instill medication into the eye without introducing pathogens.
Supplies & Conditions:	Latex or vinyl gloves, medication with dropper, tissue.
Standards:	A maximum of three attempts may be used to complete the task. The time limit for each attempt is 10 minutes, with a minimum score of 100 percent. **Scoring:** Determine student's score by dividing points awarded by total points possible and multiplying results by 100.

EVALUATION

Evaluator Signature: _____   Date: _____

Evaluator Comments:

Name: _____ Date: _____ Score: _____

Procedure 52–4 Steps

Start Time: _____ End Time: _____ Total Time: _____

	Steps	Possible Points	First Attempt	Second Attempt	Third Attempt
1.	Wash hands; apply clean gloves.	15			
2.	*Explain to the patient the rationale for performance of the procedure, showing awareness of the patient's concerns related to the procedure being performed.*	15			
3.	*Incorporate critical thinking skills when performing patient assessment.* Ask the patient whether he or she is allergic to any medications.	15			
4.	*Incorporate critical thinking skills when performing patient care.* Have the patient sit, leaning back slightly in the chair, or lie supine on exam table.	15			
5.	Tilt head slightly toward the side drops will be placed. Place gentle traction on the skin slightly below the lower eyelid and place prescribed number of drops, one at a time, in the inner canthus of the eye followed by gentle pressure. Repeat for each drop administered. Do not allow patient to rub, only dab, drops with a clean tissue that run onto the skin.	15			
6.	Document medication, time, date, and patient response to medication in the chart.	15			
	Points Awarded / Points Possible	_____/ 90			

Competency Checklist
Procedure 52–5 Instill Drops in the Ears

ABHES Curriculum

MA.A.1.4.a	Follow documentation guidelines
MA.A.1.9.f	Prepare and administer oral and parenteral medications and monitor intravenous (IV) infusions

CAAHEP Core Curriculum

I.P.7	Administer parenteral (excluding IV) medications
I.A.1	Incorporate critical thinking skills when performing patient assessment
I.A.2	Incorporate critical thinking skills when performing patient care
I.A.3	Show awareness of a patient's concerns related to the procedure being performed
V.A.4	Explain to a patient the rationale for performance of a procedure
X.P.3	Document patient care accurately in the medical record

Task: Introduce appropriate medications into the ear canal.

Supplies & Conditions: Latex or vinyl gloves, medication with dropper, tissue for dabbing external leakage of excess.

Standards: A maximum of three attempts may be used to complete the task. The time limit for each attempt is 10 minutes, with a minimum score of 100 percent. **Scoring:** Determine student's score by dividing points awarded by total points possible and multiplying results by 100.

EVALUATION

Evaluator Signature: _____ Date: _____

Evaluator Comments:

Name: _____ Date: _____ Score: _____

Procedure 52–5 Steps

Start Time: _____ End Time: _____ Total Time: _____

	Steps	Possible Points	First Attempt	Second Attempt	Third Attempt
1.	Wash hands; apply clean gloves.	15			
2.	*Explain to the patient the rationale for performance of the procedure, showing awareness of the patient's concerns related to the procedure being performed.*	15			
3.	*Incorporate critical thinking skills when performing patient assessment.* Ask the patient whether he or she is allergic to any medications.	15			
4.	*Incorporate critical thinking skills when performing patient care.* Have the patient sit, leaning back slightly in the chair or on the opposite side comfortably positioned on the exam table.	15			
5.	Have the patient turn the head so that the affected ear is facing upward. Place *gentle* upward traction on the earlobe to straighten the external canal (downward traction is used in patients under the age of three).	15			
6.	Drop prescribed number of drops into ear canal.	15			
7.	Have patient remain in position for a few minutes or as indicated by prescriber.	15			
8.	Document medication, time, date, and patient response to medication in the chart.	15			
	Points Awarded / Points Possible	_____/ **120**			

Competency Checklist
Procedure 52–6 Administer Rectal Medication

ABHES Curriculum

MA.A.1.4.a	Follow documentation guidelines
MA.A.1.9.f	Prepare and administer oral and parenteral medications and monitor intravenous (IV) infusions

CAAHEP Core Curriculum

I.P.7	Administer parenteral (excluding IV) medications
I.A.1	Incorporate critical thinking skills when performing patient assessment
I.A.2	Incorporate critical thinking skills when performing patient care
I.A.3	Show awareness of a patient's concerns related to the procedure being performed
V.A.4	Explain to a patient the rationale for performance of a procedure
X.P.3	Document patient care accurately in the medical record

Task:	Deliver medication suppository rectally.
Supplies & Conditions:	Latex or vinyl gloves, drape or sheet for protecting patient dignity, medication suppository with or without applicator as appropriate.
Standards:	A maximum of three attempts may be used to complete the task. The time limit for each attempt is 10 minutes, with a minimum score of 100 percent. **Scoring:** Determine student's score by dividing points awarded by total points possible and multiplying results by 100.

EVALUATION

Evaluator Signature: _____ Date: _____

Evaluator Comments:

661

Name: _____ Date: _____ Score: _____

Procedure 52–6 Steps

Start Time: _____ End Time: _____ Total Time: _____

	Steps	Possible Points	First Attempt	Second Attempt	Third Attempt
1.	Wash hands; apply clean gloves.	15			
2.	*Explain to the patient the rationale for the performance of the procedure, showing awareness of the patient's concerns related to the procedure being performed.*	15			
3.	*Incorporate critical thinking skills when performing patient assessment.* Ask the patient whether he or she is allergic to any medications.	15			
4.	*Incorporate critical thinking skills when performing patient care.* Position patient on left side, as tolerated, with knees drawn comfortably toward chest.	15			
5.	Remove foil wrapper on medication and insert into rectum just past the anal sphincter, holding gentle manual pressure against the suppository for a few seconds to avoid involuntary expulsion from the rectum. If medication is supplied as a cream with applicator, follow specific package directions for use, withdrawing accurate amount of medication into applicator for delivery. Advise patient to remain in the same position for a few minutes following administration.	15			
6.	Document medication, time, date, and patient response to medication in the chart.	15			
	Points Awarded / Points Possible	_____/ 90			

Competency Checklist
Procedure 53–1 Withdraw Medication from an Ampule

ABHES Curriculum

MA.A.1.9.f   Prepare and administer oral and parenteral medications and monitor intravenous (IV) infusions

CAAHEP Core Curriculum

I.P.4   Verify the rules of medication administration: (a) right patient, (b) right medication, (c) right dose, (d) right route, (e) right time, and (f) right documentation
I.A.1   Incorporate critical thinking skills when performing patient assessment
I.A.2   Incorporate critical thinking skills when performing patient care
III.P.10   Demonstrate proper disposal of biohazardous material: (a) sharps and (b) regulated waste

---

Task: To demonstrate steps required to prepare medication for injection from an ampule.

Supplies & Conditions: Medication ampule, medication tray, disposable ampule breaker or sterile gauze pads, sterile safety needle and syringe, filter needle, disposable latex or vinyl gloves, alcohol prep-pad.

Standards: A maximum of three attempts may be used to complete the task. The time limit for each attempt is 5 minutes, with a minimum score of 100 percent. **Scoring:** Determine student's score by dividing points awarded by total points possible and multiplying results by 100.

EVALUATION

Evaluator Signature: _____   Date: _____

Evaluator Comments:

Name: _____ Date: _____ Score: _____

Procedure 53–1 Steps

Start Time: _____   End Time: _____   Total Time: _____

	Steps	Possible Points	First Attempt	Second Attempt	Third Attempt
1.	Compare the label of the ampule with all the elements of the ordered medication in the chart. *Incorporating critical thinking skills when performing patient assessment and care*, calculate desired dose to be given, if applicable. Wash hands and apply gloves.	15			
2.	Clean the neck of the ampule with an alcohol prep-pad.	15			
3.	Tap the ampule to release any medication into the main part of the ampule; using sterile gauze or ampule breaker, snap off the tip of the ampule and discard in a sharps container.	15			
4.	Use a syringe fitted with a filter needle to withdraw the entire contents of the ampule into the syringe, keeping the tip of the needle below the fluid line.	15			
5.	Cap the filter needle using the one-handed scoop method and remove; discard in sharps container.	15			
6.	Attach a clean needle of appropriate gauge for the injection. Expel any air bubbles and then adjust the amount of medication in the syringe to that of the ordered dose.	15			
7.	Discard the ampule in a sharps container.	10			
	Points Awarded / Points Possible	_____/ **100**			

Competency Checklist
Procedure 53–2 Prepare Medication from a Multi- or Single-Dose Vial

ABHES Curriculum

MA.A.1.9.f   Prepare and administer oral and parenteral medications and monitor intravenous (IV) infusions

CAAHEP Core Curriculum

I.P.4   Verify the rules of medication administration: (a) right patient, (b) right medication, (c) right dose, (d) right route, (e) right time, and (f) right documentation

III.P.10   Demonstrate proper disposal of biohazardous material: (a) sharps and (b) regulated waste

---

Task:	To demonstrate steps required to prepare medication for injection from a multi- or single-dose vial.
Supplies & Conditions:	Multiple- and single-dose vials (simulation practice vials, or sterile water), alcohol-prep pads, sterile safety needle and syringe, medication tray, disposable latex or vinyl gloves, sharps container.
Standards:	A maximum of three attempts may be used to complete the task. The time limit for each attempt is 5 minutes, with a minimum score of 100 percent. **Scoring:** Determine student's score by dividing points awarded by total points possible and multiplying results by 100.

EVALUATION

Evaluator Signature: _____   Date: _____

Evaluator Comments:

Name: _____ Date: _____ Score: _____

Procedure 53–2 Steps

Start Time: _____ End Time: _____ Total Time: _____

	Steps	Possible Points	First Attempt	Second Attempt	Third Attempt
1.	Wash hands and apply gloves. Compare the vial of medication to the medication order and clean the top of the vial with an alcohol prep-pad.	5			
2.	Attach a safety needle to the syringe. Holding the syringe pointed upward, pull back on the plunger and take a volume of air into the syringe equal to the order of medication.	15			
3.	Insert the needle into the vial stopper. Invert the vial and needle and syringe unit.	15			
4.	Gently inject the air into the vial above the fluid level.	15			
5.	Withdraw the desired amount of medication into the syringe, keeping the needle below the fluid line.	15			
6.	Gently tap the barrel of the syringe to allow air bubbles to travel to the top of the syringe, and push them back in the vial.	15			
7.	Close the safety cover on the needle and remove. Discard in sharps container.	10			
8.	Using aseptic technique, attach a new safety needle of the appropriate gauge and length for the injection being given onto the tip of the syringe.	15			
9.	Label the syringe with its contents and place it on a medication tray along with the medication vial and medication order.	15			
	Points Awarded / Points Possible	_____/ 120			

Name: _____ Date: _____ Score: _____

Competency Checklist
Procedure 53–3 Reconstitute a Powder Medication

ABHES Curriculum

MA.A.1.9.f   Prepare and administer oral and parenteral medications and monitor intravenous (IV) infusions

CAAHEP Core Curriculum

I.P.4   Verify the rules of medication administration: (a) right patient. (b) right medication, (c) right dose, (d) right route, (e) right time, and (f) right documentation

III.P.10   Demonstrate proper disposal of biohazardous material: (a) sharps and (b) regulated waste

---

Task: To add a diluent to a powdered medication in a vial, preparing it for administration.

Supplies & Conditions: Powdered medication, diluent, two sterile safety needles and syringes, alcohol wipes, disposable latex or vinyl gloves, sharps container.

Standards: A maximum of three attempts may be used to complete the task. The time limit for each attempt is 5 minutes, with a minimum score of 100 percent. **Scoring:** Determine student's score by dividing points awarded by total points possible and multiplying results by 100.

EVALUATION

Evaluator Signature: _____ Date: _____

Evaluator Comments:

Name: _____ Date: _____ Score: _____

Procedure 53–3 Steps

Start Time: _____ End Time: _____ Total Time: _____

	Steps	Possible Points	First Attempt	Second Attempt	Third Attempt
1.	Assemble the safety needle and syringe units; wash hands and apply gloves.	15			
2.	Remove the tops from the diluent and powder medication vials and clean with alcohol wipes.	15			
3.	Insert the needle through the rubber stopper of the vial of diluent. The syringe should have an amount of air in it equal to the amount of diluent to be withdrawn. Invert the vial and needle and syringe unit, and withdraw the appropriate amount of diluent to be added to the powdered medication.	15			
4.	Insert the needle into the rubber stopper of the powdered medication and inject the diluent.	15			
5.	Withdraw the needle from the top of the vial, activate the safety device, and remove it from the syringe. Discard it in a sharps container.	15			
6.	Gently roll the vial of medication between your hands to mix it thoroughly.	15			
7.	Label the vial of prepared medication.	15			
8.	Prepare the syringe with a second sterile needle, and properly withdraw the medication for administration. Label the syringe or place a card with medication information on the medication tray.	15			
9.	Discard gloves and wash hands.	15			
	Points Awarded / Points Possible	_____/ 135			

Competency Checklist
Procedure 53–4 Administer an Intradermal Injection

ABHES Curriculum

MA.A.1.4.a	Follow documentation guidelines
MA.A.1.9.a	Practice standard precautions and perform disinfection/sterilization techniques
MA.A.1.9.f	Prepare and administer oral and parenteral medications and monitor intravenous (IV) infusions

CAAHEP Core Curriculum

I.P.4	Verify the rules of medication administration: (a) right patient, (b) right medication, (c) right dose, (d) right route, (e) right time, and (f) right documentation
I.P.5	Select proper sites for administering parenteral medication
I.P.7	Administer parenteral (excluding IV) medications
I.A.1	Incorporate critical thinking skills when performing patient assessment
I.A.2	Incorporate critical thinking skills when performing patient care
I.A.3	Show awareness of a patient's concerns related to the procedure being performed
III.P.2	Select appropriate barrier/personal protective equipment (PPE)
III.P.3	Perform handwashing
V.A.4	Explain to a patient the rationale for performance of a procedure
X.P.3	Document patient care accurately in the medical record
III.P.10	Demonstrate proper disposal of biohazardous material: (a) sharps and (b) regulated waste

---

Task:	To inject liquid solutions of 0.01 mL and 0.05 mL into the dermal layer of tissue for allergy and immunity testing of patients.
Supplies & Conditions:	Medication (sterile water for injection in vial), gauze pads, sterile safety needle (usually $\frac{3}{8}$ to $\frac{5}{8}$ inch, 25G to 27G) and syringe, medication tray, alcohol-prep pads, patient's chart/EHR, pen, latex or vinyl gloves.
Standards:	A maximum of three attempts may be used to complete the task. The time limit for each attempt is 15 minutes, with a minimum score of 100 percent. **Scoring:** Determine student's score by dividing points awarded by total points possible and multiplying results by 100.

EVALUATION

Evaluator Signature: _____   Date: _____

Evaluator Comments:

Name: _____ Date: _____ Score: _____

Procedure 53–4 Steps

Start Time: _____   End Time: _____   Total Time: _____

	Steps	Possible Points	First Attempt	Second Attempt	Third Attempt
1.	Wash and glove hands.	15			
2.	Prepare the syringe with the ordered amount of medication, verifying the ordered doses or dosages prior to patient administration.	15			
3.	Identify the patient and **explain the rationale for performance of the procedure**, using language the patient understands. Compare the medication order (again) with the patient's chart.	15			
4.	Allow the patient to ask questions, **and show awareness of any patient concerns related to the procedure being performed**. Respond to the patient as appropriate.	15			
5.	**Incorporate critical thinking skills when performing patient assessment and care.** Select and prepare the injection site with an alcohol-prep pad. Allow the alcohol to air-dry.	15			
6.	Hold the patient's skin taut on the anterior forearm between your thumb and fingers and insert the needle at a 10- to 15-degree angle of insertion. Slowly expel the medication from the syringe by depressing the plunger, ensuring the medication forms a wheal.	15			
7.	Remove the needle quickly by the same angle of injection and apply the safety. Do not massage the injection site.	15			
8.	Give the patient instructions on when to come back to get the test read as ordered, and answer any questions.	15			
9.	Do not cover the site.	15			
10.	Discard disposable items and gloves into a biohazard waste bag. Place the entire syringe and needle into the biohazard sharps container. Return the medication and tray to the proper storage area.	15			
11.	Document the procedure in the patient's chart or medication log.	15			
	Points Awarded / Points Possible	____/ 165			

Competency Checklist
Procedure 53–5 Administer a Subcutaneous Injection

ABHES Curriculum

MA.A.1.4.a	Follow documentation guidelines
MA.A.1.9.a	Practice standard precautions and perform disinfection/sterilization techniques
MA.A.1.9.f	Prepare and administer oral and parenteral medications and monitor intravenous (IV) infusions

CAAHEP Core Curriculum

I.P.4	Verify the rules of medication administration: (a) right patient, (b) right medication, (c) right dose, (d) right route, (e) right time, and (f) right documentation
I.P.5	Select proper sites for administering parenteral medication
I.P.7	Administer parenteral (excluding IV) medications
I.A.1	Incorporate critical thinking skills when performing patient assessment
I.A.2	Incorporate critical thinking skills when performing patient care
I.A.3	Show awareness of a patient's concerns related to the procedure being performed
III.P.2	Select appropriate barrier/personal protective equipment (PPE)
III.P.3	Perform handwashing
V.A.4	Explain to a patient the rationale for performance of a procedure
X.P.3	Document patient care accurately in the medical record
III.P.10	Demonstrate proper disposal of biohazardous material: (a) sharps and (b) regulated waste

---

Task:	To inject aqueous solutions of 0.5 to 2.0 mL into the subcutaneous tissue.
Supplies & Conditions:	Medication (sterile water for injection in vial or ampule), alcohol-prep pads, adhesive bandage or hypoallergenic tape, sterile safety needle (usually ½ to ⅝ inch, 25G) and syringe, latex or vinyl gloves.
Standards:	A maximum of three attempts may be used to complete the task. The time limit for each attempt is 15 minutes, with a minimum score of 100 percent. **Scoring:** Determine student's score by dividing points awarded by total points possible and multiplying results by 100.

EVALUATION

Evaluator Signature: _____ Date: _____

Evaluator Comments:

Name: _____   Date: _____   Score: _____

Procedure 53–5 Steps

Start Time: _____   End Time: _____   Total Time: _____

	Steps	Possible Points	First Attempt	Second Attempt	Third Attempt
1.	Wash and glove hands.	15			
2.	Prepare the syringe with the ordered amount of medication, verifying all ordered doses or dosages prior to administration.	15			
3.	Identify the patient and *explain the rationale for performance of the procedure*, using language the patient understands. Ask patient to remove clothes, if necessary.	15			
4.	Allow the patient to ask questions, *and show awareness of any patient concerns related to the procedure being performed*. Respond to the patient as appropriate.	15			
5.	*Incorporate critical thinking skills when performing patient assessment and care.* Select and prepare the injection site with an alcohol-prep pad. Allow the alcohol to air-dry.	15			
6.	Pinch the patient's skin between the thumb and finger of one hand and, with the other hand, hold the syringe securely. Insert the needle at a 45-degree angle with a steady penetration. Let go of the skin.	15			
7.	With one hand, hold the barrel of the syringe while pulling back on the plunger slightly with the other hand to make sure a blood vessel has not been penetrated. If no blood appears in the syringe, proceed by slowly pushing down on the plunger to expel medication into the tissues.	15			
8.	Remove the needle quickly by the same angle of injection, apply safety, and dispose in sharps. Wipe the site with an alcohol-prep or gauze pad. Gently massage the area.	15			
9.	Observe the patient and time the reaction if warranted. Give the patient instructions as ordered and answer any questions.	15			
10.	Apply a bandage.	15			
11.	Discard disposable items and gloves into a biohazard waste bag. Return the medication (if using a multidose vial) and tray to the proper storage area.	15			
12.	Document the procedure in the patient's chart.	15			
	Points Awarded / Points Possible	_____/ **180**			

Name: _____ Date: _____ Score: _____

Competency Checklist
Procedure 53–6 Administer an Intramuscular Injection

ABHES Curriculum

MA.A.1.4.a	Follow documentation guidelines
MA.A.1.9.a	Practice standard precautions and perform disinfection/sterilization techniques
MA.A.1.9.f	Prepare and administer oral and parenteral medications and monitor intravenous (IV) infusions

CAAHEP Core Curriculum

I.P.4	Verify the rules of medication administration: (a) right patient, (b) right medication, (c) right dose, (d) right route, (e) right time, and (f) right documentation
I.P.5	Select proper sites for administering parenteral medication
I.P.7	Administer parenteral (excluding IV) medications
I.A.1	Incorporate critical thinking skills when performing patient assessment
I.A.2	Incorporate critical thinking skills when performing patient care
I.A.3	Show awareness of a patient's concerns related to the procedure being performed
III.P.2	Select appropriate barrier/personal protective equipment (PPE)
III.P.3	Perform handwashing
V.A.4	Explain to a patient the rationale for performance of a procedure
X.P.3	Document patient care accurately in the medical record
III.P.10	Demonstrate proper disposal of biohazardous material: (a) sharps and (b) regulated waste

---

Task:	To inject large amounts of medication, 0.5 mL to 3.0 mL, and oil-based substances or irritating solutions that are more easily tolerated in the muscle tissue.
Supplies & Conditions:	Medication (sterile water for injection in vial or ampule), gauze pads, alcohol-prep pads, adhesive bandage or hypoallergenic tape, sterile safety needle (usually 1 to 3 inches, 18G to 23G), medication tray, patient's chart/EHR, pen, latex or vinyl gloves.
Standards:	A maximum of three attempts may be used to complete the task. The time limit for each attempt is 15 minutes, with a minimum score of 100 percent. **Scoring:** Determine student's score by dividing points awarded by total points possible and multiplying results by 100.

EVALUATION

Evaluator Signature: _____ Date: _____

Evaluator Comments:

673

Name: _____ Date: _____ Score: _____

Procedure 53–6 Steps

Start Time: _____   End Time: _____   Total Time: _____

	Steps	Possible Points	First Attempt	Second Attempt	Third Attempt
1.	Wash and glove hands.	15			
2.	Prepare the syringe with the ordered amount of medication, verifying all ordered doses or dosages prior to administration.	15			
3.	Identify the patient and **explain the rationale for performance of the procedure**, using language the patient understands. Ask patient to remove clothes, if necessary.	15			
4.	Allow the patient to ask questions, **and show awareness of any patient concerns related to the procedure being performed**. Respond to the patient as appropriate.	15			
5.	**Incorporate critical thinking skills when performing patient assessment and care.** Select and prepare the injection site with an alcohol-prep pad. Allow the alcohol to air-dry.	15			
6.	Secure a large area of skin (to accommodate the large amount of medication); spread the skin between the thumb and finger of one hand; and, with the other hand, hold the syringe securely. Insert the needle at a 90-degree angle with a steady penetration.	15			
7.	With one hand, hold the barrel of the syringe while pulling back on the plunger slightly with the other hand to make sure a blood vessel has not been penetrated. If no blood appears in the syringe, proceed by slowly pushing down on the plunger to expel medication into the muscle.	15			
8.	Remove the needle quickly by the same angle of injection, apply safety, and discard into the sharps. Wipe the site with an alcohol-prep or gauze pad. Gently massage the area.	15			
9.	Observe the patient and time the reaction if warranted. Give the patient instructions as ordered and answer any questions.	15			
10.	Apply a bandage.	15			
11.	Discard disposable items and gloves into a biohazard waste bag. Return the medication (if using a multidose vial) and tray to the proper storage area.	15			
12.	Document the procedure in the patient's chart.	15			
	Points Awarded / Points Possible	____/ **180**			

Competency Checklist
Procedure 53–7 Administer an Intramuscular Injection by Z-Track Method

ABHES Curriculum

MA.A.1.4. a	Follow documentation guidelines
MA.A.1.9.a	Practice standard precautions and perform disinfection/sterilization techniques
MA.A.1.9.f	Prepare and administer oral and parenteral medications and monitor intravenous (IV) infusions

CAAHEP Core Curriculum

I.P.4	Verify the rules of medication administration: (a) right patient, (b) right medication, (c) right dose, (d) right route, (e) right time, and (f) right documentation
I.P.5	Select proper sites for administering parenteral medication
I.P.7	Administer parenteral (excluding IV) medications
I.A.1	Incorporate critical thinking skills when performing patient assessment
I.A.2	Incorporate critical thinking skills when performing patient care
I.A.3	Show awareness of a patient's concerns related to the procedure being performed
III.P.2	Select appropriate barrier/personal protective equipment (PPE)
III.P.3	Perform handwashing
V.A.4	Explain to a patient the rationale for performance of a procedure
X.P.3	Document patient care accurately in the medical record
III.P.10	Demonstrate proper disposal of biohazardous material: (a) sharps and (b) regulated waste

---

Task:	To inject substances, 0.5 mL to 3.0 mL, which can be irritating or discoloring to the tissues, deep into the muscle layer of tissue.
Supplies & Conditions:	Medication (sterile water for injection in vial or ampule), gauze pads, alcohol-prep pads, adhesive bandage or hypoallergenic tape, , sterile safety needle (usually 1 to 3 inches, 18G to 23G), medication tray, patient's chart/EHR, pen, latex or vinyl gloves.
Standards:	A maximum of three attempts may be used to complete the task. The time limit for each attempt is 15 minutes, with a minimum score of 100 percent. **Scoring:** Determine student's score by dividing points awarded by total points possible and multiplying results by 100.

EVALUATION

Evaluator Signature: _____   Date: _____

Evaluator Comments:

Name: _____ Date: _____ Score: _____

Procedure 53–7 Steps

Start Time: _____ End Time: _____ Total Time: _____

	Steps	Possible Points	First Attempt	Second Attempt	Third Attempt
1.	Wash and glove hands.	15			
2.	Prepare the syringe with the ordered amount of medication, verifying all ordered doses or dosages prior to administration.	15			
3.	Identify the patient and *explain the rationale for performance of the procedure*, using language the patient understands. Ask patient to remove clothes, if necessary.	15			
4.	Allow the patient to ask questions, *and show awareness of any patient concerns related to the procedure being performed*. Respond to the patient as appropriate.	15			
5.	*Incorporate critical thinking skills when performing patient assessment and care.* Select and prepare the injection site with an alcohol-prep pad. Allow the alcohol to air-dry.	15			
6.	Use a gauze square to hold the patient's skin securely at the injection site to one side to displace skin and tissues until the injection is completed. Insert the needle at a 90-degree angle with a steady penetration.	15			
7.	The first and second fingers may be used to aspirate while the thumb and ring finger hold the syringe near the needle end. If no blood appears in the syringe, proceed by slowly pushing down on the plunger to expel medication into the muscle. Wait a few seconds before removing the needle.	15			
8.	Remove the needle quickly by the same angle of injection, apply safety, and discard. Let go of the skin quickly so that displaced tissue will cover the needle track and prevent it from leaking into the surrounding tissues. Cover the site with an alcohol or gauze pad. Do not massage the area.	15			
9.	Observe the patient and time the reaction if warranted. Give the patient instructions as ordered and answer any questions.	15			
10.	Apply a bandage.	15			
11.	Discard disposable items and gloves into a biohazard waste bag. Return the medication (if using a multidose vial) and tray to the proper storage area.	15			
12.	Document the procedure in the patient's chart.	15			
	Points Awarded / Points Possible	____ / **180**			

Competency Checklist
Procedure 54–1 Produce Up-To-Date Documentation of Provider/Professional Level CPR

CAAHEP Core Curriculum

I.P.12   Produce up-to-date documentation of provider/professional level CPR

Task: Produce up-to-date documentation of provider/professional-level CPR

Supplies & Conditions: Paper, pen, and access to resource tools (computer with Internet access).

Standards: The time limit for providing documentation is determined by the individual educational policies
                                    regarding CPR documentation. **Scoring:** Determine student's score by dividing points awarded
                                    by total points possible and multiplying results by 100.

EVALUATION

Evaluator Signature: _____   Date: _____

Evaluator Comments:

677

Name: _____ Date: _____ Score: _____

Procedure 54–1 Steps

Start Time: _____ End Time: _____ Total Time: _____

	Steps	Possible Points	First Attempt	Second Attempt	Third Attempt
1.	Complete an approved CPR training course through one of the approved organizations recognized for health care professionals including medical assistants.	15			
2.	Make a copy of your completed course certificate and CPR card to present to your instructor and/or employer.	15			
3.	Keep the original documentation on your person.	15			
	Points Awarded / Points Possible	_____/ **45**			

Competency Checklist
Procedure 54–2 Perform First Aid Procedures for Syncope (Fainting Episode)

ABHES Curriculum

M.A.A.1.4.a	Follow documentation guidelines
M.A.A.1.9.a	Practice standard precautions and perform disinfection/sterilization techniques
M.A.A.1.9.g	Recognize and respond to medical office emergencies

CAAHEP Core Curriculum

I.P.3	Perform patient screening using established protocols
I.P.8	Instruct and prepare a patient for a procedure or a treatment
I.P.13.f	Perform first aid procedures for syncope
I.A.1	Incorporate critical thinking skills when performing patient assessment
I.A.2	Incorporate critical thinking skills when performing patient care
V.P.11	Report relevant information concisely and accurately
X.P.3	Document patient care accurately in the medical record
XII.A.1	Recognize the physical and emotional effects on persons involved in an emergency situation

---

Task: Following the steps listed in the procedure, care for an individual that has had a syncope episode or fainted.

Supplies & Conditions: Blanket, pillow.

Standards: A maximum of three attempts may be used to complete the task. The time limit for each attempt is 20 minutes, with a minimum score of 70 percent. **Scoring:** Determine student's score by dividing points awarded by total points possible and multiplying results by 100.

EVALUATION

Evaluator Signature: _____   Date: _____

Evaluator Comments:

Name: _____ Date: _____ Score: _____

Procedure 54–2 Steps

Start Time: _____ End Time: _____ Total Time: _____

	Steps	Possible Points	First Attempt	Second Attempt	Third Attempt
1.	***Incorporate critical thinking skills when performing patient assessment and care.*** If individual is conscious and alerts you that he or she feels faint or dizzy, assist the person to a sitting position and help to bend forward placing head between the knees.	15			
2.	If the patient faints, lay him or her flat on his or her back and elevate the feet and legs with a pillow.	15			
3.	Loosen the patient's clothing. May supply a blanket for warmth. ***Recognize the physical and emotional effects on persons involved in an emergency situation.***	10			
4.	Alert the provider and activate EMS (call 911) if warranted or directed by the provider.	15			
5.	If individual recovers and is not transported, obtain vitals and document along with incident and care in the patient's chart.	15			
	Points Awarded / Points Possible	_____ / **70**			

Competency Checklist
Procedure 54–3 Perform First Aid Procedures for Bleeding

ABHES Curriculum

M.A.A.1.4.a   Follow documentation guidelines
M.A.A.1.9.a   Practice standard precautions and perform disinfection/sterilization techniques
M.A.A.1.9.g   Recognize and respond to medical office emergencies

CAAHEP Core Curriculum

I.P.3   Perform patient screening using established protocols
I.P.8   Instruct and prepare a patient for a procedure or a treatment
I.P.13.a   Perform first aid procedures for bleeding
I.A.1   Incorporate critical thinking skills when performing patient assessment
I.A.2   Incorporate critical thinking skills when performing patient care
III.P.2   Select appropriate barrier/personal protective equipment (PPE)
III.P.8   Perform wound care
III.P.10.b   Demonstrate proper disposal of biohazardous material: regulated wastes
V.P.11   Report relevant information concisely and accurately
X.P.3   Document patient care accurately in the medical record
XII.A.1   Recognize the physical and emotional effects on persons involved in an emergency situation

Task:	Following the steps listed in the procedure, control bleeding from a wound.
Supplies & Conditions:	Sterile gauze pads, sterile gloves, other warranted PPE, biohazardous waste container.
Standards:	A maximum of three attempts may be used to complete the task. The time limit for each attempt is 20 minutes, with a minimum score of 70 percent. **Scoring:** Determine student's score by dividing points awarded by total points possible and multiplying results by 100.

EVALUATION

Evaluator Signature: _____   Date: _____

Evaluator Comments:

Name: _____ Date: _____ Score: _____

Procedure 54–3 Steps

Start Time: _____ End Time: _____ Total Time: _____

	Steps	Possible Points	First Attempt	Second Attempt	Third Attempt
1.	Wash hands and apply sterile gloves and other PPE as needed.	15			
2.	***Incorporate critical thinking skills when performing patient assessment and care.*** Apply sterile gauze pads to the wound and press firmly. Elevate bleeding body area above heart level if possible. ***Recognize the physical and emotional effects on persons involved in an emergency situation.***	15			
3.	If bleeding does not stop, locate the closest artery between the wound and the heart and apply pressure.	15			
4.	Alert the provider if bleeding still doesn't stop, for further directions.	15			
5.	If bleeding stops, apply pressure bandage and alert provider for further directions. Dispose of soiled materials in biohazard waste container, wash hands, and document.	15			
	Points Awarded / Points Possible	_____/ **75**			

Competency Checklist
Procedure 54–4 Perform First Aid Procedures for Seizures

ABHES Curriculum

M.A.A.1.4.a	Follow documentation guidelines
M.A.A.1.9.a	Practice standard precautions and perform disinfection/sterilization techniques
M.A.A.1.9.g	Recognize and respond to medical office emergencies

CAAHEP Core Curriculum

I.P.3	Perform patient screening using established protocols
I.P.8	Instruct and prepare a patient for a procedure or a treatment
I.P.13.d	Perform first aid procedures for seizures
I.A.1	Incorporate critical thinking skills when performing patient assessment
I.A.2	Incorporate critical thinking skills when performing patient care
III.P.2	Select appropriate barrier/personal protective equipment (PPE)
V.P.11	Report relevant information concisely and accurately
X.P.3	Document patient care accurately in the medical record
XII.A.1	Recognize the physical and emotional effects on persons involved in an emergency situation

---

Task: Following the steps listed in the procedure, provide care to prevent injury during a seizure.

Supplies & Conditions: Pillow, sterile gloves, other warranted PPE, biohazardous waste container, blanket.

Standards: A maximum of three attempts may be used to complete the task. The time limit for each attempt is 20 minutes, with a minimum score of 70 percent. **Scoring:** Determine student's score by dividing points awarded by total points possible and multiplying results by 100.

EVALUATION

Evaluator Signature: _____ Date: _____

Evaluator Comments:

Name: _____ Date: _____ Score: _____

Procedure 54–4 Steps

Start Time: _____ End Time: _____ Total Time: _____

	Steps	Possible Points	First Attempt	Second Attempt	Third Attempt
1.	***Incorporate critical thinking skills when performing patient assessment and care.*** If the patient is in the upright position when the seizure starts, slowly assist him or her to the ground.	15			
2.	Move any objects out of the way that might cause injury. Use a pillow as a cushion if necessary to prevent injury.	15			
3.	Do not force any object between the patient's teeth.	15			
4.	If mucus or saliva is present, turn the head to the side to prevent choking. Apply appropriate PPE prior to cleaning up if warranted.	15			
5.	If the victim is not breathing, open the airway with the head-tilt or jaw-thrust maneuver.	15			
6.	If the seizure is due to the condition of status epilepticus (continuous seizure), EMS must be activated because this is a life-threatening condition. Administration of oxygen and antiseizure medication might be necessary; therefore, alert the provider immediately.	15			
7.	Allow the patient to rest or sleep after the seizure is over. Cover with a blanket for warmth. Document the length of the seizure and any other pertinent information in the patient's chart. ***Recognize the physical and emotional effects on persons involved in an emergency situation.***	15			
	Points Awarded / Points Possible	_____/ **105**			

Competency Checklist
Procedure 54–5 Perform an Abdominal Thrust on an Adult Victim with an Obstructed Airway

ABHES Curriculum

M.A.A.1.4.a	Follow documentation guidelines
M.A.A.1.9.a	Practice standard precautions and perform disinfection/sterilization techniques
M.A.A.1.9.g	Recognize and respond to medical office emergencies

CAAHEP Core Curriculum

I.P.3	Perform patient screening using established protocols
I.P.8	Instruct and prepare a patient for a procedure or a treatment
I.P.12	Produce up-to-date documentation of provider/professional level CPR
I.A.1	Incorporate critical thinking skills when performing patient assessment
I.A.2	Incorporate critical thinking skills when performing patient care
III.P.2	Select appropriate barrier/personal protective equipment (PPE)
V.P.11	Report relevant information concisely and accurately
X.P.3	Document patient care accurately in the medical record
XII.A.1	Recognize the physical and emotional effects on persons involved in an emergency situation

Task:	Following the steps listed in the procedure, dislodge an object obstructing the airway and restore breathing.
Supplies & Conditions:	Disposable gloves and resuscitation mouthpiece.
Standards:	A maximum of three attempts may be used to complete the task. The time limit for each attempt is 20 minutes, with a minimum score of 70 percent. **Scoring:** Determine student's score by dividing points awarded by total points possible and multiplying results by 100.

EVALUATION

Evaluator Signature: _____ Date: _____

Evaluator Comments:

Name: _____ Date: _____ Score: _____

Procedure 54–5 Steps

Start Time: _____ End Time: _____ Total Time: _____

	Steps	Possible Points	First Attempt	Second Attempt	Third Attempt
1.	***Incorporate critical thinking skills when performing patient assessment and care.*** Observe the victim using the universal distress signal.	15			
2.	Ask, "Are you choking?" If yes, ask, "Can you speak?"	15			
3.	Get into position behind the victim.	15			
4.	Extend your arms around the victim's abdomen and locate his or her umbilicus with the index finger of one hand. With the other hand, make a fist with your thumb bent outward. Place the thumb against the abdomen just above the umbilicus.	15			
5.	Place your other hand over the fist.	15			
6.	Keep your thrusts in the soft high abdominal area to avoid injury to the rib cage and sternum. Give an abdominal thrust by forcefully pulling up and back quickly.	15			
7.	If this is unsuccessful, repeat thrusts until the obstruction is expelled or the victim loses consciousness.	15			
8.	If the victim becomes unresponsive and falls to the floor, position him or her on his or her back and activate the emergency response system by calling 911, apply gloves, open the airway, remove the object if you see it, and begin CPR.	15			
9.	Every time you open the airway to give breaths, open the victim's mouth wide and look for the object. If you see it, remove it; if not, continue CPR.	15			
10.	After the victim has resumed breathing and the heart is beating or EMS services have taken over the rescue, remove your gloves and the mouthpiece and dispose of them in the biohazard waste container. ***Recognize the physical and emotional effects on persons involved in an emergency situation.***	15			
11.	Document the procedure.	15			
	Points Awarded / Points Possible	_____/ **165**			

Competency Checklist
Procedure 54–6 Perform First Aid Procedures for Shock

ABHES Curriculum

M.A.A.1.4.a	Follow documentation guidelines
M.A.A.1.9.a	Practice standard precautions and perform disinfection/sterilization techniques
M.A.A.1.9.g	Recognize and respond to medical office emergencies

CAAHEP Core Curriculum

I.P.3	Perform patient screening using established protocols
I.P.8	Instruct and prepare a patient for a procedure or a treatment
I.P.13.e	Perform first aid procedures for shock
I.A.1	Incorporate critical thinking skills when performing patient assessment
I.A.2	Incorporate critical thinking skills when performing patient care
V.P.11	Report relevant information concisely and accurately
X.P.3	Document patient care accurately in the medical record
XII.A.1	Recognize the physical and emotional effects on persons involved in an emergency situation

---

Task: Following the steps listed in the procedure, provide care when patient is suffering from shock.

Supplies & Conditions: Blanket, pillow.

Standards: A maximum of three attempts may be used to complete the task. The time limit for each attempt is 20 minutes, with a minimum score of 70 percent. **Scoring:** Determine student's score by dividing points awarded by total points possible and multiplying results by 100.

EVALUATION

Evaluator Signature: _____ Date: _____

Evaluator Comments:

687

Name: _____ Date: _____ Score: _____

Procedure 54–6 Steps

Start Time: _____ End Time: _____ Total Time: _____

	Steps	Possible Points	First Attempt	Second Attempt	Third Attempt
1.	***Incorporate critical thinking skills when performing patient assessment and care.*** Activate EMS.	15			
2.	Place the patient in a recumbent position with feet elevated unless there is a head injury, in which case the patient is kept flat.	15			
3.	It is best to place a blanket under and over the patient to maintain body warmth but not to overheat.	15			
4.	Stay with patient and monitor vitals until EMS arrives for patient transfer to the hospital. ***Recognize the physical and emotional effects on persons involved in an emergency situation.***	15			
5.	Document in the patient's chart.	15			
	Points Awarded / Points Possible	_____/ **75**			

Competency Checklist
Procedure 54–7 Develop Safety Plans for Emergency Preparedness

ABHES Curriculum

M.A.A.1.4.a   Follow documentation guidelines

CAAHEP Core Curriculum

XII.A.1   Recognize the physical and emotional effects on persons involved in an emergency situation

---

Task:	Following the steps listed in the procedure, develop safety plans for an environmental event (such as a tornado or flood), for personal safety on the job, and for personal safety at home.
Supplies & Conditions:	Paper, pen, and access to resource tools (computer with Internet access).
Standards:	A maximum of three attempts may be used to complete the task. The time limit for each attempt is 20 minutes, with a minimum score of 70 percent. **Scoring:** Determine student's score by dividing points awarded by total points possible and multiplying results by 100.

EVALUATION

Evaluator Signature: _____   Date: _____

Evaluator Comments:

689

Name: _____ Date: _____ Score: _____

Procedure 54–7 Steps

Start Time: _____ End Time: _____ Total Time: _____

	Steps	Possible Points	First Attempt	Second Attempt	Third Attempt
1.	Develop a personal plan for yourself and your family in case of environmental emergency, such as tornado or flood. ***Recognize the physical and emotional effects on persons involved in an emergency situation.***	15			
2.	Find local telephone numbers of organizations and include them in your personal plan.	15			
3.	Verbalize (explain) an evacuation plan out of your home in case of fire.	15			
4.	Develop a typed safety plan in the case of a chemical spill in the office.	15			
5.	Verbalize (explain) an evacuation plan for a medical office in the event of an emergency.	15			
	Points Awarded / Points Possible	_____/ 75			

Competency Checklist
Procedure 55–1 Perform First Aid Procedures for Fractures

ABHES Curriculum

MA.A.1.4.a	Follow documentation guidelines
MA.A.1.9.a	Practice standard precautions and perform disinfection/sterilization techniques
MA.A.1.9.g	Recognize and respond to medical office emergencies

CAAHEP Core Curriculum

I.P.8	Instruct and prepare a patient for a procedure or a treatment
I.P.9	Assist provider with a patient exam
I.P.13.c	Perform first aid procedures for fractures
I.A.1	Incorporate critical thinking skills when performing patient assessment
I.A.2	Incorporate critical thinking skills when performing patient care
I.A.3	Show awareness of a patient's concerns related to the procedure being performed
III.P.2	Select appropriate barrier/personal protective equipment (PPE)
V.A.4	Explain to a patient the rationale for performance of a procedure
V.P.11	Report relevant information concisely and accurately
X.P.3	Document patient care accurately in the medical record

Task: Following the steps listed in the procedure, provide care for an individual who has a fracture.

Supplies & Conditions: Latex or vinyl gloves, ice pack, gauze pads, splint, padding, patient chart/EHR.

Standards: A maximum of three attempts may be used to complete the task. The time limit for each attempt is 15 minutes, with a minimum score of 70 percent. **Scoring:** Determine student's score by dividing points awarded by total points possible and multiplying results by 100.

EVALUATION

Evaluator Signature: _____ Date: _____

Evaluator Comments:

Name: _____ Date: _____ Score: _____

Procedure 55–1 Steps

Start Time: _____ End Time: _____ Total Time: _____

	Steps	Possible Points	First Attempt	Second Attempt	Third Attempt
1.	Introduce yourself, identify the patient, and *explain the rationale for performance of the procedure*, using language the patient can understand. Don't move the person unless necessary to avoid further injury. Alert the provider and activate EMS (call 911) if warranted or directed by the provider.	15			
2.	*Incorporate critical thinking skills when performing patient assessment and care.* If bleeding is occurring, apply gloves and apply pressure to the wound with a sterile bandage, a clean cloth or a clean piece of clothing.	15			
3.	Immobilize the injured area. Do not try to realign the bone or push a bone that's sticking out back in. Apply a splint to the area above and below the fracture sites. Padding the splints can help reduce discomfort.	15			
4.	Apply ice packs to limit swelling and help relieve pain until emergency personnel arrive or until patient is released and sent to orthopedics.	15			
5.	Treat for shock. *Show awareness of the patient's concerns related to the procedure being performed.* If the person feels faint or is breathing in short, rapid breaths, lay him or her down with the head slightly lower than the trunk and, if possible, elevate the legs.	15			
6.	Document care in the patient's medical record.	15			
	Points Awarded / Points Possible	_____/ 90			

Competency Checklist
Procedure 55–2 Perform wound care

ABHES Curriculum

MA.A.1.4.a	Follow documentation guidelines
MA.A.1.9.a	Practice standard precautions and perform disinfection/sterilization techniques
MA.A.1.9.g	Recognize and respond to medical office emergencies

CAAHEP Core Curriculum

I.P.8	Instruct and prepare a patient for a procedure or a treatment
I.P.9	Assist provider with a patient exam
I.A.1	Incorporate critical thinking skills when performing patient assessment
I.A.2	Incorporate critical thinking skills when performing patient care
I.A.3	Show awareness of a patient's concerns related to the procedure being performed
III.P.2	Select appropriate barrier/personal protective equipment (PPE)
III.P.8	Perform wound care
V.P.11	Report relevant information concisely and accurately
V.A.4	Explain to a patient the rationale for performance of a procedure
X.P.3	Document patient care accurately in the medical record

Task: Following the steps listed in the procedure, remove blood, debris, and surface microorganisms from the area of injury.

Supplies & Conditions: Basin, antibacterial solution (Betadine), warm water, sterile gauze sponges, sterile sponge forceps, latex or vinyl gloves, sterile water, irrigation syringe, biohazard and regular waste receptacle, bandage and tape, patient chart/EHR, pen.

Standards: A maximum of three attempts may be used to complete the task. The time limit for each attempt is 15 minutes, with a minimum score of 70 percent. **Scoring:** Determine student's score by dividing points awarded by total points possible and multiplying results by 100.

EVALUATION

Evaluator Signature: _____ Date: _____

Evaluator Comments:

Name: _____ Date: _____ Score: _____

Procedure 55–2 Steps

Start Time: _____ End Time: _____ Total Time: _____

	Steps	Possible Points	First Attempt	Second Attempt	Third Attempt
1.	Assemble the equipment and materials, wash hands, and put on gloves.	15			
2.	Introduce yourself, identify the patient, and *explain the rationale for performance of the procedure*, using language the patient can understand. *Show awareness of the patient's concerns related to the procedure being performed*.	15			
3.	*Incorporate critical thinking skills when performing patient assessment and care.* Grasp several gauze sponges with sponge forceps.	15			
4.	Dip the sponges into warm detergent water.	15			
5.	Wash the wound and wound area to remove microorganisms and any foreign matter.	15			
6.	Discard the sponges in proper waste receptacle.	15			
7.	Irrigate the wound thoroughly with sterile water.	15			
8.	Blot the wound dry with sterile gauze and dispose of the gauze in the proper waste receptacle.	15			
9.	Call the provider to inspect the wound and assist as needed with treatment.	15			
10.	Apply a sterile dressing and bandage it in place.	15			
11.	Instruct patient in how to care for the bandage and to watch for signs of circulation impairment and infection.	15			
12.	Clean up the work area; disinfect.	15			
13.	Wash hands.	15			
14.	Document in the patient's chart.	15			
	Points Awarded / Points Possible	_____/ **210**			

Competency Checklist
Procedure 55–3 Apply a Tube Gauze Bandage

ABHES Curriculum

MA.A.1.4.a	Follow documentation guidelines
MA.A.1.9.a	Practice standard precautions and perform disinfection/sterilization techniques
MA.A.1.9.g	Recognize and respond to medical office emergencies

CAAHEP Core Curriculum

I.P.8	Instruct and prepare a patient for a procedure or a treatment
I.P.9	Assist provider with a patient exam
I.A.1	Incorporate critical thinking skills when performing patient assessment
I.A.2	Incorporate critical thinking skills when performing patient care
I.A.3	Show awareness of a patient's concerns related to the procedure being performed
III.P.2	Select appropriate barrier/personal protective equipment (PPE)
V.A.4	Explain to a patient the rationale for performance of a procedure
X.P.3	Document patient care accurately in the medical record

Task:	Following the steps listed in the procedure, cover a wound or hold a bandage in place on an appendage such as a finger, toe, arm, or leg.
Supplies & Conditions:	Scissors, dressing, adhesive tape, tube gauze bandage, applicator, latex or vinyl gloves, a waste container, patient chart/EHR, pen
Standards:	A maximum of three attempts may be used to complete the task. The time limit for each attempt is 15 minutes, with a minimum score of 70 percent. **Scoring:** Determine student's score by dividing points awarded by total points possible and multiplying results by 100.

EVALUATION

Evaluator Signature: _____ Date: _____

Evaluator Comments:

Name: _____ Date: _____ Score: _____

Procedure 55–3 Steps

Start Time: _____ End Time: _____ Total Time: _____

	Steps	Possible Points	First Attempt	Second Attempt	Third Attempt
1.	Assemble the equipment and materials, wash hands, and put on gloves.	15			
2.	Introduce yourself, identify the patient, and *explain the rationale for the procedure being performed*, using language the patient can understand. *Show awareness of the patient's concerns related to the procedure being performed*.	15			
3.	*Incorporate critical thinking skills when performing patient assessment and care.* Choose an applicator that is larger than the appendage to be bandaged.	15			
4.	Cut an appropriate amount of tubular bandage to be applied and slide onto the applicator.	15			
5.	Slide the applicator over the appendage. (*Apply first layer.*)	15			
6.	Turn the bandage gauze one complete turn.	15			
7.	Next, slide the applicator toward the proximal end of the appendage.	15			
8.	Repeat application process until area is completely covered.	15			
9.	Anchor bandage at the proximal end and secure with tape.	15			
10.	Instruct patient in how to care for the bandage and to watch for signs of circulation impairment and infection.	15			
11.	Clean up area; disinfect and dispose of used supplies.	15			
12.	Wash hands.	15			
13.	Document in the patient chart.	15			
	Points Awarded / Points Possible	_____/ **195**			

Competency Checklist
Procedure 55–4 Apply a Spiral Bandage

ABHES Curriculum

MA.A.1.4.a   Follow documentation guidelines
MA.A.1.9.a   Practice standard precautions and perform disinfection/sterilization techniques
MA.A.1.9.g   Recognize and respond to medical office emergencies

CAAHEP Core Curriculum

I.P.8   Instruct and prepare a patient for a procedure or a treatment
I.P.9   Assist provider with a patient exam
I.A.1   Incorporate critical thinking skills when performing patient assessment
I.A.2   Incorporate critical thinking skills when performing patient care
I.A.3   Show awareness of a patient's concerns related to the procedure being performed
III.P.2   Select appropriate barrier/personal protective equipment (PPE)
V.A.4   Explain to a patient the rationale for performance of a procedure
X.P.3   Document patient care accurately in the medical record

---

Task: Following the steps listed in the procedure, apply a spiral bandage. *Note: This procedure describes how to apply a dressing to a wound and then cover it with a bandage. Omit Step 3 to eliminate dressing application.*

Supplies & Conditions: Bandage, adhesive tape, scissors, sterile dressing, latex or vinyl gloves, a waste container, patient chart/ EHR, pen.

Standards: A maximum of three attempts may be used to complete the task. The time limit for each attempt is 15 minutes, with a minimum score of 70 percent. **Scoring:** Determine student's score by dividing points awarded by total points possible and multiplying results by 100.

EVALUATION

Evaluator Signature: _____   Date: _____

Evaluator Comments:

Name: _____ Date: _____ Score: _____

Procedure 55–4 Steps

Start Time: _____ End Time: _____ Total Time: _____

	Steps	Possible Points	First Attempt	Second Attempt	Third Attempt
1.	Assemble the equipment and materials, wash hands, and put on gloves.	15			
2.	Introduce yourself, identify the patient, and *explain the rationale for performance of the procedure*, using language the patient can understand. *Show awareness of the patient's concerns related to the procedure being performed*.	15			
3.	*Incorporate critical thinking skills when performing patient assessment and care.* Carefully open a dressing, without contaminating it, and place it over the wound area.	15			
4.	Anchor the bandage by placing the end of the bandage on a bias at the starting point.	15			
5.	Encircle the part, allowing the corner of the bandage end to protrude.	15			
6.	Turn down the protruding tip of the bandage.	15			
7.	Encircle the part again.	15			
8.	Continue to encircle the area to be covered with spiral turns spaced so that they do not overlap.	15			
9.	If a closed spiral bandage is desired, overlap spiral turns until the dressing is completely covered.	15			
10.	Complete the bandage by taping it in place.	15			
11.	Instruct patient in how to care for the bandage and to watch for signs of circulation impairment and infection.	15			
12.	Clean the area; disinfect and discard contaminated materials and gloves in a proper waste receptacle.	15			
13.	Wash hands.	15			
14.	Document in the patient's chart.	15			
	Points Awarded / Points Possible	____/ **210**			

Competency Checklist
Procedure 55–5 Apply a Figure-Eight Bandage

ABHES Curriculum

MA.A.1.4.a	Follow documentation guidelines
MA.A.1.9.a	Practice standard precautions and perform disinfection/sterilization techniques
MA.A.1.9.g	Recognize and respond to medical office emergencies

CAAHEP Core Curriculum

I.P.8	Instruct and prepare a patient for a procedure or a treatment
I.P.9	Assist provider with a patient exam
I.A.1	Incorporate critical thinking skills when performing patient assessment
I.A.2	Incorporate critical thinking skills when performing patient care
I.A.3	Show awareness of a patient's concerns related to the procedure being performed
III.P.2	Select appropriate barrier/personal protective equipment (PPE)
V.A.4	Explain to a patient the rationale for performance of a procedure
X.P.3	Document patient care accurately in the medical record

Task: Following the steps listed in the procedure, demonstrate application of a figure-eight bandage.

Supplies & Conditions: Sterile dressing, bandage, latex or vinyl gloves, scissors, tape, a proper waste receptacle, patient chart/EHR, pen.

Standards: A maximum of three attempts may be used to complete the task. The time limit for each attempt is 15 minutes, with a minimum score of 70 percent. **Scoring:** Determine student's score by dividing points awarded by total points possible and multiplying results by 100.

EVALUATION

Evaluator Signature: _____ Date: _____

Evaluator Comments:

Name: _____ Date: _____ Score: _____

Procedure 55–5 Steps

Start Time: _____ End Time: _____ Total Time: _____

	Steps	Possible Points	First Attempt	Second Attempt	Third Attempt
1.	Assemble the equipment and materials, wash hands, and put on gloves.	15			
2.	Introduce yourself, identify the patient, and *explain the rationale for performance of the procedure*, using language the patient can understand. *Show awareness of the patient's concerns related to the procedure being performed*.	15			
3.	*Incorporate critical thinking skills when performing patient assessment and care.* Apply a dressing over the wound if necessary or proceed to Step 4 if applying to a sprained area.	15			
4.	Anchor the bandage with one or two turns around the palm of the hand.	15			
5.	Roll the gauze diagonally across the front of the wrist and in a figure-eight pattern around the hand.	15			
6.	Cut the gauze and tape at the wrist.	15			
7.	Instruct patient in how to care for the bandage and to watch for signs of circulation impairment and infection.	15			
8.	Disinfect, discard contaminated materials and gloves in a proper waste receptacle.	15			
9.	Wash hands.	15			
10.	Document in patient chart.	15			
	Points Awarded / Points Possible	____/ **150**			

Competency Checklist
Procedure 55–6 Apply a Cravat Bandage to Forehead, Ear, or Eyes

ABHES Curriculum

MA.A.1.4.a	Follow documentation guidelines
MA.A.1.9.a	Practice standard precautions and perform disinfection/sterilization techniques
MA.A.1.9.g	Recognize and respond to medical office emergencies

CAAHEP Core Curriculum

I.P.8	Instruct and prepare a patient for a procedure or a treatment
I.P.9	Assist provider with a patient exam
I.A.1	Incorporate critical thinking skills when performing patient assessment
I.A.2	Incorporate critical thinking skills when performing patient care
I.A.3	Show awareness of a patient's concerns related to the procedure being performed
III.P.2	Select appropriate barrier/personal protective equipment (PPE)
V.A.4	Explain to a patient the rationale for performance of a procedure
X.P.3	Document patient care accurately in the medical record

Task: Following the steps listed in the procedure, demonstrate application of a cravat bandage to the head. *Note: This procedure describes how to apply a dressing to a wound and then cover it with a bandage. Omit Step 3 to eliminate dressing application.*

Supplies & Conditions: Sterile dressing, cravat bandage, latex or vinyl gloves, a proper waste receptacle, patient chart/EHR, pen.

Standards: A maximum of three attempts may be used to complete the task. The time limit for each attempt is 15 minutes, with a minimum score of 70 percent. **Scoring:** Determine student's score by dividing points awarded by total points possible and multiplying results by 100.

EVALUATION

Evaluator Signature: _____ Date: _____

Evaluator Comments:

Name: _____ Date: _____ Score: _____

Procedure 55–6 Steps

Start Time: _____ End Time: _____ Total Time: _____

	Steps	Possible Points	First Attempt	Second Attempt	Third Attempt
1.	Assemble the equipment and materials, wash hands, and put on gloves.	15			
2.	Introduce yourself, identify the patient, and *explain the rationale for performance of the procedure*, using language the patient can understand. *Show awareness of the patient's concerns related to the procedure being performed*.	15			
3.	*Incorporate critical thinking skills when performing patient assessment and care.* Apply a dressing over the wound.	15			
4.	Place the center of the cravat over the dressing.	15			
5.	Take the ends around to the opposite side of the head and cross them. Do not tie.	15			
6.	Bring the ends back to the starting point and tie them.	15			
7.	Instruct patient in how to care for the bandage and to watch for signs of circulation impairment and infection.	15			
8.	Disinfect, discard the contaminated materials and gloves in a proper waste receptacle.	15			
9.	Wash hands.	15			
10.	Document in the patient chart.	15			
	Points Awarded / Points Possible	_____/ **150**			

Competency Checklist
Procedure 56–1 Use Proper Body Mechanics

ABHES Curriculum

MA.A.1.4.a	Follow documentation guidelines
MA.A.1.9.j	Make adaptations with patients with special needs

CAAHEP Core Curriculum

I.P.8	Instruct and prepare a patient for a procedure or a treatment
I.P.9	Assist provider with a patient exam
I.A.1	Incorporate critical thinking skills when performing patient assessment
I.A.2	Incorporate critical thinking skills when performing patient care
V.P.4	Coach patients regarding: (b) health maintenance, and (c) disease prevention
V.A.4	Explain to a patient the rationale for performance of a procedure
X.P.3	Document patient care accurately in the medical record

Task: Following the steps listed in the procedure, demonstrate proper techniques when lifting or moving objects to prevent back injury.

Supplies & Conditions: Will vary based on object or person selected.

Standards: A maximum of three attempts may be used to complete the task. The time limit for each attempt is 10 minutes, with a minimum score of 70 percent. **Scoring:** Determine student's score by dividing points awarded by total points possible and multiplying results by 100.

EVALUATION

Evaluator Signature: _____ Date: _____

Evaluator Comments:

Name: _____ Date: _____ Score: _____

Procedure 56–1 Steps

Start Time: _____ End Time: _____ Total Time: _____

	Steps	Possible Points	First Attempt	Second Attempt	Third Attempt
1.	If a patient is involved, introduce yourself and identify the patient. ***Explain to the patient the rationale for performance of the procedure*** and what you are going to do, using language the patient can understand.	15			
2.	***Incorporate critical thinking skills when performing patient assessment and care.*** Before lifting anything or anyone, determine whether it is possible for one person to do; if a patient or object is too heavy, obtain help.	15			
3.	Make sure the path is clear, the floor is clean and dry, and the area is ready to receive the patient or object before lifting or moving.	15			
4.	Face the patient or object; keep the back as straight as possible and feet shoulder-width apart to provide a good base of support.	15			
5.	Always bend from the hips and knees.	15			
6.	Pivot the entire body instead of twisting it.	15			
7.	Hold heavy objects close to the body and use the body's weight to push or pull any heavy object.	15			
8.	Document procedure (if appropriate).	15			
	Points Awarded / Points Possible	_____ / **120**			

Competency Checklist
Procedure 56–2 Apply an Arm Sling

ABHES Curriculum

MA.A.1.4.a	Follow documentation guidelines
MA.A.1.9.d	Assist provider with specialty examination
MA.A.1.9.h	Teach self-examination, disease management and health promotion
MA.A.1.9.j	Make adaptations with patients with special needs

CAAHEP Core Curriculum

I.P.8	Instruct and prepare a patient for a procedure or a treatment
I.P.9	Assist provider with a patient exam
I.A.1	Incorporate critical thinking skills when performing patient assessment
I.A.2	Incorporate critical thinking skills when performing patient care
I.A.3	Show awareness of a patient's concerns related to the procedure being performed
V.P.4	Coach patients regarding: (b) health maintenance, and (c) disease prevention
V.A.4	Explain to a patient the rationale for performance of a procedure
X.P.3	Document patient care accurately in the medical record

Task: Following the steps listed in the procedure, apply an arm sling to provide support for an injured arm or shoulder.

Supplies & Conditions: Commercial, buckle-type arm sling, patient's chart/EHR, and pen.

Standards: A maximum of three attempts may be used to complete the task. The time limit for each attempt is 10 minutes, with a minimum score of 70 percent. **Scoring:** Determine student's score by dividing points awarded by total points possible and multiplying results by 100.

EVALUATION

Evaluator Signature: _____ Date: _____

Evaluator Comments:

Name: _____ Date: _____ Score: _____

Procedure 56–2 Steps

Start Time: _____ End Time: _____ Total Time: _____

	Steps	Possible Points	First Attempt	Second Attempt	Third Attempt
1.	Introduce yourself, identify the patient, and *explain the rationale for performance of the procedure*, using language the patient can understand. *Show awareness of the patient's concerns related to the procedure being performed.*	15			
2.	Wash hands.	15			
3.	*Incorporate critical thinking skills when performing patient assessment and care.* Select the proper size arm sling.	15			
4.	For patient safety, support the injured arm above and below the injury site.	15			
5.	Position the arm into a 90-degree angle and slide it into the pouch-like opening of the sling.	15			
6.	Bring the adjustable strap around the back of the neck on the side of the uninjured arm and slide into the ring attached to the end of the sling, fasten, and tighten strap.	15			
7.	Check arm for circulation impairment.	15			
8.	Document procedure in patient's chart.	15			
	Points Awarded / Points Possible	____/ 120			

Competency Checklist
Procedure 56–3 Use a Cane

ABHES Curriculum

MA.A.1.4.a	Follow documentation guidelines
MA.A.1.9.d	Assist provider with specialty examination
MA.A.1.9.h	Teach self-examination, disease management and health promotion
MA.A.1.9.j	Make adaptations with patients with special needs

CAAHEP Core Curriculum

I.P.8	Instruct and prepare a patient for a procedure or a treatment
I.P.9	Assist provider with a patient exam
I.A.1	Incorporate critical thinking skills when performing patient assessment
I.A.2	Incorporate critical thinking skills when performing patient care
I.A.3	Show awareness of a patient's concerns related to the procedure being performed
V.P.4	Coach patients regarding: (b) health maintenance, and (c) disease prevention
V.A.4	Explain to a patient the rationale for performance of a procedure
X.P.3	Document patient care accurately in the medical record

Task: Following the steps listed in the procedure, adjust a cane for proper height, and teach a patient its correct and safe use.

Supplies & Conditions: Cane, patient's chart/EHR, and pen.

Standards: A maximum of three attempts may be used to complete the task. The time limit for each attempt is 10 minutes, with a minimum score of 70 percent. **Scoring:** Determine student's score by dividing points awarded by total points possible and multiplying results by 100.

EVALUATION

Evaluator Signature: _____ Date: _____

Evaluator Comments:

Procedure 56–3 Steps

Start Time: _____ End Time: _____ Total Time: _____

	Steps	Possible Points	First Attempt	Second Attempt	Third Attempt
1.	Introduce yourself, identify the patient, and *explain the rationale for performance of the procedure*, using language the patient can understand. *Show awareness of the patient's concerns*.	15			
2.	*Incorporate critical thinking skills when performing patient assessment and care.* Wash hands and assemble the equipment. Check the cane for an intact rubber tip.	15			
3.	Adjust the height of the cane so that the patient's elbow is flexed comfortably at approximately a 25- to 30-degree angle and check that the handle of the cane is positioned just below the hip level of the uninjured or strong side.	15			
4.	Demonstrate for the patient the gait ordered for safe ambulation.	15			
5.	Move the cane and injured extremity forward simultaneously.	15			
6.	Then move the strong or uninjured extremity forward.	15			
7.	Allow the patient to practice the procedure.	15			
8.	Demonstrate going up stairs. Move the uninjured extremity up first and then move the injured extremity up.	15			
9.	Demonstrate going down stairs. Move the uninjured extremity down first. Then move the injured extremity down.	15			
10.	Instruct the patient to take small, slow steps.	15			
11.	Ensure that the cane height is correct and that the patient is using the cane correctly.	15			
12.	Document procedure in the patient's chart.	15			
	Points Awarded / Points Possible	____/ **180**			

Name: _____   Date: _____   Score: _____

Competency Checklist
Procedure 56–4 Use Crutches

ABHES Curriculum

MA.A.1.4.a	Follow documentation guidelines
MA.A.1.9.d	Assist provider with specialty examination
MA.A.1.9.h	Teach self-examination, disease management and health promotion
MA.A.1.9.j	Make adaptations with patients with special needs

CAAHEP Core Curriculum

I.P.8	Instruct and prepare a patient for a procedure or a treatment
I.P.9	Assist provider with a patient exam
I.A.1	Incorporate critical thinking skills when performing patient assessment
I.A.2	Incorporate critical thinking skills when performing patient care
I.A.3	Show awareness of a patient's concerns related to the procedure being performed
V.P.4	Coach patients regarding: (b) health maintenance, and (c) disease prevention
V.A.4	Explain to a patient the rationale for performance of a procedure
X.P.3	Document patient care accurately in the medical record

Task: Following the steps listed in the procedure, adjust crutches' length and teach a patient to use crutches correctly and safely.

Supplies & Conditions: Crutches, hand pads, rubber tips, patient's chart/EHR, and pen.

Standards: A maximum of three attempts may be used to complete the task. The time limit for each attempt is 20 minutes, with a minimum score of 70 percent. **Scoring:** Determine student's score by dividing points awarded by total points possible and multiplying results by 100.

EVALUATION
Evaluator Signature: _____   Date: _____
Evaluator Comments:

Name: _____ Date: _____ Score: _____

Procedure 56–4 Steps

Start Time: _____ End Time: _____ Total Time: _____

	Steps	Possible Points	First Attempt	Second Attempt	Third Attempt
1.	Introduce yourself, identify the patient, and *explain the rationale for performance of the procedure*, using language the patient can understand. *Show awareness of the patient's concerns*.	15			
2.	Wash hands and assemble the equipment.	15			
3.	*Incorporate critical thinking skills when performing patient assessment and care.* For patient safety, stabilize the patient upright near a wall or chair for support. Apply a gait belt to the patient.	15			
4.	Adjust the length of the crutches for the patient so that the handles are comfortable, with a 30-degree angle bend of the elbows and two inches between the axilla and the top of the crutches.	15			
5.	Explain to the patient to support his or her weight at the handles and not under the arm. Tell the patient to take small steps slowly to avoid losing balance and possibly falling.	15			
6.	Instruct the patient to stand on his or her uninjured foot while swinging the injured leg forward with crutches.	15			
7.	Demonstrate the proper use of crutches.	15			
8.	Allow the patient to practice the procedure to ensure correct use.	15			
9.	Document the procedure in the patient's chart.	15			
	Points Awarded / Points Possible	____/ **135**			

Competency Checklist
Procedure 56–5 Use a Walker

ABHES Curriculum

MA.A.1.4.a	Follow documentation guidelines
MA.A.1.9.d	Assist provider with specialty examination
MA.A.1.9.h	Teach self-examination, disease management and health promotion
MA.A.1.9.j	Make adaptations with patients with special needs

CAAHEP Core Curriculum

I.P.8	Instruct and prepare a patient for a procedure or a treatment
I.P.9	Assist provider with a patient exam
I.A.1	Incorporate critical thinking skills when performing patient assessment
I.A.2	Incorporate critical thinking skills when performing patient care
I.A.3	Show awareness of a patient's concerns related to the procedure being performed
V.P.4	Coach patients regarding: (b) health maintenance, and (c) disease prevention
V.A.4	Explain to a patient the rationale for performance of a procedure
X.P.3	Document patient care accurately in the medical record

Task: Following the steps listed in the procedure, adjust the walker's height and teach a patient the proper and safe use of a walker.

Supplies & Conditions: Walker, handles, rubber tips, patient's chart or EHR, and pen.

Standards: A maximum of three attempts may be used to complete the task. The time limit for each attempt is 10 minutes, with a minimum score of 70 percent. **Scoring:** Determine student's score by dividing points awarded by total points possible and multiplying results by 100.

EVALUATION

Evaluator Signature: _____   Date: _____

Evaluator Comments:

Name: _____ Date: _____ Score: _____

Procedure 56–5 Steps

Start Time: _____ End Time: _____ Total Time: _____

	Steps	Possible Points	First Attempt	Second Attempt	Third Attempt
1.	Introduce yourself, identify the patient, and *explain the rationale for performance of the procedure*, using language the patient can understand. *Show awareness of the patient's concerns*.	15			
2.	Wash hands and assemble the equipment.	15			
3.	*Incorporate critical thinking skills when performing patient assessment and care.* For patient safety, stabilize the patient upright near a wall or chair for support. Apply a gait belt to the patient.	15			
4.	The height of the walker should be adjusted so that the handles are at the patient's hip level and the bend of the patient's elbows is at a comfortable 25- to 30-degree angle.	15			
5.	Position the walker around the patient.	15			
6.	Instruct the patient to pick up the walker, move it slightly forward, and walk into it. Instruct the patient to keep all four feet of the walker on the floor. Explain to the patient not to slide the walker. Instruct the patient not to step too close to the walker.	15			
7.	Demonstrate the correct use of a walker.	15			
8.	Have the patient practice the procedure.	15			
9.	Observe the patient and be ready to assist in case of a fall.	15			
10.	Document the procedure in the patient's chart.	15			
	Points Awarded / Points Possible	_____/ **150**			

Competency Checklist
Procedure 57–1 Instruct a Patient According to Special Dietary Needs

ABHES Curriculum

MA.A.1.2.d	Apply a system of diet and nutrition: (1) Explain the importance of diet and nutrition, (2) Educate patients regarding proper diet and nutrition guidelines, (3) Identify categories of patients that require special diets or diet modifications
MA.A.1.4.a	Follow documentation guidelines
MA.A.1.9.h	Teach self-examination, disease management and health promotion

CAAHEP Core Curriculum

IV.P.1	Instruct a patient according to patient's special dietary needs
IV.A.1	Show awareness of patient's concerns regarding a dietary change
V.A.4	Explain to a patient the rationale for performance of a procedure

---

Task:	Following the steps listed in the procedure, to create an individualized nutritional plan for a patient and instruct them according to their needs.
Supplies & Conditions:	Access to a computer and Internet.
Standards:	A maximum of three attempts may be used to complete the task. The time limit for each attempt is 10 minutes, with a minimum score of 70 percent. **Scoring:** Determine student's score by dividing points awarded by total points possible and multiplying results by 100.

EVALUATION

Evaluator Signature: _____   Date: _____

Evaluator Comments:

Name: _____ Date: _____ Score: _____

Procedure 57–1 Steps

Start Time: _____ **End Time:** _____ **Total Time:** _____

	Steps	Possible Points	First Attempt	Second Attempt	Third Attempt
1.	Introduce yourself and identify the patient. ***Explain the rationale for the procedure being performed*** and what you are going to do, using language the patient can understand.	15			
2.	Obtain the dietary order and instructions from the provider.	15			
3.	Access the federal government's food icon at www.ChooseMyPlate.gov and select the appropriate plan.	15			
4.	***Showing awareness of the patient's concerns regarding a dietary change***, discuss with the patient any obstacles that may prevent them from following the plan ordered by the provider.	15			
5.	Instruct the patient how to access additional tools on the MyPlate site such as menu options, recipes, and exercise suggestions.	15			
6.	Instruct the patient on the guidelines and specifics of the plan chosen by the provider.	15			
7.	Allow the patient time to ask questions and have them repeat back to you the instructions provided for clarity and acknowledgment of understanding.	15			
8.	Document patient education provided.	15			
	Points Awarded / Points Possible	_____ / **120**			

Competency Checklist
Procedure 58–1 Prepare a Résumé

ABHES Curriculum

MA.A.1.11.a   Perform the essential requirements for employment such as résumé writing, effective interviewing, dressing professionally, and following up appropriately

MA.A.1.11.b   Demonstrate professional behavior

CAAHEP Core Curriculum

V.C.7   Recognize elements of fundamental writing skills

V.P.8   Compose professional correspondence utilizing electronic technology

---

Task:	Prepare a résumé, following the steps in the procedure and documenting information concerning education, experience, and abilities for employment consideration.
Supplies & Conditions:	High-quality paper, dictionary, thesaurus, telephone book, computer, and printer. The résumé must be without errors, organized attractively on the page, and printed on appropriate paper. Alternatively, the résumé may be saved as a PDF.
Standards:	A maximum of three attempts may be used to complete the task. The time limit for each attempt is 30 minutes, with a minimum score of 100 percent. **Scoring:** Determine student's score by dividing points awarded by total points possible and multiplying results by 100.

EVALUATION

Evaluator Signature: _____   Date: _____

Evaluator Comments:

Procedure 58–1 Steps

Start Time: _____   **End Time:** _____   **Total Time:** _____

	Steps	Possible Points	First Attempt	Second Attempt	Third Attempt
1.	Determine the résumé style appropriate for your needs.	5			
2.	Write your complete legal name, address, phone number, and email address. This information may be arranged flush left or centered at the top of the page.	15			
3.	List your educational background, beginning with the most recent or present date.	15			
4.	List all pertinent employment experience, beginning with the most recent or present date, or enter information in an alternative résumé style.	15			
5.	List other information that might be relevant: memberships and affiliations in professional organizations; community service, including volunteer programs; and activities as might be appropriate	10			
6.	Print the completed résumé and proofread it for errors. Make any necessary edits.	15			
7.	Prepare the résumé for distribution: a. Print copies of the résumé on quality paper. b. If possible, convert the résumé into PDF format for electronic distribution.	5			
	Points Awarded / Points Possible	_____/ 80			

Competency Checklist
Procedure 58–2 Prepare a Cover Letter

ABHES Curriculum

MA.A.1.11.a   Perform the essential requirements for employment such as résumé writing, effective interviewing, dressing professionally, and following up appropriately

MA.A.1.11.b   Demonstrate professional behavior

CAAHEP Core Curriculum

V.C.7   Recognize elements of fundamental writing skills

V.P.8   Compose professional correspondence utilizing electronic technology

---

Task: Write an error-free cover letter as an indication of interest in being interviewed for a desired position.

Supplies & Conditions: Computer, printer, high-quality paper, addressee's name and address, dictionary, thesaurus. The cover letter must be without errors, formatted appropriately on the page, and printed on appropriate paper. The letter must express your skills and qualifications that would be an asset to the desired position and should be personalized to gain attention.

Standards: A maximum of three attempts may be used to complete the task. The time limit for each attempt is 30 minutes, with a minimum score of 85 percent. **Scoring:** Determine student's score by dividing points awarded by total points possible and multiplying results by 100.

EVALUATION

Evaluator Signature: _____   Date: _____

Evaluator Comments:

Name: _____ Date: _____ Score: _____

Procedure 58–2 Steps

Start Time: _____ End Time: _____ Total Time: _____

	Steps	Possible Points	First Attempt	Second Attempt	Third Attempt
1.	Assemble the needed information and equipment.	5			
2.	Enter your name and address in a letterhead format.	5			
3.	Enter the date.	5			
4.	Enter the addressee information and salutation.	10			
5.	Write the first paragraph, expressing your skills and qualifications that make you an asset to the position desired.	15			
6.	Write the second paragraph, making it clear when and how you can be reached.	15			
7.	Enter the closing and then your typed name four spaces below.	10			
8.	Print the cover letter and proofread it for errors. Make any necessary edits.	15			
9.	Save, print, and sign the letter and make a copy. Send the cover letter in answer to an ad or at the request of an individual.	5			
	Points Awarded / Points Possible	____/ 85			

Competency Checklist
Procedure 58–3 Complete a Job Application

ABHES Curriculum

MA.A.1.11.a   Perform the essential requirements for employment such as résumé writing, effective interviewing, dressing professionally, and following up appropriately

MA.A.1.11.b   Demonstrate professional behavior

CAAHEP Core Curriculum

V.C.7   Recognize elements of fundamental writing skills

Task: Complete a job application, following all directions and entering all information neatly and without error.

Supplies & Conditions: Job application; pen; copy of résumé; list of necessary names, addresses, and phone numbers; and copies of educational achievements. Procedure Form 58–3 can be used to complete this activity.

Standards: A maximum of three attempts may be used to complete the task. The time limit for each attempt is 20 minutes, with a minimum score of 85 percent. **Scoring:** Determine student's score by dividing points awarded by total points possible and multiplying results by 100.

Forms: Procedure 58–3 Form. Procedure forms can be downloaded from the Student Companion website.

EVALUATION

Evaluator Signature: _____   Date: _____

Evaluator Comments:

719

Name: _____ Date: _____ Score: _____

Procedure 58–3 Steps

Start Time: _____ End Time: _____ Total Time: _____

	Steps	Possible Points	First Attempt	Second Attempt	Third Attempt
1.	Assemble all necessary equipment and supporting documents.	5			
2.	Read the application, noting the instructions for completion.	15			
3.	Neatly enter your personal information.	15			
4.	Enter your educational information, including names, addresses, and phone numbers.	15			
5.	Enter work experience information, including employers' names, addresses, and phone numbers.	15			
6.	Enter any other information requested.	5			
7.	List the names and phone numbers of personal references.	15			
8.	Review the application, checking for missed or incorrectly entered information. Check for accuracy of spelling and general appearance. Make any necessary edits.	15			
9.	Present or mail the application to the prospective employer.	5			
	Points Awarded / Points Possible	____/ **105**			

Competency Checklist
Procedure 58–4 Write an Interview Follow-Up Letter

ABHES Curriculum

MA.A.1.11.a   Perform the essential requirements for employment such as résumé writing, effective interviewing, dressing professionally, and following up appropriately

MA.A.1.11.b   Demonstrate professional behavior

CAAHEP Core Curriculum

V.C.7   Recognize elements of fundamental writing skills

V.P.8   Compose professional correspondence utilizing electronic technology

---

Task: Write an error-free interview follow-up letter or thank-you note as an indication of interest and appreciation following an employment interview.

Supplies & Conditions: Computer, printer, high-quality paper, addressee's name and address, dictionary, and thesaurus. The cover letter must be without errors, formatted appropriately on the page, and printed on appropriate paper. The letter must express appreciation for the interview, restate desire and capability for position, and request notification of decision.

Standards: A maximum of three attempts may be used to complete the task. The time limit for each attempt is 20 minutes, with a minimum score of 85 percent. **Scoring:** Determine student's score by dividing points awarded by total points possible and multiplying results by 100.

EVALUATION

Evaluator Signature: _____ Date: _____

Evaluator Comments:

Name: _____ Date: _____ Score: _____

Procedure 58–4 Steps

Start Time: _____ End Time: _____ Total Time: _____

	Steps	Possible Points	First Attempt	Second Attempt	Third Attempt
1.	Assemble the needed information and equipment.	5			
2.	Enter your name, address, telephone number, and email address in a letterhead format.	5			
3.	Enter the date.	5			
4.	Enter the addressee information and salutation.	10			
5.	Write the first paragraph, expressing appreciation for the interview.	15			
6.	Write the second paragraph, restating your preparation for and confidence in your ability to perform in the position.	15			
7.	Write a closing paragraph, again expressing appreciation and requesting notification of the decision.	15			
8.	Enter the closing and then your typed name four spaces below.	10			
9.	Print the letter and proofread it for errors. Make any necessary edits.	15			
10.	Sign the letter, make a copy, and place the original in an addressed envelope to be mailed.	5			
	Points Awarded / Points Possible	____/ 100			

Competency Checklist
Procedure 59–1 Conduct a Staff Meeting

ABHES Curriculum

MA.A.1.8.f   Display professionalism through written and verbal communications
MA.A.1.11.b   Demonstrate professional behavior

CAAHEP Core Curriculum

V.P.11   Report relevant information concisely and accurately

---

Task: Schedule and conduct a staff meeting. Prepare an agenda, take notes, and follow up as needed.

Supplies & Conditions: In a simulated medical office, conduct a staff meeting. The following equipment and supplies are needed: meeting room, pen, paper, printer, computer with word processing and PowerPoint presentation programs, and a screen.

Standards: A maximum of three attempts may be used to complete the task. The time limit for each attempt is 90 minutes, with a minimum score of 70 percent. **Scoring:** Determine student's score by dividing points awarded by total points possible and multiplying results by 100.

EVALUATION

Evaluator Signature: _____   Date: _____

Evaluator Comments:

Name: _____ Date: _____ Score: _____

Procedure 59–1 Steps

Start Time: _____ End Time: _____ Total Time: _____

	Steps	Possible Points	First Attempt	Second Attempt	Third Attempt
1.	Discuss the purpose, objectives, and general expectations of the meeting with managing provider (and vendor or other interested parties).	10			
2.	Gather information.	10			
3.	Make schedule/calendar notation.	5			
4.	Reserve the meeting room and order any equipment necessary.	5			
5.	Notify participants.	5			
6.	Prepare the agenda.	15			
7.	Prepare materials for attendees and managing provider.	10			
8.	Order food and beverages to be served.	5			
9.	Create a sign-in sheet for all attendees to sign with date, time, and agenda noted.	5			
10.	Greet provider(s), staff, and introduce guest. Call meeting to order.	10			
11.	Take notes and minutes.	10			
12.	Handle special problems and questions as they arise.	10			
13.	Thank the staff, provider(s), and guest(s) for attending the meeting. Adjourn the meeting.	10			
14.	Return all equipment; clean up.	5			
15.	Prepare the notes or minutes.	10			
16.	Perform routine follow-up duties.	5			
17.	Evaluate the meeting.	5			
18	File the minutes.	5			
	Points Awarded / Points Possible	_____ / **140**			